THE STATE OF THE WORLD'S CHILDREN 2023

For Every Child, Vaccination

Acknowledgements

Report team
Brian Keeley, *Editor in Chief*; Juliano Diniz de Oliveira, *Research and Policy Specialist*; Tara Dooley, *Editor*; Moira Herbst, *Editor Special Projects*; Rouslan Karimov, *Data Specialist*; Sahiba Turgesen, *Assistant Editor/Coordinator*; Kathleen Edison, *Design Specialist*; Dennis Gayanelo, *Programme Associate*; John McIlwaine, *Photo Writer and Editor*; and Amanda Marlin, *Chief, Editorial and Flagships*, UNICEF Innocenti – Office of Global Research and Foresight.

Technical Report Team
Ephrem T. Lemango, *Associate Director, Immunization*; Viorica Berdaga, *Deputy Chief, Immunization*; Deepa Risal Pokharel, *Team Leader – Demand, Immunization*; Ulla Griffiths, *Team Leader – Financing, Immunization*; Niklas Danielsson, *Senior Advisor, Immunization*; and Jennifer Requejo, *Senior Advisor, Statistics and Monitoring.*

External Advisory Group
Aluísio Barros, Filimona Bisrat, Tim Crocker-Buque, Thomas B. Cueni, Tom Davis, Gaurav Garg, Githinji Gitahi, Anuradha Gupta, Randa Sami Hamadeh, Firas J. Hashim, Richard Hatchett, Sarah Hawks, Heidi Larson, Orin Levine, Violane Mitchell, Christopher Morgan, Christopher Murray, Kate O'Brien, Anna Ong-Lim, Walter Orenstein, Henry B. Perry, Pavani Ram, Helen Rees, Roberta Rughetti, Faisal Shuaib, Robert Steinglass, Mesfin Tessema, Naveen Thacker, Angus Thomson, Oyewale Tomori, Cesar Victora and Fredrick N. Were.

Internal Advisory Group
Lily Caprani, Liz Case, Lauren Francis, Christopher Gregory, Peter Hawkins, Benjamin Hickler, S.M. Moazzem Hossain, Alison Jenkins, Andrew Owain Jones, Sowmya Kadandale, Aboubacar Kampo, Priyanka Khanna, Ralph Midy, Padraic Murphy, Daniel Ngemera, Luwei Pearson and Ahmadu Yakubu.

Editorial and production
Samantha Wauchope, *Head of Production (Global Communication and Advocacy)*; Ahmed Al Izzi Alnaqshbandi, *Arabic Editor*; Maud Combier-Perben, *French Editor*; Elena Munoz-Vico, *Spanish Editor*; Yasmine Hage and Baishalee Nayak, *Fact Checkers*; and Guy Manners (Green Ink), *Copy Editor.*

Media, communications and advocacy
Imad Aoun, Kurtis Cooper, Tess Ingram and Laura Kerr.

Design
Blossom

Photography and reporting
VII Photo Agency

Statistical tables
Statistical tables prepared by the Data and Analytics team in the **Division of Data, Analytics, Planning and Monitoring**: Vidhya Ganesh, *Director*; Claudia Cappa, *Senior Adviser Statistics and Monitoring*; Karen Avanesyan, Jan Beise, Jorge Bica, Savvy Brar, Antonio Canaviri, Samuel Chakwera, Joel Conkle, Ayca Donmez, Joao Pedro Wagner De Azevedo, Chika Hayashi, Lucia Hug, Robert Johnston, Munkhbadar Jugder, Yoshito Kawakatsu, Julia Krasevec, Yang Liu, Chibwe Lwamba, Vrinda Mehra, Suguru Mizunoya, Colleen Murray, Nicole Petrowski, Tyler A. Porth, David Sharrow, Tom Slaymaker, Liliana Carvajal Velez, Dee Wang and Danzhen You.

The State of the World's Children is produced by UNICEF Innocenti – Global Office of Research and Foresight
Bo Viktor Nylund, *Director.*

Research and policy development
This report draws on background papers prepared by:

Tim Crocker-Buque and Sandra Mounier-Jack; Ève Dubé, Pippa McDermid and Robert Böhm; Holly Seale; Alyssa Sharkey; Sarah Tougher; and Maliha Ahmad.

Cesar Victora and Aluísio Barros, with Bianca O. Cata-Preta, Andrea Wendt, Luisa Arroyave and Thiago M Santos, at the International Center for Equity in Health at the Federal University of Pelotas carried out a special study of within-country inequalities in zero-dose prevalence.

PATH carried out a survey of innovations in immunization, with inputs from Deborah Atherly, Emily Carnahan, Allison Clifford, Yvette Collymore, Steven Diesburg, Collrane Frivold, Heidi Good, Miren Iturriza-Gomara, Monica Graham, Courtney Jarrahian, Laura Kallen, Manjari Lal, Pat Lennon, Joe Little, Kelsey Mertes, Mercy Mvundura, Lauren Newhouse, Eileen Quinn, Maya Rivera, Joanie Robertson, Laurie Werner and Jessica White.

Policy recommendations in this report draw on discussions at For every child, vaccines: UNICEF convening event on immunization, Florence, Italy on 9–10 June 2022, facilitated by Matter Solutions and hosted by then-Director of UNICEF Innocenti, Gunilla Olsson.

This report is the result of collaboration among many individuals and institutions. The report team thanks all who gave so willingly of their time, expertise and energy – in particular:

UNICEF Country Offices and National Committees
Cambodia: Foroogh Foyouzat, *Representative, retired*; Jaime Gill, Rathmony Hong, Hedy Ip, Raveesha Mugali and Rudina Vojvoda; **Ecuador**: Luz Ángela Melo, *Representative*; Juan Enrique Quiñonez, *Deputy Representative*; Andrea Apolo, Cristina Arboleda, Magdalena Chávez and Katherine Silva; **Haiti**: Carine Exantus, Therloune Guerrier, Herold Joseph, Lydie Maoungou Minguiel, Rachel Opota and Ndiaga Seck; **India**: Luigi d'Aquino, Zafrin Chowdhury, Madhulika Jonathan, Purvi Malhotra and Sonia Sarkar; **Indonesia**: Allison Brown-Knight, Brian Clark, Sugiarto Hiu, Jimmy Kruglinski, Abdul Khalil Noorzad, Jana Kartika Sari, Ardila Syakriah and Ria Nurrachman (IndoXplore); **Iraq**: David Hipgrave, Miguel Mateos Muñoz, Alaa Rahi, Anmar Rfaat and Falah Wadi; **Kyrgyzstan**: Christine Jaulmes, *Representative*; Asylgul Akimjanova, Mavliuda Dzhaparova, Tomiris Orozoeva and Galina Solodunova; **Nicaragua**: Antero Almeida de Pina, *Representative*; Eduardo Gallardo, *Deputy Representative*; María Delia Espinoza, Bomar Méndez, Ana Gretchen Robleto and FACTSTORY; **Nigeria**: Folashade Adebayo, Ijeoma Agbo, Blessing Ejiofor, Geoffrey Njoku and Bolanle Orefejo; **Pakistan**: Sheeba Afghani, Shoukat Ali, Mehdi Bokhari, Mariam Iqbal, Tarana Jahanuddin, Hayat Khan, Mahim Maher and Arifa S. Sharmin; **Somalia**: Mohamed Jama Fahiye, Abdirizak Abdullahi Haga, Mohamed Hiirad, Lisa Hill, Yodit Hiruy, Abdinasir Adan Ibrahim, Monsen Owusu-Aboagye and Yakub Yahye Khalif; **Uzbekistan**: Umidjon Khudaykulov and Yuriya Pak; **Yemen**: Shawki Alabasi, Paul Conner and Malak Shaher.

UNICEF Regional Offices
East Asia and the Pacific: Khin Devi Aung; **Europe and Central Asia**: Svetlana Stefanet; **Eastern and Southern Africa**: Antoinette Eleonore Ba and Paul Ngwakum; **Latin America and Caribbean**: Maaike Arts and Leysin De Leon; **Middle East and North Africa**: Saba Al Abbadi; **South Asia**: Gunter Boussery and Lalita Gurung; **West and Central Africa**: Rokhaya Diop and Ulrike Gilbert.

Division of Global Communication and Advocacy
Naysan Sabha, *Director*; Germain Ake, Hemawathy Balasundaram, Marissa Buckanoff, Merva Faddoul, Nicole Foster, Selma Hamouda, Jacob Hunt, William Jones, Debbie Toskovic Kavanagh, Mary Lynn Lalonde, Maria Lauret, Nicholas Ledner, Pragya Mathema, Mahak Morsawala, Harriet Riley and Alona Volinsky.

Private Fund Raising and Partnerships Division
Carla Haddad Mardini, *Director*; Christine Murugami.

Programme Group
Sanjay Wijesekera, *Director*; Steven Lauwerier, *Director – Health* (ai); Natalia Winder-Rossi, *Director – Social Policy*; Surangani Abeyesekera, Jennifer Asman, Sanjay Bhardwaj, Genevieve Boutin, Myungsoo Choo, Stanislaus Joseph D'Souza, Vivian Lopez, Shahira Malm, Nikhil Mandalia, Phoebe Meyer, Miraj Pradhan, Shalini Rosario, Lauren Rumble, Nateetong Tandideeravit, Sarah Tougher and Sarah Wilbanks.

Public Partnerships Division
June Kunugi, *Director*; Valentina Buj, Megan Gilgan and Barbara Renamy.

Supply Division
Etleva Kadilli, *Director*; Jean-Pierre Amorij, Anthony Bellon, Michaela Briedova, Hans Christiansen, Kristoffer Gandrup-Marino, Soren Munk Hansen, Ian Lewis, Antonia Naydenov, Ann Ottosen and Lilia Velinova-de Boever.

UNICEF Innocenti – Global Office of Research and Foresight
Claire Akehurst, David Anthony, Patricia Arquero Caballero, Evan Easton Calabria, Arno Johnstone, Josiah Kaplan, Laura Meucci, Daniele Regoli and Ramya Subrahmanian.

Special thanks to:
Cinzia Iusco Bruschi, Laurence Chandy, Paloma Escudero and Robin Nandy.

From Gavi, the Vaccine Alliance: Anamaria Bejar, Seth Berkley, Olly Cann, Amanda Fazzone Tschopp and Hamzah Zekrya.

From the Government of India:
Talo Herang.

From Lagos State and Lagos State Primary Healthcare Board: Akin Emmanuel and Ibrahim Akinwumi Mustafa.

From the Ministry of Health of Uzbekistan: Shoira Khalilova, Nasiba Tairova, Dilorom Tursunova and Bakhodir Yusupaliev.

From the Vaccine Confidence Project: Alex De Figueiredo, Rachel Eagan, Heidi Larson and Martin Wiegand.

From the World Health Organization: Raymond Hutubessy and So Yoon Sim.

Contents

Foreword i

Key messages iii

Introduction: One in five children 1

    Case study: Somalia **12**

Chapter 1. How the COVID-19 pandemic set back vaccination **15**

    How the pandemic set back immunization **16**

        Rising risk of measles 19

        HPV losses 19

        Understanding the pandemic's impact 20

    Case study: Indonesia **22**

    Making up lost ground **24**

        Catch-up and recovery 24

    Learning from the pandemic **25**

        The urgency of routine immunization 25

        A sped-up, coordinated response 26

        Integrate health crisis response with routine immunization 27

    Longer-term challenges **27**

    Case study: Cambodia **28**

Chapter 2. Zero-dose children matter **31**

    Left behind: socioeconomic determinants of immunization **32**

        Poverty 32

        Location 33

        Marginalization 35

        Crisis 37

    Case study: Nigeria **38**

    Availability, accessibility and affordability **40**

        Solutions 41

    Why it matters **42**

        Survive and thrive 42

        The value of vaccination 42

        Making the case 43

    Case study: Nicaragua **44**

Chapter 3. Immunization and primary health care **47**

    Structures and challenges **48**

        Weak primary health care 48

        Health workforce 49

    Case study: Yemen **50**

    Solutions **53**

        Strengthen primary health care 53

        Integrate immunization in primary health care 53

        Community engagement 55

    Case study: Pakistan **56**

Support for health workers 58

Next steps.. 59

Case study: India **60**

Chapter 4. How can we build vaccine confidence? **63**

Shaken trust.. **65**

The impact of COVID-19....................................... 69

Motivation and hesitancy 69

The toll 71

Case study: Kyrgyzstan **72**

Building vaccine confidence **74**

Community engagement, dialogue and ownership................. 74

Social data and social listening 76

Pro-vaccine education and public messaging........................... 77

Applying a gender lens 78

Case study: Ecuador... **80**

Chapter 5. Funding and innovation for the future....................................... **83**

Funding: The current situation **84**

Economic instability 84

Government budgets 85

Financing immunization's future **86**

Funding 87

Partnerships 87

Challenges 87

Solutions 88

Commitment.. 89

Case study: Uzbekistan **90**

New vaccines and products...................................... **92**

Recent vaccine developments.............................. 92

Vaccine product developments 94

Logistics and supply chain innovations................. 95

Digital tools 95

Strengthening local manufacturing 97

Case study: Haiti.. **98**

Chapter 6. For every child, vaccination: An equity agenda **101**

Introduction **102**

For every child, vaccination: An equity agenda **103**

1. Vaccinate every child, everywhere 103

2. Strengthen demand for – and confidence in – vaccination................ 104

3. Spend more and spend better on immunization and health.............. 105

4. Build resilient systems and shockproof them for the future.............. 106

Endnotes.. **108**

Statistical tables.. **115**

Foreword

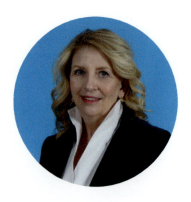

Catherine Russell
UNICEF Executive Director

Human history is full of stories of disease and pestilence. But the story of vaccines has radically altered the course of human survival and development.

Almost 80 years ago, Europe struggled to recover from a catastrophic war.

Millions of people crowded into wrecked buildings and dugouts – conditions that were ripe for outbreaks of infectious disease. Tuberculosis (TB) was particularly infectious and virulent in communities across the continent. Children were especially vulnerable, with thousands suffering debilitating fever, weight loss, chest pain, even death.

Until then, diseases like smallpox, measles and polio frequently ravaged large segments of the human population, claiming the lives of countless children in the process.

But this time was different. Equipped with vials of BCG, the vaccine that helps protect against TB, teams of medical workers fanned out across Europe to save lives. By 1950, some 11.4 million children had been vaccinated against the disease through the UNICEF-supported campaign. It marked the beginning of a new era in which the lives of millions of children would be protected from vaccine-preventable diseases.

Fast forward to 1980. The first-ever edition of *The State of the World's Children* report stated that "in the poorest countries only one child in ten will ever see a trained health worker or be immunized in its first year against diphtheria, tetanus, measles, tuberculosis, pertussis or poliomyelitis – the six most common preventable diseases of childhood." This finding was deeply troubling, but there were signs of hope and progress in immunization. That same year, smallpox was finally declared eradicated, demonstrating the remarkable power of vaccines to save lives.

That success helped inspire a global programme to protect more of the world's children against other life-threatening diseases – measles, diphtheria, pneumonia and more. By the end of the 1980s, about 7 in 10 of the world's children were protected by vaccines, and that number continued to climb, albeit more slowly, in subsequent decades. UNICEF played its part, and we still do. Today, we supply vaccines that reach 45 per cent of the world's children under 5 years of age.

In 2020, the COVID-19 virus continued to spread around the world – lives were lost and put on hold, schools closed, health systems were pushed to their limits and beyond. But in an extraordinarily short period of time, vaccines were developed, and mass vaccination campaigns began. Again, UNICEF was there. With our partners Gavi, the Vaccine Alliance, the World Health Organization (WHO) and the Coalition for Epidemic Preparedness Innovations (CEPI), we are part of the largest vaccine supply operation in history, providing almost two billion vaccine doses to 146 countries and territories. In addition, we have supported the development of technology that keeps vaccines cold as we move them to the most remote regions of the world, and we have worked hard to increase trust in the safety and efficacy of vaccines.

For almost 80 years, UNICEF has worked with international partners, national governments and many others to protect children against vaccine-preventable diseases. But, in a world slowly recovering from the COVID-19 pandemic, we know that the approaches we have taken in the past may not always be suited for current or future circumstances.

Despite decades of progress in childhood immunization, our collective efforts are falling short. Put simply, we are not meeting our goal to vaccinate every child. While new vaccines have been introduced that broaden protection against disease, none have managed to reach more than 9 out of 10 children. Many are not even coming close – only one in eight girls has received the HPV vaccine, which protects against cervical cancer.

The pandemic has only darkened this picture. In the past three years, more than a decade of hard-earned gains in routine childhood immunization have been eroded. Getting back on track will be challenging. The shadow of the pandemic will hang over economies for years to come, forcing tough choices in spending and investment. Another challenge looms too: Confidence in vaccines seems to be waning in many countries. While vaccine confidence is far from being the most important determinant of vaccine demand in most communities, the apparent rise in hesitancy cannot be ignored.

Reaching our goal – to vaccinate every child – will require a real commitment by governments.

Some of this change will be technical – making better use of data, improving communication and outreach, and strengthening cold chains.

Some will require difficult conversations about financing and challenging trade-offs, including by national governments, donors and others, on how best to fund primary health care and immunization services and how to make them more resilient to future shocks.

And some will force societies and communities to examine their fundamental values. Children from marginalized communities are among the least likely to be vaccinated. Whether or not they are vaccinated is often a result of deep inequities – between rich and poor, between men and women, between communities at the centre of power and communities on the margins.

Achieving the change needed to vaccinate every child will not be easy. But the achievements of the past 80 years should give us hope. Time and again, the world has made remarkable progress in immunization, often in the most difficult and challenging circumstances.

Those achievements have transformed our world. They have allowed millions of children to survive and to live lives free of the lingering effects of illness. They have relieved families of the heartache and financial burden of caring for sick children. And they have added to the human capital, talent and energy of our societies.

In the years to come, we can achieve even more. New vaccines are already helping in the war against malaria. There will likely be more soon, including against chronic diseases such as cancer and Alzheimer's disease.

Our journey has been long but, in many ways, it is only just beginning.

KEY MESSAGE 1

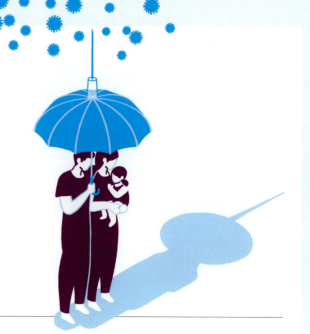

Vaccines save lives

Vaccines save lives, but far too many children in the world are not being vaccinated. The COVID-19 pandemic only added to their numbers. The children who are missing out live in the poorest, most remote and most marginalized communities. To reach them, it is vital to prioritize investment in primary health care and in the health workers – mostly women – who deliver services. It is essential, too, to build confidence in vaccines and to make the most of a host of new ideas and technologies that can boost the power of vaccines and ensure they reach every child.

Over the past decade or so, despite growing efforts to expand immunization, there has been little progress in reducing the number of zero-dose children. Reaching every child remains a challenge.

Figure 1. Zero-dose children globally, 2000–2021

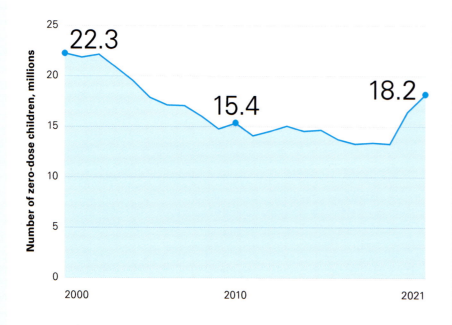

Source: World Health Organization and United Nations Children's Fund, 'Estimates of National Immunization Coverage (WUENIC), 2021 revision', July 2022.

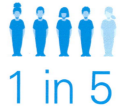

1 in 5

children are **zero-dose** (unvaccinated) and **under-vaccinated**, leaving them vulnerable to a range of vaccine-preventable diseases.

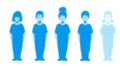

Around

1 in 5

children have no protection at all against measles, a childhood killer.

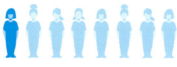

Around

7 in 8

eligible girls are not vaccinated against human papillomavirus (HPV), which can cause cervical cancer.

THE STATE OF THE WORLD'S CHILDREN 2023

KEY MESSAGE 2

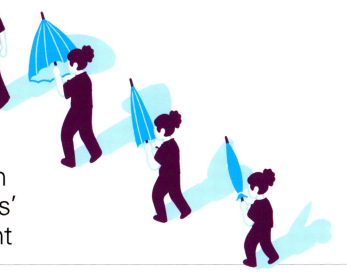

When we don't vaccinate children, we risk their lives and health – as well as our societies' growth and development

Vaccines save

4.4 million lives

every year, a figure that could rise to

5.8 million

by 2030 if the goals of the Immunization Agenda 2030 (IA2030) are met.

Before the introduction of a vaccine in 1963, measles killed an estimated 2.6 million people globally every year, mostly children. By 2021, that had fallen to 128,000 – still too high, but a remarkable improvement.

Vaccines help children thrive, support families and caregivers, and benefit the health of the wider community

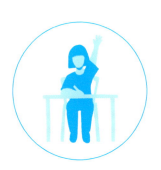 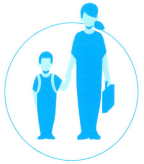

Being immunized protects children against illness. That helps prevent absences from school, which improves **learning outcomes**.

When children are protected against illness, parents and caregivers – mostly mothers – need to take less **time off work** to care for sick children.

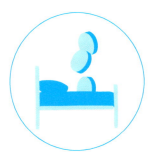 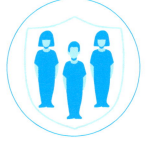

Families are also less likely to face the emotional pain and sometimes **catastrophic costs** of caring for a sick child.

Vaccinating children supports the health of the wider community by promoting **herd immunity** and helping to limit the spread of antimicrobial resistance.

Vaccines deliver an unrivalled return on investment

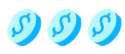
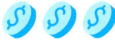
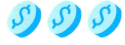

US$26

Every dollar spent on vaccination delivers a return on investment of US$26.

KEY MESSAGE 3

The COVID-19 pandemic set back childhood immunization around the world

UNICEF estimates that

67 million children

missed out entirely or partially on routine immunization between 2019 and 2021;

48 million

of them missed out entirely.

Disruptions caused by the pandemic interrupted childhood vaccination almost everywhere, setting back vaccination rates to levels not seen since 2008.

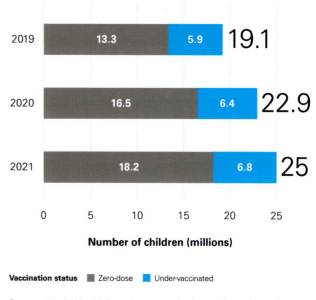

Figure 2. **The number* of children who missed vaccination rose during the COVID-19 pandemic**

Year	Zero-dose	Under-vaccinated	Total
2019	13.3	5.9	19.1
2020	16.5	6.4	22.9
2021	18.2	6.8	25

Number of children (millions)

Vaccination status: Zero-dose ■ Under-vaccinated ■

Source: World Health Organization and United Nations Children's Fund, 'Estimates of National Immunization Coverage (WUENIC), 2021 revision', July 2022. *Numbers are rounded.

Why did the pandemic set back childhood immunization?

It placed huge new demands on **health systems**, which they were often ill-equipped to cope with.

It exacerbated existing **shortages** of health workers.

It placed **heavy strains** on front-line health workers, mostly women, who were also coping with additional care burdens at home.

Stay-at-home recommendations and the fear of contracting the virus from health-care facilities led families to put off vaccinating children.

What can be done?
Catch-up and recovery: Children born just before or during the pandemic are now moving past the age when they would normally be vaccinated. Urgent action is now needed to catch up on those who missed out on vaccination and to support the recovery of immunization services set back during the pandemic.

KEY MESSAGE 4

But even before the pandemic, far too many children missed out on vaccination. Many live in the poorest and most marginalized communities

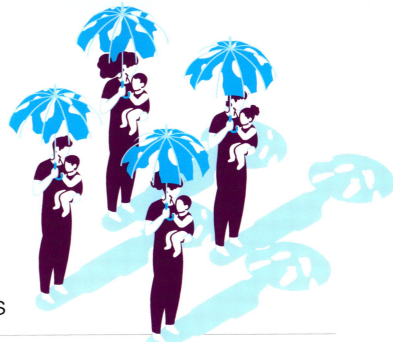

The story of the children who are not being vaccinated is a story of inequity, poverty, underserved communities and unempowered women

Poverty

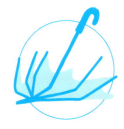

In the poorest households, just over 1 in 5 children are zero-dose; in the wealthiest, it is just 1 in 20.

In some regions, the gap is even greater: In West and Central Africa, almost 1 in 2 children in the poorest households are zero-dose, compared with around 1 in 16 in the wealthiest.

Unempowered women
Children of mothers with no or little education are much less likely to be vaccinated

Mothers with:	Proportion of zero-dose children
No education	23.5%
Primary school education	13.1%
At least secondary school education	6.9%

Source: Victora, Cesar, and Aluísio Barros, 'Within-Country Inequalities in Zero-Dose Prevalence: Background paper for *The State of the World's Children 2022*', International Center for Equity in Health, Federal University of Pelotas, Brazil, December 2022.

Underserved communities face challenges of availability, access and affordability

Availability
Are vaccines delivered to health centres or outreach campaigns and are health workers there to administer them?

Accessibility
Are vaccines and services located in a place and offered at a time where and when children and families can get to them?

Affordability
Can families afford health service, pay for bus fares or skip a day's work to get to the health centre?

Underserved communities

 Many zero-dose and under-vaccinated children live in challenging settings, such as remote rural communities, built-up urban settlements, and areas experiencing conflict and crises.

 These challenges are greatest in low- and middle-income countries, where about 1 in 10 children in urban areas are zero-dose; the figure is just under 1 in 6 in rural areas. In upper-middle-income countries, there is almost no gap in between urban and rural children.

 2 in 5 of the children in the world who had not been immunized lived in conflict-affected or fragile settings (in 2018).

FOR EVERY CHILD, VACCINATION

KEY MESSAGE 5

To vaccinate every child, it is vital to strengthen primary health care and provide its mostly female front-line workers with the resources and support they need

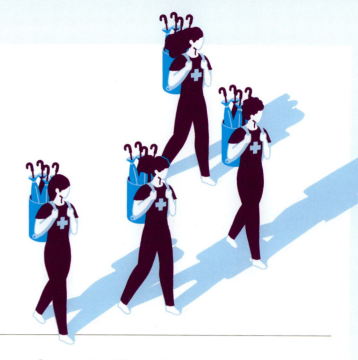

- Many children miss out on vaccination because they live in places where there is no or limited primary health care – a health-care approach that includes health promotion, disease prevention and treatment.

- Vaccine campaigns play a powerful role in reaching many of these children, and they will continue to do so. But campaigns are, by definition, short-lived, and they have inherent limitations because they do not necessarily offer continuous and predictable services.

- Integrating childhood immunization into strengthened primary health is essential to sustainably reach the goal of vaccinating every child.

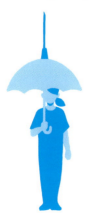

Support health workers
As health workers and community health workers, women are at the front line of delivering vaccinations, but they face low pay, informal employment, lack of career opportunities and threats to their security. Far too few are in leadership positions. Responses need to include:

- Offering full-time jobs with good and regular pay and decent working conditions
- Providing career development and training opportunities, including in the integrated management of childhood illness
- Recognizing and regularizing the role of community health workers.

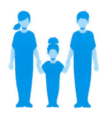

Integrate services
As a well-established point of contact with families, vaccination services can be an entry-point for providing additional essential health services. Equally, strong primary health-care systems can contribute to vaccination efforts, providing platforms to reach those left behind.

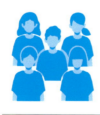

Engage with communities
Vaccination interventions designed, delivered and evaluated by members of the communities they serve can increase equity and efficacy.

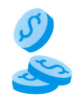

Prioritize financing immunization
Even in a time of tight budgets, the high returns on investment from immunization underscore the benefits of prioritizing funding.

KEY MESSAGE 6

Parents and communities need to believe in the value of vaccination; there are worrying signs that confidence in vaccines is slipping in some countries

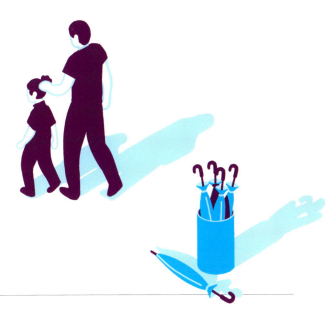

To bolster vaccine confidence, strong efforts are needed to:

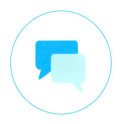

Engage with communities and promote dialogue
Engagement can also stem the influence of rumour and misinformation and bolster widespread support for immunization. Dialogue can help foster trust, opening the door for people to share their feelings and concerns about vaccination.

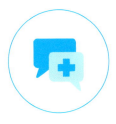

Support health-care providers to make an impact
Health-care providers are a trusted voice on vaccines. Motivating and equipping immunization providers – and the community health workers supporting them – to have impactful conversations about vaccination is essential.

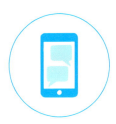

Carry out social listening
Social listening – investing in understanding people's attitudes to vaccines in real time – is vital. Approaches can include carrying out regular surveys and monitoring debates and discussions on social media.

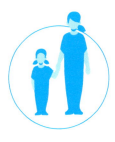

Empower women and girls
Understanding how gender impacts vaccine uptake can help with the design of more effective programmes, as well as education and information campaigns.

Trends in vaccine confidence

- Data collected before and during the COVID-19 pandemic indicate **declines in the perception of the importance** of vaccines for children in many (but not all) countries for which data are available *(see Figure 3)*.

- Confidence levels appear to have declined more in **younger** than in older age groups.

- Vaccine confidence is notoriously **volatile**, and any trends are time and location specific. But any signs of broader loss of confidence need to be taken seriously.

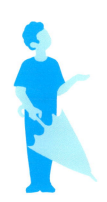

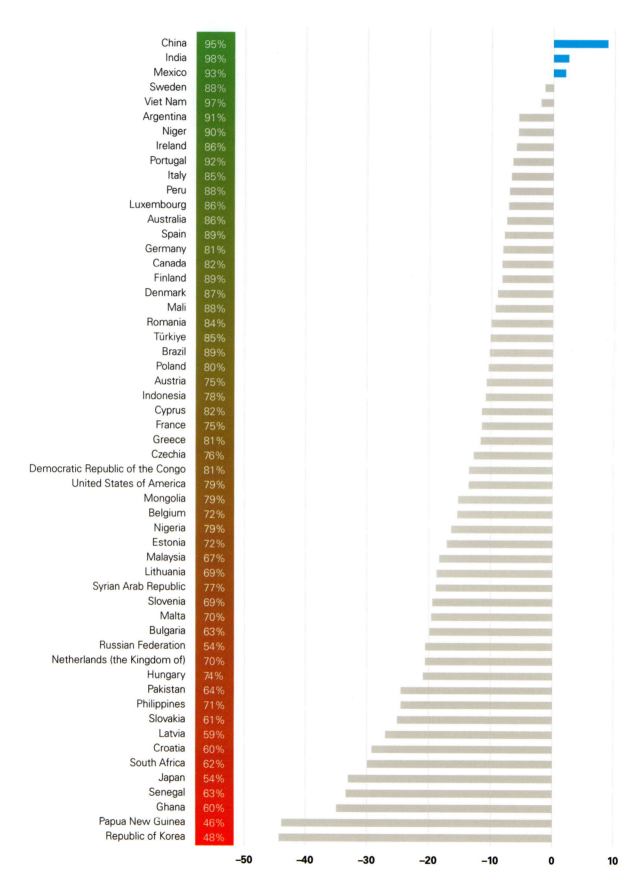

Figure 3. Confidence that vaccines are important for children dropped after the start of the pandemic
Percentage of population that currently (most recent year) perceive vaccines as important for children and percentage point change before and after the start of the pandemic.

Source: UNICEF analysis based on data from The Vaccine Confidence Project, London School of Hygiene & Tropical Medicine, 2022.

KEY MESSAGE 7

Vaccinating every child means investing in new approaches to strengthen financing and make the most of scientific and technological innovations

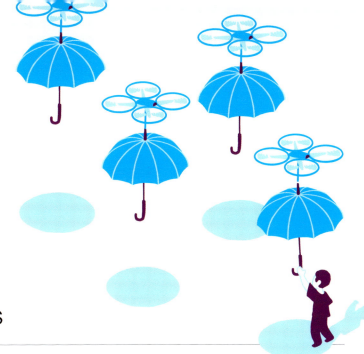

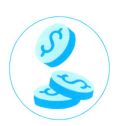

Overcoming fiscal constraints in low- and middle-income countries is essential to remove significant obstacles to providing vaccination services
- Overall, governments are the largest contributors to immunization, but donors provide other essential funds.
- The amount governments allocate is not always the same as what is actually spent. Problems can include revenue projections falling short, shifting of funds to meet other needs, delays in procurement, and coordination issues.
- Further strengthening of health and finance systems is essential to ensure funds are spent efficiently.

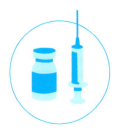

The COVID-19 pandemic helped change the landscape for vaccine development
- The speed with which vaccines were developed and produced during the pandemic offers important lessons for faster vaccine development and approval.
- Several new vaccines are emerging – and one has already been approved – to protect children against malaria, which kills nearly half a million children each year.
- Innovations in producing a new pneumococcal conjugate vaccine (PCV), which helps protect children from pneumonia, look set to cut the cost of the vaccine and improve supplies.

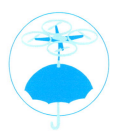

Innovations in vaccine supply chains will help improve access to vaccines in remote areas
- Small temperature-sensitive indicators on vaccine vials allow health workers to monitor vaccines for heat exposure.
- Drones are being successfully used to deliver health commodities in some African countries.

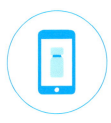

Digital technologies are helping to improve the quality and timeliness of data
- Electronic immunization registries can ensure the right child receives the right vaccination at the right time.
- Mapping systems using 'big data' from vaccinators' phones can help ensure communities in need are being identified.
- Sending text-message reminders to parents can help raise vaccination rates.

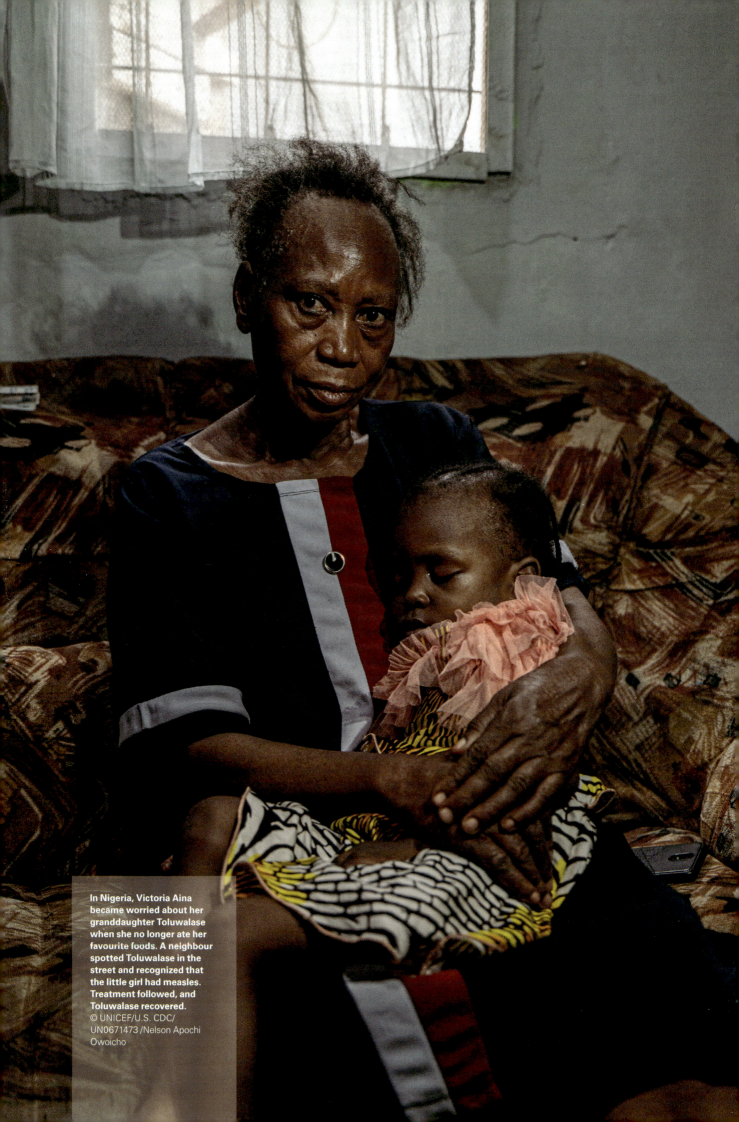

In Nigeria, Victoria Aina became worried about her granddaughter Toluwalase when she no longer ate her favourite foods. A neighbour spotted Toluwalase in the street and recognized that the little girl had measles. Treatment followed, and Toluwalase recovered.
© UNICEF/U.S. CDC/UN0671473/Nelson Apochi Owoicho

INTRODUCTION

One in five children

On a mat in a tenement in Lagos, a little girl is sleeping. Her forehead and arms are covered with fading scars. A few months earlier, the girl fell ill with a high fever and developed a skin rash. Her grandmother, Victoria Aina, who cares for her, was concerned ...

Box 1
Understanding zero-dose

'Zero-dose' and 'under-vaccinated' have become key concepts in explaining immunization coverage, in aligning global efforts to improve vaccine coverage, and for monitoring success. What do they mean?

Zero-dose refers to children who have not received any vaccinations. Most live in communities that experience multiple deprivations (see Chapter 2).

Under-vaccinated refers to children who have received some, but not all, of their recommended schedule of vaccinations.

To calculate the numbers of zero-dose and under-vaccinated children, a proxy measure is used. Children who have not received the first dose of the diphtheria, tetanus and pertussis (DTP1) vaccine are described as zero-dose. Children who have received DPT1 but not the third dose (DTP3) are described as under-vaccinated.

Children typically receive these vaccines in the first year of life. In general terms, therefore, where data for zero-dose and under-vaccinated children are presented in percentage terms, these numbers represent percentages of surviving infants (rather than the entire child population).

"I became worried when she stopped eating her favourite meals," she said. "Toluwalase loves bread and beverage. I was alarmed when she shunned them."

Someone in the neighbourhood spotted Toluwalase in the street and diagnosed her illness: measles. Treatment followed, and the girl recovered.

Toluwalase was lucky. Many other children are not. Measles is a killer. Often dismissed as just one of those things that children get – a rash and a fever that clears in a few days – measles claims around 351 lives every day, mostly children.[1] Children who catch the highly contagious disease are at risk of pneumonia and of longer-term consequences such as brain damage, deafness and blindness.[2]

Since the introduction of a vaccine in 1963, infections and deaths from measles have been preventable.

That vaccine has helped to transform childhood. Before its introduction, measles claimed around 2.6 million lives every year and was the leading cause of childhood blindness in low-income countries.[3] Over the past two decades, immunization against measles is estimated to have saved more than 31 million lives.[4]

But far too many children are still not getting the protection they need against measles and a raft of other serious diseases.

For the little girl's grandmother, the lesson is simple: "Children should be vaccinated."

The children left behind

Toluwalase is not alone.

In remote rural villages, in city slums, in conflict and fragile settings, and in many other places around the world, far too many children are not getting the vaccines they need to protect them against serious disease. In 2021, just over 25 million children were estimated to be either unvaccinated – **zero-dose** – or under-vaccinated (see Box 1).[5] Like Toluwalase, many of these children come from the poorest families and communities. Their lives are often marked by multiple deprivations, with limited access to basic services, such as clean water, education and – crucially – primary health care (see Chapter 2).

Just as it did with so many other aspects of life, the COVID-19 pandemic severely disrupted childhood immunization. Between 2019 and 2021, UNICEF estimates that **67 million children** missed out entirely or partially on routine immunization; 48 million of them missed out entirely.[6]

In percentage terms, the share of vaccinated children fell 5 percentage points to 81 per cent. In other words, **around one in five children worldwide were not fully protected against vaccine-preventable diseases**.[7] Worryingly, the backsliding during the pandemic came at the end of a decade when, in broad terms, growth in childhood immunization had stagnated (see Figure 1).

For the sake of children like Toluwalase, and children everywhere, we must do better.

Figure 1. Backsliding in vaccination coverage during the pandemic came at the end of a decade that saw little growth

Percentages of under-vaccinated children, 1980–2021

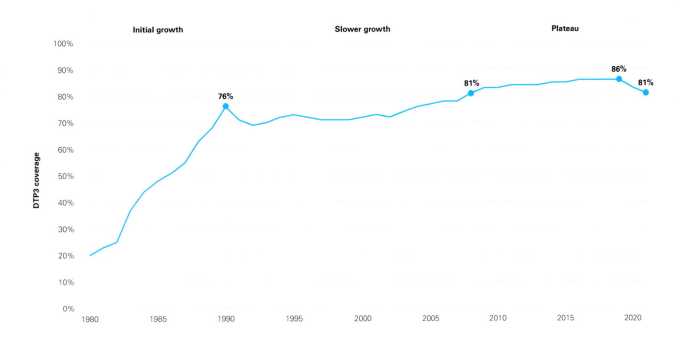

Source: World Health Organization and United Nations Children's Fund, 'Estimates of National Immunization Coverage (WUENIC), 2021 revision', July 2022.

Figure 2. Children in parts of Africa and South Asia are at higher risk of not being vaccinated

Zero-dose and under-vaccinated children by UNICEF programme regions, 2021

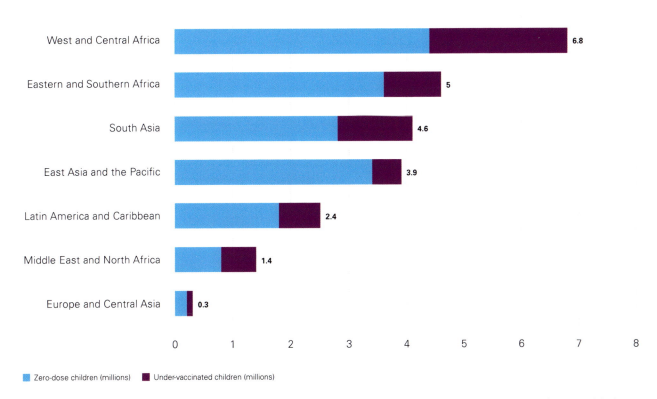

Source: World Health Organization and United Nations Children's Fund, 'Estimates of National Immunization Coverage (WUENIC), 2021 revision', July 2022.

In countries around the world, governments, donors and partners are working with communities on solutions: They are reaching out to immunize the most marginalized children and provide essential primary health care services.

1 NICARAGUA

Reynilda Cramer, part of a team of community nurses from the Miskito community who visit children in their homes.

"Children are given routine vaccines according to their schedule, their height and weight. Furthermore, heights are taken, deworming and vitamins are administered if appropriate. If anyone else in the family has health problems, we also take care of that other person."

3 HAITI

Mona Yvrose Jean Claude, a nurse at Sacré Coeur Health Centre for more than 10 years.

"To improve immunization in our health centre, it would be helpful to renew our multi-skilled community health workers and have the possibility of creating assembly stations and carry out mobile clinics."

2 ECUADOR

Maria Catucuago, part of a corps of indigenous volunteers who keep watch over the health and well-being of children under the age of 5.

"I feel passionate about helping others. For many years, I have been involved in community activities that promote the well-being and health of families."

4 YEMEN

Ghada Ali Obaid, midwife and vaccinator, who has witnessed needless suffering when children are not vaccinated.

"The essence of our work is saving peoples' lives and reducing the suffering of women and children. Personally, this is the most significant indicator of success in my work and life."

5 UZBEKISTAN

Umida Djuraeva, a nurse who administers the HPV vaccine at the Central Multidisciplinary Policlinic of Kibray.

"Nowadays, people come voluntarily. They have realized the vaccine is safe and tolerated well."

6 KYRGYZSTAN

Mirlan Dezhyusubekov, an imam who works with the Kaiyrma village community health committee.

"From a religious point of view, we cannot judge parents' decisions to vaccinate or not to vaccinate their children. But I tell families that I was vaccinated, as well as my children, and we have all been well."

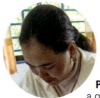

7 CAMBODIA

Pyun Kunthea, a government health worker who immunizes children in a remote community.

"Just 20 years ago, preventable diseases were still common ... Things got better, but it was still difficult to reach villages like this, which were distant from health centres. Also, people lacked confidence in vaccines because they weren't always given information in their own language. That's changed."

9 INDIA

Dematso Khamblai, a health worker who is part of the Alternative Delivery System, which brings vaccines to remote areas by foot.

"It becomes dangerous during the monsoon season as rains make the trek slippery. There are also frequent landslides during the monsoon season, which make the trek tough."

10 SOMALIA

Maimuna Hussein, a nurse and head of the Jilab Health Centre, part of the Jilab camp for internal displaced persons.

"[Antenatal care] is very, very important. It is the entry-point when the mothers get a private consultation. That is why you need to give them more time."

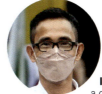

8 INDONESIA

Irwan Hakim, a community clinic nurse who works on routine immunization outreach in a remote island community.

"Fathers are the decision makers of the household here... I'm lucky I'm from a neighbouring island and I can speak local dialect so it's easier to communicate with them."

Most often, the goals are realized by health workers, especially women.

Box 2
Immunization Agenda 2030

The *Immunization Agenda 2030* (IA2030) is the international community's vision and strategy to ensure that immunization leaves no one behind over the next decade. This ambitious global strategy aims to halve the number of children who miss out on essential vaccines and to achieve 90 per cent coverage for key life-saving vaccines. Overall, if the agenda is met, it will save an estimated 50 million lives in this decade.[16]

The strategy also targets a major increase in the introduction of new vaccines in individual countries. Between 2010 and 2017, some 116 low- and middle-income countries introduced at least one new vaccine.[17] Worryingly, however, none of the newer vaccine introductions, such as the second dose of measles vaccine and the vaccine against rotavirus (a virus that can cause diarrhoea and vomiting in children and lead to death), have achieved global coverage above 90 per cent.[18] The pandemic set progress back still further, with marked slowdowns in vaccine introductions in 2020 (other than COVID-19 vaccines), followed by only a slight pick-up in 2021.[19] The IA2030 sets a target of 500 introductions of new or under-used vaccines.[20]

Strengthening the role of health systems in immunization is a key pillar of IA2030. The global strategy also emphasizes the role of immunization as a key part of people-centred primary health care services. And it places countries at the centre of the strategy, emphasizing the core role of national governments in ensuring citizens are immunized.[21]

We *can* do better

Immunization is one of humanity's most remarkable success stories. It has saved countless lives. Many more lives will be saved if the ambitious – but realizable – goals of the *Immunization Agenda 2030* (IA2030) are achieved. This global strategy for increasing vaccination coverage aims for a world where "everyone, everywhere, at every age, fully benefits from vaccines for good health and well-being" *(see Box 2).*[8]

By helping to protect against some of humanity's greatest scourges, immunization allows children everywhere to live lives free of many forms of disability. Immunization has led to the eradication of smallpox, a disfiguring and often fatal disease that in the twentieth century alone claimed an estimated 300 million lives.[9] There has been remarkable progress, too, on the long road to eradicating polio: Today, most of us live in countries that are free of a disease that once robbed so many people of the ability to walk.[10]

The power of immunization was demonstrated again in the COVID-19 pandemic. The disease claimed 14.9 million lives – directly and indirectly – in 2020 and 2021, according to the World Health Organization (WHO), and disrupted many more lives around the world, especially children's.[11] The development of vaccines against COVID-19, many using innovative technologies *(see Chapter 5)*, has essentially allowed life to return to normal in much of the world. While it has taken far too long to get those vaccines to people living in the poorest countries, the global impact is still astounding: Already, at least two thirds of the world's population has been immunized against COVID-19.[12] Those vaccines have prevented an estimated 20 million deaths globally.[13]

The achievements of mass immunization and the development of the COVID-19 vaccines are all the more remarkable considering how quickly they happened. Following the identification of the COVID-19 virus in December 2019, it took only a year for the first vaccine against COVID-19 to be authorized.[14] Within another year, it is estimated that more than half of the global population had received at least one dose of a COVID-19 vaccine.[15]

These examples demonstrate that public demand, scientific innovations and – perhaps above all – political will can drive rapid change.

We *must* do more, and we must do better, now

That change is needed, and it is needed now.

The backsliding in immunization during the pandemic should sound an alarm bell. As the 67 million children who missed out on vaccines over the past three years pass the age when they would routinely be immunized, it will require a dedicated effort to ensure that they catch up with their vaccinations *(see Chapter 1).*

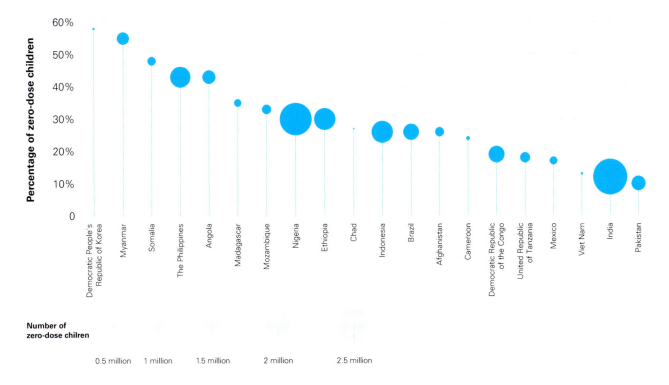

Figure 3. Top 20 countries with the largest numbers of zero-dose children
Zero-dose children by number and percentage of the country's child population, 2021

Source: World Health Organization and United Nations Children's Fund, 'Estimates of National Immunization Coverage (WUENIC), 2021 revision', July 2022.

The backsliding is worrying not just in itself, but also for what it represents.

It highlighted the reality that the story of zero-dose and under-immunized children is overwhelmingly a story of inequities. In Angola, Nigeria and Papua New Guinea, a child from the wealthiest group in society is at least five times more likely to be vaccinated than one from the poorest group *(see Chapter 2)*. The children who are not vaccinated are also often the children of mothers who have not been able to go to school and who are given little say in family and spending decisions.

The pandemic also exposed – and exacerbated – persistent weaknesses in health systems and primary health care, which are key to ensuring children are vaccinated. Key resources were diverted to respond to the pandemic, which, along with many other factors *(see Chapter 1)*, contributed to the backslide in routine immunization. But even before the pandemic, far too many primary health care systems suffered from a lack of skilled health workers, limited access to essential supplies and equipment, weak capacity for collecting and using data and conducting disease surveillance, and shortages of key medicines and vaccines at the local level. These systems also faced barriers to using available resources efficiently and effectively.

The pandemic highlighted the difficulties facing women working in health-care and immunization programmes. Although they form the bulk of the health workforce, they have long been underrepresented in leadership roles, denied opportunities for training and professional advancement, and have faced the risk of violence and gender-based violence in doing their jobs. The pandemic only exacerbated these challenges. Many women health workers faced the additional burden of balancing an increased workload with extra family responsibilities, such as looking after children locked out from school.

If primary health care is to become more resilient, the needs and potential of women health workers must be better recognized. They need more opportunities for full-time – rather than short-term and ad hoc – employment and for training and professional development. They also need to be better represented in leadership roles, so that decisions at the top of health systems better reflect the realities faced by the people who account for the vast majority of health workers on the ground.

The pandemic also brought fresh attention to vaccine hesitancy. A multifaceted challenge, vaccine hesitancy – or the state of being undecided or uncertain about vaccination – is only one of many barriers to families seeking out vaccines for children.[22] But it is a challenge that new data presented in this report show needs greater attention. The data, from the Vaccine Confidence Project, show that confidence in the importance of vaccines for children was lower after the emergence of the pandemic than before in most countries for which data are available *(see Chapter 4)*. The declines were generally greater among younger people than older people. Even before the pandemic, vaccine hesitancy was identified as one of the top ten threats to global health.[23] The influence of a number of factors, including growing access to misleading information on social media, declining trust in authority in some parts of the world, and political polarization,[24] suggest this threat may only be growing.

The consequences of failure

Failure to protect children against disease has serious consequences. Put bluntly, children die, and many more suffer lifelong disabilities. Unfortunately, the world continues to see far too many outbreaks of vaccine-preventable diseases. In 2022, for example, the number of measles outbreaks was double the total in the previous year *(see Chapter 1)*.[25] Meanwhile, the discovery of poliovirus in Israel, the United Kingdom of Great Britain and Northern Ireland, and the United States of America in 2022 was a reminder that even remarkable progress against a disease like polio can be put at risk if we fail to vaccinate every child.

In other words, **no one is safe until everyone is safe.**[26]

The consequences of failing to vaccinate children may become more severe in years to come. Climate change risks exposing new communities to infectious diseases such as malaria, dengue and cholera, and may alter seasonal disease patterns. Increasing risk of overlapping climate crises, including droughts, heatwaves and floods, will put further strain on children's access to essential services, including clean water and primary health care.[27] Also of long-term concern is the rise of drug-resistant infections *(see Chapter 2)*.[28]

Failure to immunize children undermines their right to what the Convention on the Rights of the Child describes as "the enjoyment of the highest attainable standard of health and to facilities for the treatment of illness and rehabilitation of health."[29]

And it sets back still further the prospects of attaining the Sustainable Development Goals (SDGs). Immunization is key to achieving SDG 3, which aims to "ensure healthy lives and promote well-being for all at all ages." But it is also linked to 13 of the other SDGs. For example, by supporting children's cognitive development and education attainment, it can drive progress on SDG 4 – delivering quality education.[30] In that sense, immunization is at the heart of our collective commitment to achieve a better and more sustainable future for us all.

A time for political will

Much will have to happen if we are to protect *every* child against vaccine-preventable disease. The needs are complex, even daunting. They will become even more so if vaccines are to reach children in those places that are often overlooked – the remote village miles from the nearest road, the urban slum where newly arrived families live in anonymity, the warzone where families do not know where they will be sleeping tomorrow night.

But overriding them all is one single necessity: political will. Nothing will happen unless we garner the political will – globally, nationally and locally – to protect children against vaccine-preventable diseases.

That will should be grounded in optimism. The emergence of mass immunization in the 1980s and the development of COVID-19 vaccines show we can make progress, and we can make progress quickly. Encouragingly, and despite the setbacks it caused to childhood immunization, the pandemic may also have helped lay the groundwork in some countries for faster progress. For example, investment in cold chains to distribute COVID-19 vaccines, the emergence of innovative approaches to vaccine development and delivery, and the use of advanced data collection techniques to keep track of vaccine doses and vaccinations – all have the potential to support childhood immunization in the years to come.

Political will should also be grounded in the realization that immunizing children makes economic sense. At an average cost of about US$58 per child in low- and middle-income countries, the standard course of vaccines can contribute enormously to protecting against disease and lifelong disability.[31] But it does much more than that. For example, it can help to protect families' livelihoods: Families, especially the poorest, can face catastrophic costs if parents have to take time off work to care for a sick child or pay for health care. Longer term, protecting children against disease can result in huge savings in spending on health care, and can support societies and economies in developing human capital and productivity.[32] Despite shrinking national budgets in some countries, immunization must remain a priority because it is a proven strategy for reducing future health-care costs and it supports economic growth.[33] Continued and sustainable investment in immunization as part of health budgets is essential. But governments and donors need to work together to improve the efficiency and effectiveness of planning, budgeting and service delivery.[34]

Now is a time for determination.

Now is a time for political will.

Now is the time to protect the health of *every* child.

> Despite shrinking national budgets in some countries, immunization must remain a priority because it is a proven strategy for reducing future health-care costs and it supports economic growth

About this report

The State of the World's Children 2023 examines what needs to happen to ensure that every child, everywhere is protected against vaccine-preventable diseases. In the wake of the COVID-19 pandemic, which set back progress in childhood immunization globally, it focuses on the role of poverty, marginalization and gender in determining whether or not children are vaccinated. Drawing on lessons learned during the pandemic and from UNICEF's decades-long expertise and experience in vaccinating children, it examines the ways in which primary health care can be strengthened to better support immunization services. It looks, too, at concerns around trust in vaccines. And examines a range of innovations in vaccine development and delivery and in financing.

Chapter 1 looks at how and why the COVID-19 pandemic set back childhood immunization. It examines what needs to happen to make up the ground that was lost during the pandemic and explores some of the lessons the pandemic offers for making routine immunization more resilient.

Chapter 2 examines which children are missing out on immunization – and why it matters. It presents new data and analysis that help to explain the role that a range of social, cultural, economic and gender-related factors play in shaping immunization outcomes.

Chapter 3 explores the vital links between immunization and primary health care. A key focus of IA2030 is the need to make immunization services sustainable and resilient by integrating them into strong and well-resourced primary health care systems that put the needs of communities at their heart.

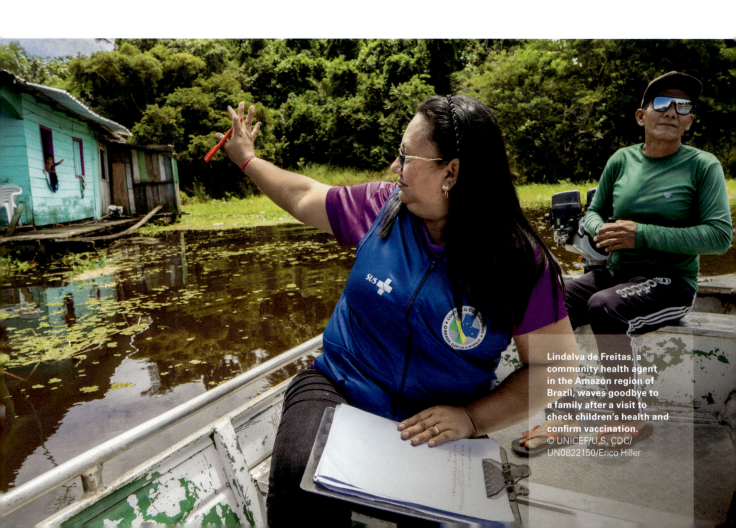

Lindalva de Freitas, a community health agent in the Amazon region of Brazil, waves goodbye to a family after a visit to check children's health and confirm vaccination.
© UNICEF/U.S. CDC/UN0822150/Erico Hiller

Chapter 4 looks at the role of vaccine confidence in shaping families' decisions to vaccinate children. It explores a range of approaches, including community engagement, social listening and empowering women and girls, that can help counter some worrying signs of declines in confidence.

Chapter 5 examines innovative approaches in vaccine development and delivery, as well as promising new approaches to improve funding for immunization services.

And **Chapter 6** proposes an action agenda for equity in immunization. It offers four key recommendations for global, national and local stakeholders to help ensure life-saving vaccines reach every child.

1. **Vaccinate every child, everywhere** by, first, catching up on children who were not vaccinated during the pandemic and helping disrupted services to recover fully. Longer term, an even more determined effort is needed to tackle the bottlenecks in health and other systems that have persistently prevented children in marginalized and underserved communities from being vaccinated.

2. **Strengthen demand for – and confidence in – vaccination** by engaging with communities, to ensure their evolving needs help to shape programmes, and by focusing on interventions that target the role of women. Health workers, especially women working on the front lines of primary health care, can be helped to play an even stronger role in advocating for and building confidence in vaccination, while strengthened accountability in health-system governance can help ensure communities' needs are better met. These efforts will ultimately boost trust in health systems.

3. **Spend more and spend better in immunization and health.** In times of fiscal pressure, the high return on investment means that immunization needs to remain a priority for governments. However, investment in immunization needs to be coupled with more effective and efficient planning, budgeting and service delivery. Developing innovative financing mechanisms is also important. In addition, donors need to increase their support, harmonize it with country contexts, and centre it on strengthening primary health care.

4. **Build resilient systems and shockproof them for the future** by expanding the health workforce, especially community health workers, and by offering them training, support and predictable payments. Focus especially on supporting, motivating and retaining the many women working in health systems, and offer clear paths for career development. Adopt innovations in vaccines, supply chains, delivery, data collection and disease surveillance to reach every child, which will help build the foundations to meet the challenges of disease outbreaks and future pandemics.

SOMALIA
Measles: Health centre outreach provides personal link to vaccination

When all else fails, Maryam Mohamud and her team at Gargaar Health Centre turn to the experts on the importance of immunization: mothers who have lived through the tragedy of measles.

"We conduct awareness campaigns, and we explain to the moms about the importance of the measles vaccine," Mohamud said.

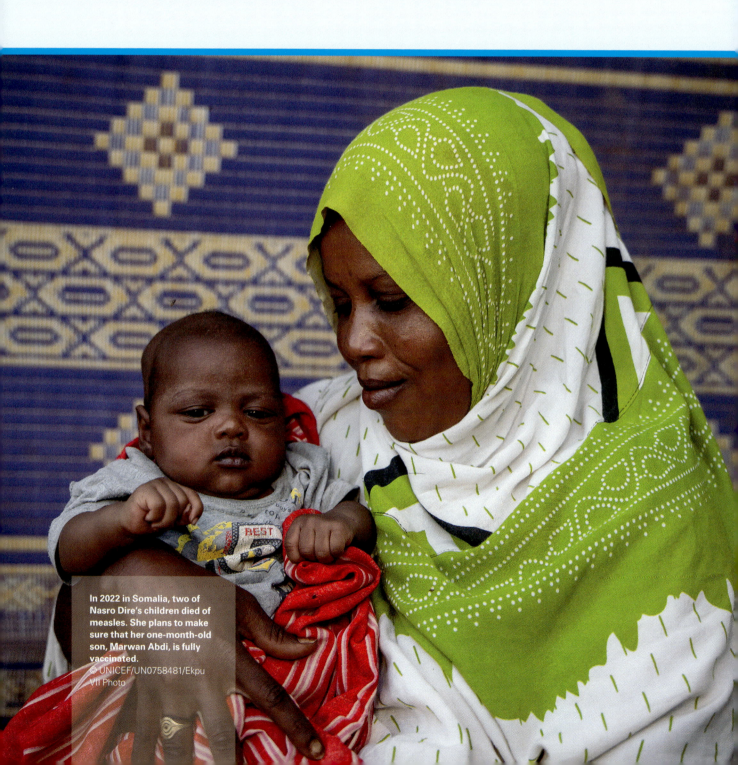

In 2022 in Somalia, two of Nasro Dire's children died of measles. She plans to make sure that her one-month-old son, Marwan Abdi, is fully vaccinated.
© UNICEF/UN0758481/Ekpu VII Photo

Then, Mohamud and her team allow a mother whose child died from measles to explain the importance.

"That's when they accept the vaccine," she said.

It is a difficult lesson, one laced with loss and tragedy. In Somalia, the effects of drought and food insecurity have left children at great risk of disease including measles. Indeed, from January to October 2022, Somalia had more than 15,000 suspected cases of measles – 79 per cent in children under age 5.

Nasro Dire knows the sorrow of measles.

Dire, 23, lives in the Jawle camp for internally displaced persons, a labyrinth of metal shacks on the northern outskirts of Garowe, in central Somalia. At the beginning of 2022, two of Dire's children – Aanas, age 2, and Masude, age 1 – fell ill. First they had fever, then a rash. She took them to Jawle Medical Centre, near the camp where she lives. But Aanas and Masude died a month apart.

"As a parent I felt very bad," Dire said. "But I still believe God has taken them."

Under the guidance of Luul Agani, a midwife and vaccine volunteer in the Jawle community, Dire made sure her surviving children – ages 3, 4 and 6 – were fully vaccinated. And she will do the same for her one-month-old boy, Marwan. Dire also helps Agani convince other mothers to do the same.

"The experience I went through with the death of my children made me want to vaccinate others," Dire said.

In general, most parents in the Jawle camp want their children immunized, said Mohud Hassan, the manager of Jawle Medical Centre. But getting these children vaccinated takes work. It means reaching out to some of the world's most vulnerable communities – internally displaced persons, host communities and families who live in the dusty dirt-road settlements of metal on the outskirts of Garowe. UNICEF provides support in Somalia by procuring vaccines, supporting the cold chain and conducting social mobilization campaigns for routine and supplementary immunization activities.

Jawle Medical Centre, like many health centres that serve marginalized communities in the Garowe area, mobilizes workers who reach out by text messages, phone or in person to make sure children have access to vaccination. At Jilab Health Centre, for example, health workers set up 'fixed temporary outreach' three times a week in parts of the community where mothers and children do not make use of the central facility.

"Outreach is very important to reach the child who cannot come to the health centre and the mother who cannot come," said Kowther Abdikadir, a 24-year-old clinical health worker and social worker at Jilab Health Centre. "It is important as well for the health workers. It is very important to check exactly what is going on at home."

Fixed temporary outreach efforts are also part of the services Mohamud and her staff offer from Gargaar Health Centre. But one-on-one interaction, a critical part of the centre's newborn delivery programme, also plays a critical role in establishing an ongoing relationship with newborns and mothers. Mohamud and staff members make sure they have contact information for the mothers of newborns delivered at the health centre and the mothers who come to the health centre for services. Most mothers have mobile phones, Mohamud said. But when they do not, health workers take a neighbour's number or the number of the local store owner.

This personalized outreach paid off for multiple mothers who recently came to Gargaar Health Centre for vaccinations. Amina Said, a mother of four children, walked for an hour to have Kafio vaccinated – she was responding to a message she received from the health centre.

"That's why I always vaccinate my children," Said said. "I don't write and I don't read but they give me calls on the phone." ■

FOR EVERY CHILD, VACCINATION

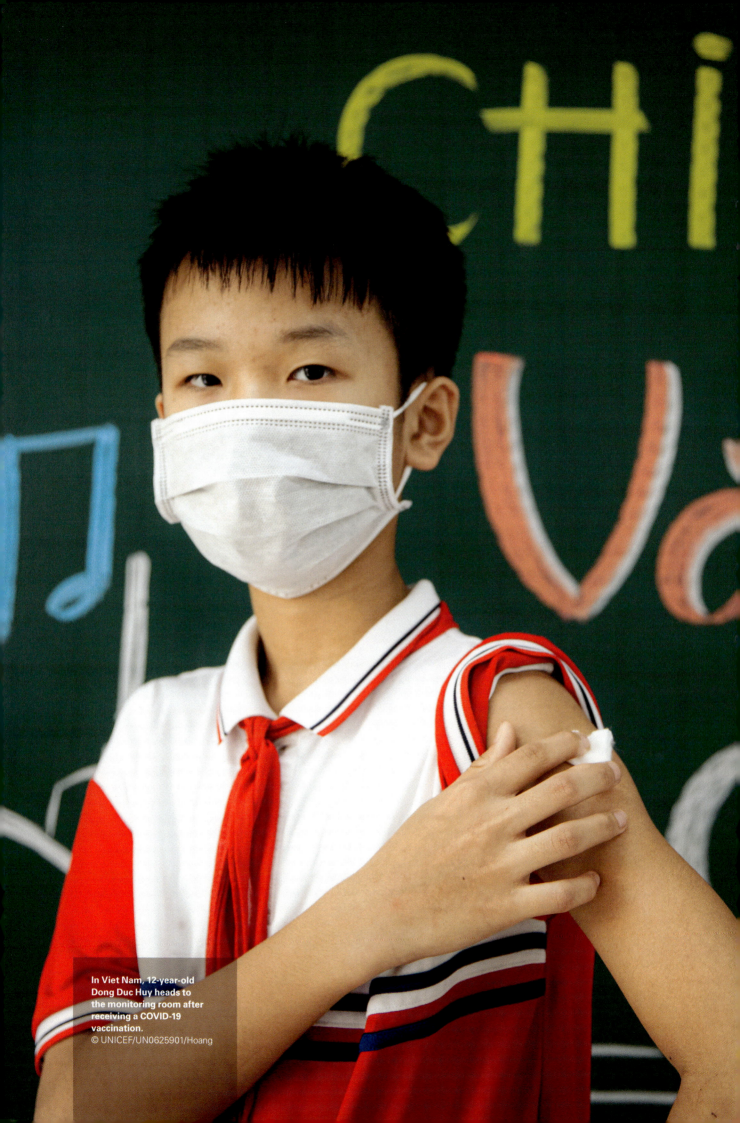

In Viet Nam, 12-year-old Dong Duc Huy heads to the monitoring room after receiving a COVID-19 vaccination.
© UNICEF/UN0625901/Hoang

CHAPTER 1

How the COVID-19 pandemic set back vaccination

The world is facing a red alert for children's health: Vaccination coverage dropped sharply during the COVID-19 pandemic, leaving millions more children unprotected against some of childhood's most serious diseases. Catch-up and recovery are urgently needed to vaccinate the children missed and to avoid further backsliding. But encouragingly, the pandemic also provided some useful lessons on how to do immunization better.

The COVID-19 pandemic has been a disaster for childhood immunization. It set immunization back to levels last seen in 2008. In just two years, the world lost more than a decade's progress in ensuring every child is adequately immunized.

The COVID-19 pandemic has been a disaster for childhood immunization. It set immunization back to levels last seen in 2008. In just two years, the world lost more than a decade's progress in ensuring every child is adequately immunized. This backsliding reflected some issues specific to the pandemic, particularly the impact of lockdowns and service disruption. But it also cast a powerful spotlight on longer-term issues, including the weakness of far too many primary health care systems, which has long undermined efforts to vaccinate every child.

Catching up on the children who missed out entirely or partly on vaccination during the pandemic will be a major challenge, and it will require substantial investment to design and implement appropriate catch-up interventions. In the face of difficult economic headwinds, there is also a need to support health and immunization services to prevent continued backsliding.

The pandemic also provided important lessons for the future of immunization, including highlighting the role of the health workforce as a key component of resilient primary health care systems. It also led to the development of new approaches to vaccine development, production and delivery, which have the potential to greatly reduce the time it takes to develop vaccines in the future and to speed up responses to future health emergencies.

How the pandemic set back immunization

The numbers are stark. Between 2019 and 2021, the number of zero-dose children rose from 13 million to 18 million globally, an increase of more than a third. There was a sharp increase, too, in the number of under-vaccinated children, which rose by 6 million to 25 million. The increases in the numbers of zero-dose children were especially notable in India, Indonesia, Myanmar and the Philippines.

In terms of coverage, the percentage of children fully vaccinated against diphtheria, tetanus and pertussis – a key measure of vaccine coverage – fell from 86 per cent to 81 per cent. There was a similar fall in measles vaccine coverage.

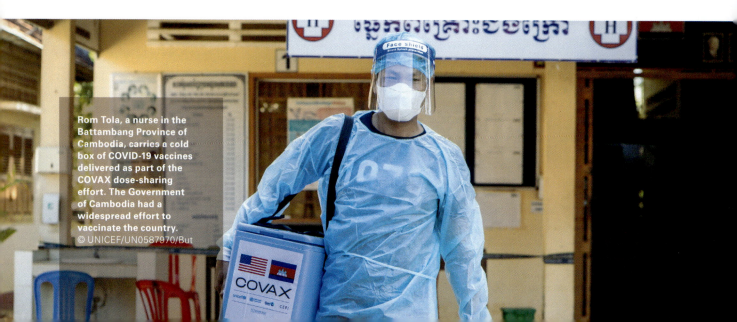

Rom Tola, a nurse in the Battambang Province of Cambodia, carries a cold box of COVID-19 vaccines delivered as part of the COVAX dose-sharing effort. The Government of Cambodia had a widespread effort to vaccinate the country.
© UNICEF/UN0587970/But

Figure 1.1. **East Asia and the Pacific region experienced particularly large declines in vaccine coverage**
DTP3 vaccination coverage by UNICEF programme region, 2019–2021

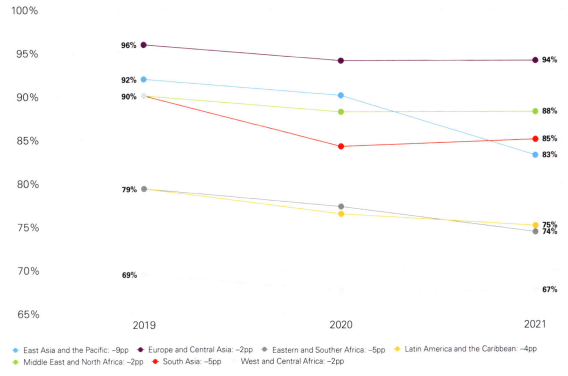

Source: World Health Organization and United Nations Children's Fund, 'Estimates of National Immunization Coverage (WUENIC), 2021 revision', July 2022.

Figure 1.2. **Vast regional differences exist for the 67 million children who missed out on vaccination**
Zero-dose and under-vaccinated children from 2019 to 2021 by UNICEF programme region in millions

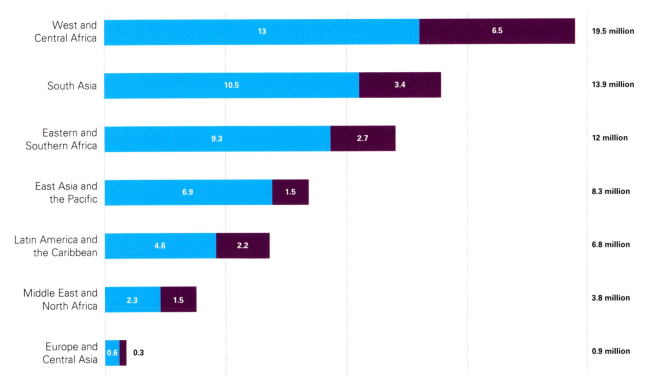

Source: World Health Organization and United Nations Children's Fund, 'Estimates of National Immunization Coverage (WUENIC), 2021 revision', July 2022.
Note: Numbers may not add up to 67 million because of rounding.

FOR EVERY CHILD, VACCINATION

Figure 1.3. **The COVID-19 pandemic brought a drop in vaccination coverage**
Percentages of children globally who received DTP1, DTP3 and measles vaccines

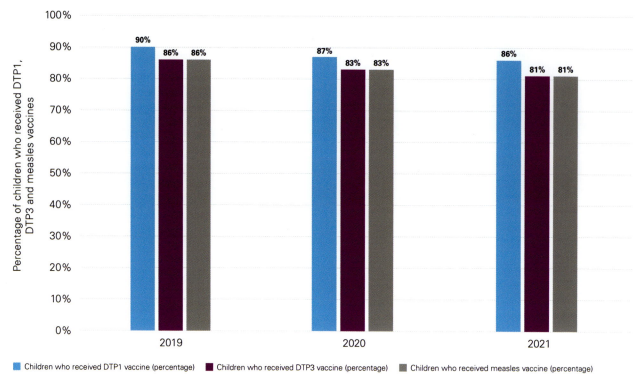

Source: World Health Organization and United Nations Children's Fund, 'Estimates of National Immunization Coverage (WUENIC), 2021 revision', July 2022.

Figure 1.4. **The pandemic set back already-low rates of HPV vaccine coverage**
Percentage of girls who received the first dose of the HPV vaccine (HPV1) by UNICEF programme region, 2019–2021

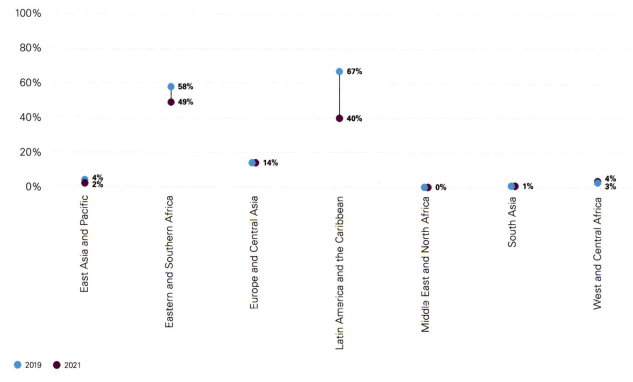

Source: World Health Organization estimates of human papillomavirus (HPV) immunization coverage, 2010–2021, 15 July 2022.

THE STATE OF THE WORLD'S CHILDREN 2023

Rising risk of measles

These figures, for zero-dose and under-vaccinated children, are based on vaccination against diphtheria, tetanus and pertussis, or DTP *(see Introduction)*. But vaccinations against other diseases also dropped sharply during the pandemic.

Two years of decline during the pandemic saw a 5-percentage point fall in the number of children receiving their first measles shot. Because measles is so contagious, around 95 per cent of a community needs to be immunized in order to reach herd immunity.[1] As a result, any decline in coverage is worrying and raises the risk of significant outbreaks of the disease.

The number of measles cases doubled in 2022 compared with the previous year,[2] and UNICEF and the World Health Organization (WHO) warned of a "perfect storm" of conditions for outbreaks of the disease.[3] There have also been concerns about the risk of outbreaks of other vaccine-preventable diseases.[4]

This deteriorating situation reflects not just disruptions to immunization during the pandemic, but also disruptions caused by conflict, fragility and extreme weather events in countries including Afghanistan, Ethiopia, Myanmar, Somalia and Ukraine. As a result, many families have been forced to leave their homes, leaving children with limited access to clean water and sanitation, and exposing them to overcrowding, all of which raise the risk of outbreaks of vaccine-preventable disease.

There are also worrying signs on children's nutrition. Poor diets can make children more vulnerable to infections. Since 2016, some countries have seen a rise of at least 40 per cent in wasting, a life-threatening condition characterized by a child being too thin for their height.[5] The number of people globally affected by hunger has risen by about 150 million since the pandemic began, while there have also been increases in the numbers facing food insecurity.[6]

HPV losses

The pandemic had a particularly severe impact on the effort to vaccinate children against human papillomavirus (HPV). Over the course of the pandemic, the world lost more than a quarter of global coverage of HPV vaccination. That large fall reflected in part the closure of schools, where many children receive their vaccinations.[7] The HPV vaccine helps protect against a number of cancers, notably cervical cancer, which is estimated to be the fourth-biggest cause of cancer deaths among women worldwide.[8] Almost three out of five cervical cancer cases occur in countries that have yet to introduce HPV vaccination.[9] Currently, only around 12 per cent of eligible girls are fully vaccinated against HPV.[10]

Understanding the pandemic's impact

Why did the pandemic set back immunization? A number of factors led to the decline, including strains on overstretched health systems and health workers, and especially on overworked women health workers, as well as confusing communication to parents.

Overstretched health systems
Perhaps the most significant factor was the impact of the pandemic on primary health care and health systems. As previous crises have shown, countries with already weak health systems are especially vulnerable to the impacts of conflict, major disease outbreaks and natural disasters.[11] The COVID-19 pandemic was no exception.

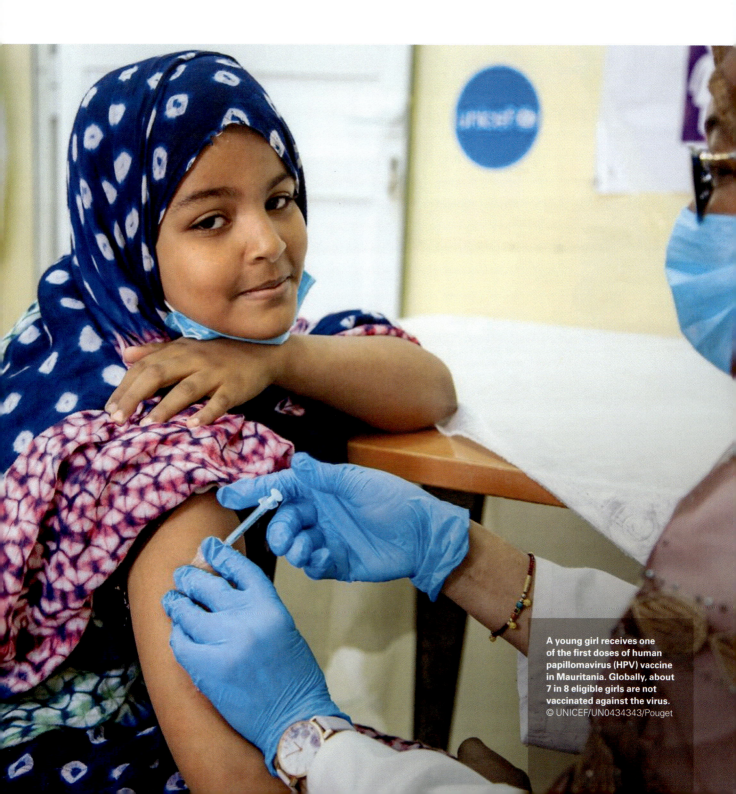

A young girl receives one of the first doses of human papillomavirus (HPV) vaccine in Mauritania. Globally, about 7 in 8 eligible girls are not vaccinated against the virus.
© UNICEF/UN0434343/Pouget

The pandemic forced many health systems to divert scarce resources away from providing routine care, including immunization.[12] For example, at the end of 2021, nearly half of 72 countries in a WHO survey said that routine vaccination programmes were being disrupted by the need to respond to the pandemic.[13]

In addition, the pandemic badly interrupted vaccination campaigns, which, unlike routine immunization, are usually targeted efforts to vaccinate large numbers of people in relatively short periods of time. In May 2020, for example, 57 per cent of campaigns in 57 countries had to be cancelled or postponed, representing the loss of 796 million vaccine doses. Although the situation began to improve in mid-2020, disruptions continued: At the end of 2021, stalled campaigns in African countries still meant the loss of 382 million doses.[14]

There was also a serious impact on the health workforce. Even before the pandemic, many countries were short of skilled health workers, particularly in disadvantaged areas. The pandemic exacerbated this problem and added to the challenges facing health workers, especially women in the health workforce *(see Chapter 3)*. Many could not access essential equipment, including personal protective equipment. They also faced the risk of infection, social discrimination and attacks. As well as being expected to handle a huge increase in their workload, most also had their own responsibilities to care for friends and family, including children locked out from school. Burn-out became a critical issue.

The pandemic also affected countries' capacities to gather health information and data and carry out surveillance of disease outbreaks. For example, following the alarming detection of a case of wild poliovirus in February 2022, Malawi struggled to determine how polio had arrived and how long it had spread undetected.[15] Even by mid-2022, disease surveillance across many countries had not returned to pre-pandemic levels.

Vaccine supply chains also came under strain, for a time at least, amid global restrictions on international travel and limits on movement within borders.[16] It is estimated that early on in the pandemic, in April 2020, global vaccine sales fell by about a third.[17] The global picture varied but, overall, these supply constraints seem to have been relatively short-lived.

Family fears

A final factor is the impact the pandemic had on families' abilities and willingness to get their children vaccinated. Even where health-care facilities remained open, travel restrictions or tight family budgets may have led families to put off getting children vaccinated. 'Stay-at-home' recommendations may have led some parents to see routine vaccination as non-essential care, which underlines the need for careful, nuanced communication with families during major disease outbreaks.[18] Significantly, parents may also have been wary of visiting clinics for fear of contracting COVID-19.[19]

INDONESIA

In the Wake of COVID-19: Catching up on childhood immunization

The sun had just risen on a Sunday morning in August as Irwan Hakim, a community clinic nurse, strode through the streets of Kerayaan, a remote village in Kalimantan, the Indonesian part of Borneo.

With a megaphone pressed to his mouth, Irwan broadcast his message: Immunize your children today.

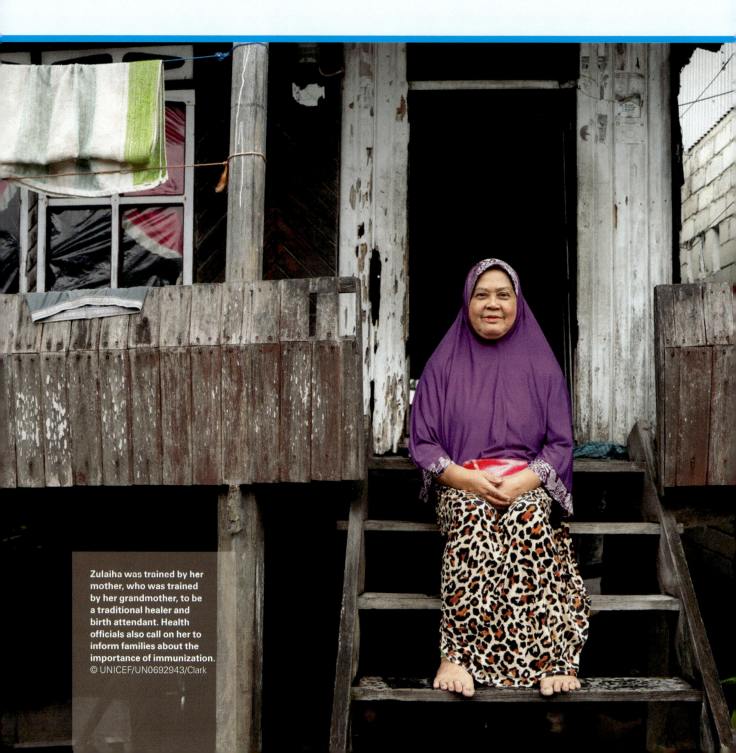

Zulaiha was trained by her mother, who was trained by her grandmother, to be a traditional healer and birth attendant. Health officials also call on her to inform families about the importance of immunization.
© UNICEF/UN0692943/Clark

By 8:30 a.m., 381 children aged 5–12 years and their parents had heeded his call and gathered at the Rusung Raya Public Primary School for vaccines against potentially deadly diseases, such as measles and rubella.

"The turnout is usually not this high," Irwan said, surveying the front yard of the school where the children and their families assembled. "This morning is an exception."

The major reason for this success is efforts by Irwan and a network of nurses, midwives and traditional birth attendants who work closely with the community to build trust, dispel myths and encourage parents to immunize their children.

Irwan and his network were activated as part of the National Child Immunization Month (BIAN). With support from partners including UNICEF, BIAN campaigns had been launched throughout Indonesia. The goal: to reverse a backslide in routine childhood vaccinations linked to the COVID-19 pandemic.

COVID-19 took a significant toll on routine immunization services for children throughout Indonesia. Full vaccination coverage dropped from 93.7 per cent in 2019 to 84.5 per cent in 2021, according to the Ministry of Health. In part, the drop was caused by disrupted supply chains, regulations that limited vaccination activities and a lack of available health workers.

Nationwide, parents and caregivers were reluctant to bring children to health-care facilities for fear of infection, according to a 2020 survey by the Indonesia Ministry of Health and UNICEF.

In Kerayaan, an area that already had a small health workforce, the virus sidelined many health workers. Vaccines were also not delivered and locations that provide vaccinations were closed. Vaccination has been particularly low in Kerayaan, where only 10 out of 45 newborns were vaccinated as of April 2022. Its remote location is a major barrier.

"It takes about 13 hours by motorized vehicles, ferry and wooden boat to reach Kerayaan from the provincial capital," said Dr. Suprapti Tri Astuti, head of Kotabaru District Health Office, which oversees immunization services in Kerayaan. "So the pandemic exacerbated this situation."

In addition to the geographic difficulties, scepticism about vaccines is also common. To address these concerns, the health network turns to traditional healers such as Zulaiha.

Zulaiha was trained by her mother, who was trained by her grandmother. She attends women who are in labour and provides guidance to people who come to her for traditional healing, including incantation and application of herbs.

But she also knows the power of immunization. As part of the BIAN campaign, Zulaiha continued her work going house to house to encourage parents and caregivers to take their children to the health centre for vaccinations.

"I do house visits to get children to be vaccinated," Zulaiha said. "I explain to their parents, get them to go to posyandu [health post]. I told them to not be afraid. Side effects like fever are normal."

Thanks to Irwan, Zulaiha and the wider network of which they are a part, nearly 90 per cent of newborns in Kerayaan were vaccinated during BIAN. UNICEF has supported health workers through workshops, monitoring and coordinating with village officials to identify unvaccinated children and encourage families to bring their children for immunization.

"Increasing understanding and awareness of the importance of immunization for children is critical for families and needs to be continuously instilled in the whole community," Irwan said. "It is our dream that all children on Kerayaan Island can have the right to live a healthy life free from illness, disability and death from diseases that can be prevented through immunization." ■

Making up lost ground

In total, UNICEF estimates that some 67 million children missed out entirely or partially on routine immunization from 2019 to 2021. The challenge of reaching these children will be substantial. While some will eventually be vaccinated through catch-up campaigns, most will not receive full vaccination, and some will receive none. And as they pass the age when children are typically vaccinated, it will become ever harder to reach them through conventional campaigns and routine immunization programmes. Encouragingly, however, there were some early signs of recovery in childhood immunization services in a number of countries in 2022.

Catch-up and recovery

As this report states, investments in areas such as primary health care, vaccine development and delivery, and innovations are required to reach the global immunization goals.

In the short term, there is also an urgent need to reach the children who missed out on vaccination because of the pandemic – and other factors including conflict – with intensified catch-up initiatives. These initiatives will need to identify and locate zero-dose and under-vaccinated children and missed communities. This will allow the development of specific plans and strategies to ensure catch-up initiatives reach the communities and children with the greatest needs. A key component of this work is engaging with communities to help identify barriers to children being vaccinated and to develop approaches that meet the needs of their families.

But catch-up alone will not be enough. In countries where the pace of recovery in immunization services is slow, and where there is a risk of continued backsliding, there is a need to ensure services are fully restored to at least pre-pandemic levels as quickly as possible. Key priorities will include tailoring strategies to specific settings that have been identified as priority areas for reaching zero-dose children.

In urban settings, this will involve ensuring immunization services respond to families' needs and recovering human resources lost due to the need to respond to the pandemic. There will also be a need in many urban settings to address the social exclusion of displaced and refugee populations. In remote rural areas, a focus will be needed on outreach activities to communities and on better integrating services. And in fragile and conflict-affected settings, restoring health workforces and infrastructure is a key priority, as is negotiating access to communities and bundling immunization with delivery of humanitarian and other essential services.

Success in both these catch-up and recovery approaches is essential to sustainably make up ground lost during the pandemic and to lay the foundations for the longer-term goals set out in the *Immunization Agenda 2030*.

> Catch-up alone will not be enough. In countries where the pace of recovery in immunization services is slow, and where there is a risk of continued backsliding, there is a need to ensure services are fully restored to at least pre-pandemic levels as quickly as possible.

Learning from the pandemic

Calamitous as it has been, the COVID-19 pandemic has brought changes in the vaccine landscape that the global community must capitalize on to boost childhood immunization. The experience of the pandemic revealed that, with political will and leadership, vast resources can be mobilized, and new vaccines can be developed rapidly and introduced around the world. These included the worldwide COVID-19 Vaccines Global Access (COVAX) initiative, which aimed at equitable access, and which has shipped just under 1.9 billion vaccine doses around the world.[20] The establishment of the COVID-19 Vaccine Delivery Partnership (CoVDP) to coordinate, harmonize and streamline support for vaccine delivery is another testimony to the political will and institutional agility needed in times of crisis *(see Box 3)*. With millions of children's lives at stake, we need the same urgency around routine child immunization.

The urgency of routine immunization

While an emergency in itself, the pandemic underscored another one: the pressing need to maximize uninterrupted, high-quality health care for children as a fundamental human right. Routine immunization is a central component of such life-saving care. Ensuring that it continues amid emergencies will require improved governance and enhanced financing, both at global level to ensure better pandemic preparedness and responses, and at national level to enable a strong health system with access to quality health care and surge capacity to accommodate heightened need during crises.

To adequately fund health systems, low-income countries would need to dramatically increase their health spending beyond what they have ever done in the past, according to the World Bank.[21] Not doing so would compromise their ability to strengthen and maintain public-health preparedness and response capabilities and may force countries into difficult zero-sum choices regarding which health services deserve investments.

Unfortunately, many countries are facing these choices amid worsening fiscal constraints. While some countries may be able to increase the share of spending on health, it may not always be possible to achieve adequate levels of health financing from governments' domestic resource investments alone.[22] A key pandemic lesson is that failures in one country's health system contribute to suffering beyond that country's borders. Collaborative efforts, including increases in development assistance for health and debt relief for countries facing debt distress, can bolster countries' abilities to immunize every child. These efforts thus represent a public good that can improve health outcomes globally.

Box 3

Partnerships to tackle COVID

The COVID-19 pandemic brought to light the urgent need for governments and partners to work together to accelerate vaccination to protect children and families.

Key among these partnerships was COVID-19 Vaccines Global Access (COVAX), a global initiative to ensure equitable access to COVID-19 vaccines. COVAX is directed by the Coalition for Epidemic Preparedness Innovations (CEPI), Gavi, the Vaccine Alliance and the World Health Organization (WHO), with UNICEF as the delivery partner.

In 2020, COVAX initiated a COVAX Country Readiness and Delivery workstream, which provided global guidance and technical support for introducing COVID-19 vaccination initiatives. Building on this work, UNICEF, Gavi, WHO and other partners founded the COVID-19 Vaccine Delivery Partnership (CoVDP) in January 2022.

CoVDP's goal is to provide support to 92 low- and middle-income countries. →

→ The particular focus is on 34 countries with COVID-19 vaccination coverage at or below 10 per cent.

Since CoVDP was founded, coverage in the 34 countries increased from 3 per cent to 25 per cent in January 2023. As of January 2023, the number of countries at or below 10 per cent coverage had decreased from 34 to 7, with 13 of the original 34 reaching over 20 per cent coverage. In addition, six countries recorded coverage above 40 per cent.

CoVDP has contributed to this progress by combining high-level advocacy and technical country missions to 27 countries. It also facilitated the urgent release of US$145 million in funding for vaccine delivery, provided specialized technical assistance, and coordinated cooperation among the partners.

As the pandemic made clear, health systems are only as strong as their health workforces. WHO has released guidance on health workforce policy to support and protect health workers so that they can maintain essential health care at all times.[23] Infection prevention and control, proper and timely remuneration, and mental health support are all essential supports for health workers.[24]

A number of countries stepped up in the face of health worker burn-out and other difficulties during the pandemic. For example, Peru established procedures for mental health care and self-care of health-care providers, along with psychosocial support teams in facilities.

A sped-up, coordinated response

The COVID-19 response accelerated norms and practices around vaccine development and approval. Advancements such as messenger RNA (mRNA), a breakthrough vaccine platform with wide applicability that had been in development on the margins for decades, suddenly had proof-of-concept with vaccinations around the globe. Approval processes by many governments for COVID vaccines were also sped up, laying the groundwork for more rapid approval of forthcoming vaccines against infectious diseases such as influenza (flu) and respiratory syncytial virus (RSV). Governments and non-governmental organizations (NGOs) also stepped in to remove risks from the research and development (R&D) process, incentivizing pharmaceutical companies to compete to develop vaccines. The global community can capitalize on these developments to hasten discoveries of new vaccines to protect children against diseases such as malaria, HIV and tuberculosis.

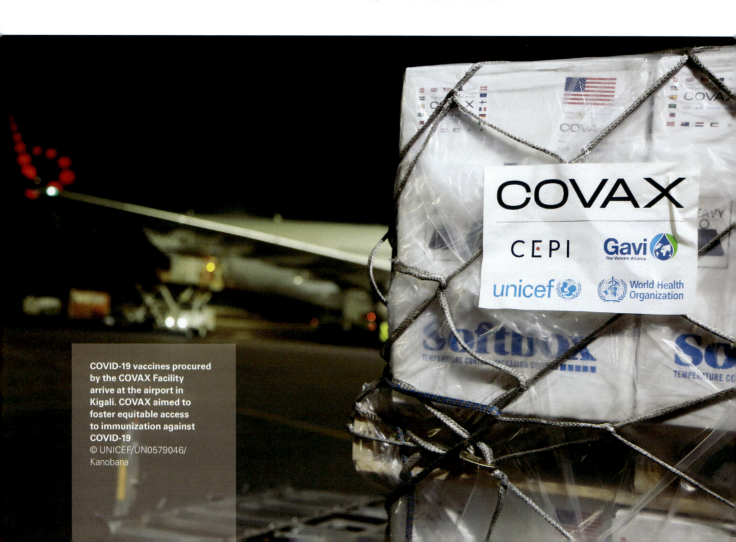

COVID-19 vaccines procured by the COVAX Facility arrive at the airport in Kigali. COVAX aimed to foster equitable access to immunization against COVID-19
© UNICEF/UN0579046/Kanobana

The benefits of digital technologies also became more evident during the pandemic. Many low- and middle-income countries have made significant investments in digital health systems and were able to expand these to provide substantial support to the COVID-19 response and beyond for critical activities including planning the distribution of diagnostics, treatments and vaccines, and monitoring coverage. The pandemic also spurred innovations such as greater use of qualitative data; remote data collection technologies; and improved communication, collaboration and data-sharing across international agencies.[25]

Integrate health crisis response with routine immunization

The pandemic underscored the importance of integrating crisis-related responses and routine immunization. Too often, supplementary immunization activities (SIAs) have redirected people, money, supplies and time from under-resourced primary health care services, which hurts routine immunization outreach and the primary service. For example, and as already noted, in many countries COVID-19 immunization campaigns were undertaken at the expense of routine vaccination programmes. During outbreaks, epidemics or pandemics, governments need to ensure that routine immunization is not interrupted. Ideally, governments can deliver routine immunization along with crisis-related vaccination and health services. In addition, routine immunization services should also be ready to adopt new vaccines that evolve because of crisis.

Integration strategies yielded results in campaigns in both Ghana and Nigeria *(see Box 4)*. Building on the success of its National Immunization Days for polio, Child Health Promotion Weeks and outbreak responses, Ghana has offered national COVID-19 vaccination combined with routine immunization during the pandemic. In November 2021, vaccination outreach teams carried yellow fever and COVID-19 vaccines and administered both to eligible people. This effort, which had a strong focus on risk communication and community engagement, stopped the yellow fever outbreak.

Longer-term challenges

Even if rapid progress is made to catch up on ground lost during the pandemic, the longer-term challenge of reaching every child with vaccines will not be solved overnight. As the next chapter shows, zero-dose and under-vaccinated children live in some of the world's most challenging settings. Identifying them and understanding the barriers they and their families face on the journey to vaccination is essential if every child is to benefit from protection against vaccine-preventable diseases.

Box 4
Nigeria's family approach

During the pandemic, Nigeria launched what is known as a 'whole family' approach, combining COVID-19 vaccination with health services such as childhood vaccination, malnutrition, family planning, antenatal and delivery services, and screening for non-communicable diseases. With this integrated model, Lagos State reported it was able to mitigate a third wave of COVID-19, prevent polio and cholera outbreaks while still curbing communicable and non-communicable diseases.

The pandemic underscored the importance of integrating crisis-related responses and routine immunization.

CAMBODIA

Progress from the Pandemic: COVID-19 inspires innovation in immunization for children

On a sweltering day in June 2022, three generations of women in the same family arrived outside a small rural grocery store where a team of vaccinators had temporarily set up a one-stop shop for protection against disease.

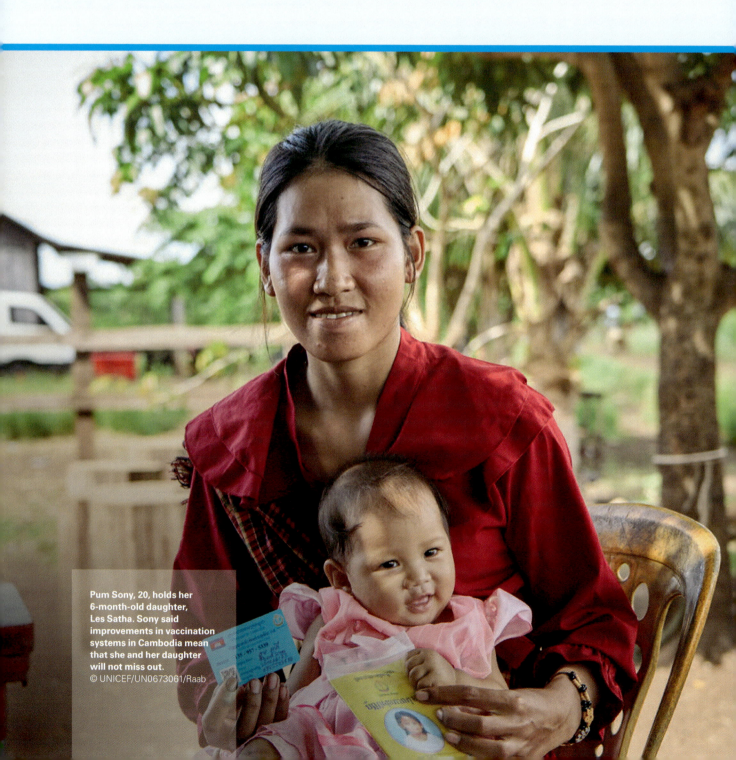

Pum Sony, 20, holds her 6-month-old daughter, Les Satha. Sony said improvements in vaccination systems in Cambodia mean that she and her daughter will not miss out.
© UNICEF/UN0673061/Raab

Beneath a shady tree, Satha, the baby, was immunized against measles and rubella. Her mother, Pum Sony, and grandmother, Krak Nhuong, received booster shots to protect them from COVID-19.

For mother and grandmother, the store-front vaccination service was a sign of progress for Mondulkiri, a remote region in the north-east of Cambodia, home to the Bunong indigenous community.

"There's more information on all vaccines, and they're delivered right here in our community," Sony said. "Before, we had to travel on 15 kilometres of dirt roads to get vaccinated at a health centre."

The progress that has benefited Nhuong, Sony and Satha resulted from investments that the Royal Government of Cambodia has made in the country's health system over the course of decades.

"Immunization improved even before the pandemic," said Pyun Kunthea, the government health worker who vaccinated the family. "Just 20 years ago, preventable diseases were still common. ... Things got better, but it was still difficult to reach villages like this, which were distant from health centres."

However, the Government's response to COVID-19 has inspired innovations in communication, technology and social behaviour change that are being applied to the national childhood vaccination programme. At the start of the pandemic, the Cambodian Government, with the support of partners including UNICEF and the World Health Organization, launched an intensive communications and social behaviour change campaign aimed at reaching the entire adult population with COVID-19 vaccinations.

Health officials adapted tools from successful polio and measles campaigns to design and conduct rapid community assessments. These adapted tools provided up-to-date information on where people were not vaccinated and why. Consequently, health workers could provide targeted outreach services and communication campaigns in local languages to communities where coverage was low. The tools were used in eight provinces with low immunization rates.

In addition, the Government of Cambodia launched the country's first digital immunization registration system, KhmerVacc. The mobile application, which has 15.8 million registered users, allows people to sign up for vaccination and sends reminders for follow up.

For children, Cambodia generally has high routine vaccination coverage rates, with only about 6 per cent considered zero-dose children. However, in communities with large populations of ethnic minorities in remote areas, such as Mondulkiri, far too many children miss out.

In 2022, the Government of Cambodia committed to building on the success of KhmerVacc and began incorporating its features into a new, improved platform. Families will be able to register for the service and record routine vaccinations including those that protect children against measles, polio and tuberculosis. This new Electronic Immunization Record, designed by the Ministry of Health with UNICEF support, will help health officials and families keep track of children's immunization status and send appointment alerts to caregivers via SMS. The improvements to these systems were also focused on reaching zero-dose children and enhancing primary health care. Next year, these innovations will be rolled out, as the Cambodian Government introduces the new human papillomavirus (HPV) vaccine that protects against cervical cancer.

For Sony, the improvements in routine immunization services mean that her daughter will benefit from a full range of immunizations that are supported by better registration, targeted communications and expanded integrated outreach services.

"Previously, children from poor families who couldn't afford to travel to health centres missed out on vaccinations," Sony said. "I'm so happy my children won't miss out and will be properly protected." ■

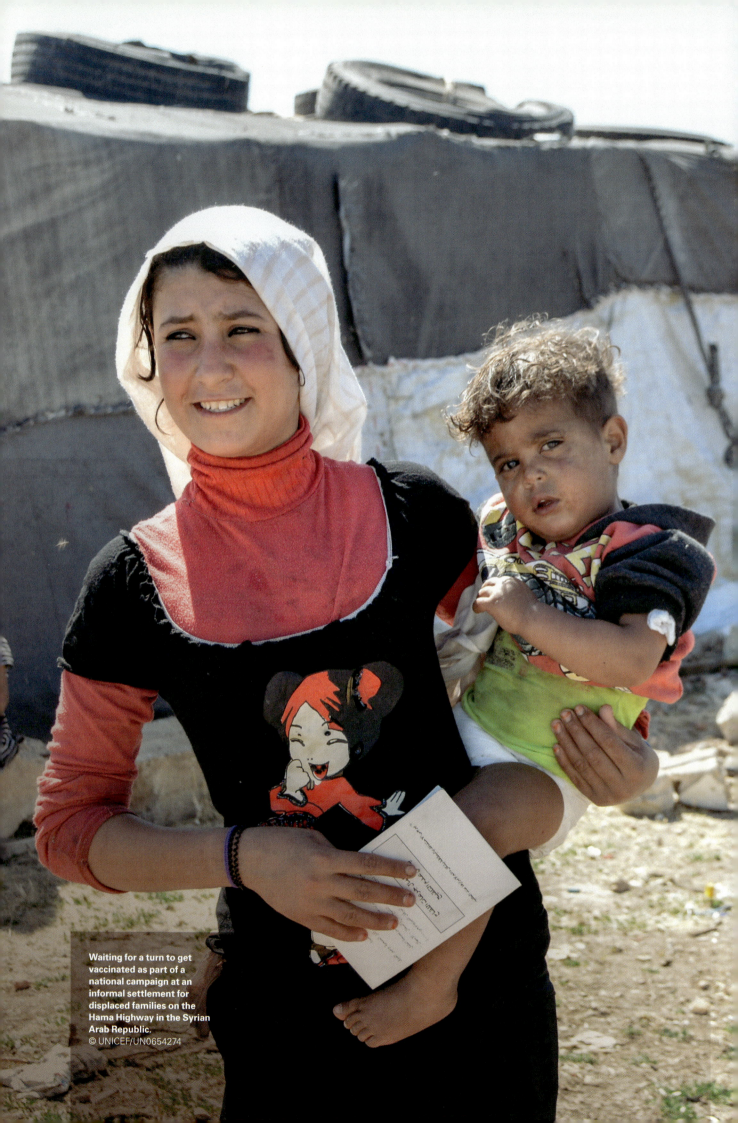

Waiting for a turn to get vaccinated as part of a national campaign at an informal settlement for displaced families on the Hama Highway in the Syrian Arab Republic.
© UNICEF/UN0654274

CHAPTER 2

Zero-dose children matter

The trusted methods that were so successful for so many children failed to immunize many of the world's most vulnerable. For these children, social and economic barriers including poverty, location, marginalization and crisis have prevented vaccines from being available, accessible and affordable. The cost of not reaching these children can be calculated in lives lost and fragile health for children, families, communities and economies.

For the most part, the children left behind live in complex contexts and face multiple deprivations.

They live in the remotest of rural areas, urban slums, peripheral urban settlements, crisis-affected areas, and migrant and refugee communities. They are confronted daily by socioeconomic barriers to immunization: poverty, gender and ethnic marginalization, migration and crisis.

Left behind: socioeconomic determinants of immunization

An analysis for *The State of the World's Children 2023* puts numbers to the link between zero-dose and under-vaccinated children and socioeconomic determinants associated with immunization.[1] The numbers make the connection between inequity and children who miss out on vaccination.

Poverty

> Poverty sits at the centre of a complex interplay of deprivations that determine whether a child is immunized against vaccine-preventable diseases – or not.

Poverty sits at the centre of a complex interplay of deprivations that determine whether a child is immunized against vaccine-preventable diseases – or not.

In the analysis for *The State of the World's Children 2023* report, data showed that children from the very poorest households – households with income in the bottom 10 per cent of the population – were less likely to be immunized than children in the wealthiest 10 per cent *(see Figure 2.1)*. For example, in the poorest households, 22.6 per cent of children were zero-dose children. In contrast, in the wealthiest group, just 4.9 per cent were zero-dose children. The data also indicated that the gaps between the wealthiest and poorest were widest in low-income countries *(see Figure 2.1)* and narrowest in upper-middle-income countries.

West and Central Africa presented the largest gap between rich and poor: 48.6 per cent of children from the poorest households were zero-dose children compared with 6.3 per cent of children in the wealthiest *(see Figure 2.2)*. The narrowest gaps occurred in Latin America and the Caribbean, where 11.3 per cent of children in the poorest households were zero-dose children compared with 5 per cent in the wealthiest.

Interestingly, in Eastern Europe and Central Asia, the situation was reversed: 4.5 per cent of children in the poorest households were zero-dose children compared with 8.1 per cent in the wealthiest.

The analysis also showed great disparities within countries: Among the ten countries with the highest gaps in vaccination coverage between rich and poor, seven were in sub-Saharan Africa.

Location

In addition to poverty, location plays a significant role in whether a child is immunized *(see Figure 2.2)*. In the 74 low- and middle-income countries analysed for UNICEF, 9.4 per cent of children in urban areas were zero-dose children and 15.1 per cent of children in rural areas were zero-dose children.

As with poverty, the greatest gap in immunization by location was in West and Central Africa, where the prevalence of zero-dose children was 16.2 per cent in urban areas and 34.6 per cent in rural areas. In general, the gaps between rural and urban were widest in low-income countries and negligible in upper-middle-income countries.

Figure 2.1. Vast inequities exist for children in poor communities and countries
In 74 low- and middle-income countries, percentage of zero-dose children, percentage in highest and lowest wealth decile, percentage in urban and rural locations organized by World Bank income classification

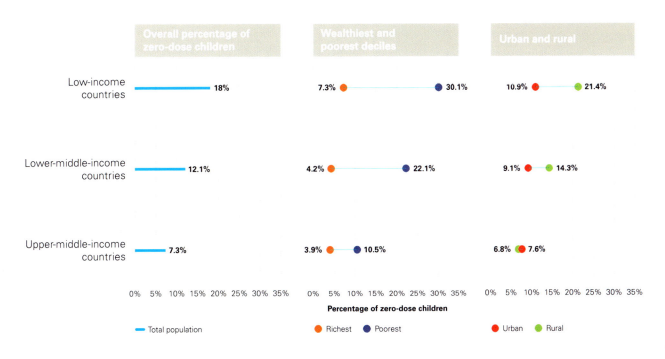

Source: Victora, Cesar, and Aluísio Barros, 'Within-country Inequalities in Zero-dose Prevalence: Background paper for *The State of the World's Children 2023*', International Center for Equity in Health at the Federal University of Pelotas, Brazil, December 2022.

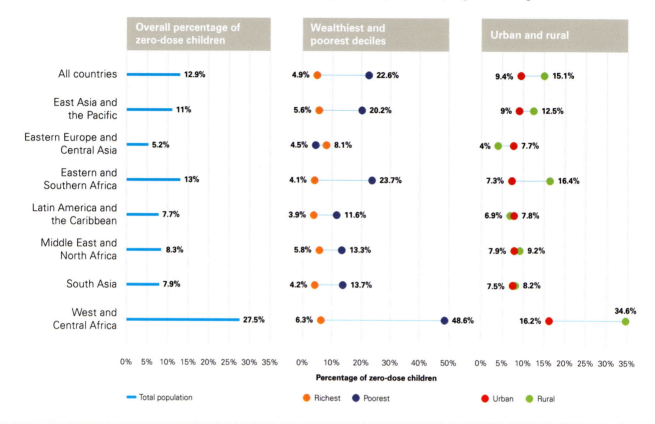

Figure 2.2. West and Central Africa has some of the greatest inequities in children's vaccination coverage
In 74 low- and middle-income countries, percentage of zero-dose children, percentage in highest and lowest wealth decile, percentage in urban and rural locations organized by UNICEF programme regions

Figure 2.3a. In 10 countries, children in poor households are less likely to be vaccinated than children in wealthy households
Ten countries with the largest gap in zero-dose children between the poorest and wealthiest deciles of households

Country	Zero-dose prevalence %	
	Poorest	Wealthiest
Nigeria	65.2	3.8
Angola	54.6	5.5
Papua New Guinea	58.6	10.1
Central African Republic	62.9	12.7
Guinea	59.9	12.7
Ethiopia	46.9	21.5
Democratic Republic of the Congo	50.7	4.8
Lao People's Democratic Republic	45.6	11.4
Pakistan	33.4	13.6
Madagascar	38.3	12.5

Figure 2.3b. Some countries have great inequities between children in urban and rural areas
Ten countries with the largest gap in zero-dose children between urban and rural locations

Country	Zero-dose prevalence %	
	Poorest	Wealthiest
Angola	50.6	18.5
Nigeria	45.0	18.8
Central African Republic	52.5	28.3
Guinea	44.7	21.4
Papua New Guinea	38.7	17.8
Ethiopia	29.7	10.0
Democratic Republic of the Congo	41.8	22.6
Cameroon	22.5	9.1
Mali	20.6	7.9
Afghanistan	29.9	18.0

Source: Victora, Cesar, and Aluísio Barros, 'Within-country Inequalities in Zero-dose Prevalence: Background paper for *The State of the World's Children 2023*', International Center for Equity in Health at the Federal University of Pelotas, Brazil, December 2022.

Marginalization

Multiple forms of marginalization also serve as a barrier to childhood immunization. Though the data show an overall gender balance in immunization rates among girls and boys, there are other ways that gender disparities become barriers to immunization.

The data analysed for the report focused on two categories: a mother's lack of education and her lack of empowerment. The analysis also looked at the connection between ethnic communities and zero-dose children.

Gender

In most communities, mothers have the primary responsibility for children's health.[2] However, social and cultural norms in homes and communities can limit their status and decision-making authority, which can interfere with their ability to act on their own and on their children's behalf. Therefore, women most often have the burden of overcoming barriers of time and distance to immunize their children; they are the family members required to take time from work and travel to have a child immunized. They carry this responsibility despite a lack of status, economic stability and information.[3]

> Multiple forms of marginalization also serve as a barrier to childhood immunization.

The analysis of data in the 74 countries puts common wisdom into numbers: The prevalence of zero-dose children declined as a mother's level of education increased. For example, the data show a:

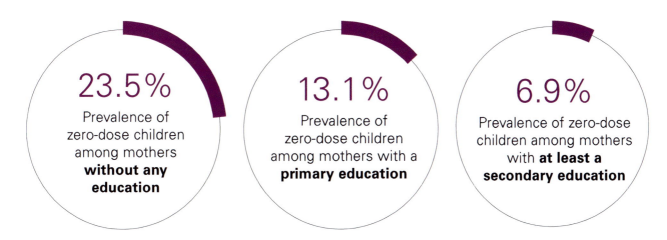

23.5% Prevalence of zero-dose children among mothers **without any education**

13.1% Prevalence of zero-dose children among mothers with a **primary education**

6.9% Prevalence of zero-dose children among mothers with **at least a secondary education**

Though lack of education may limit some mothers, others may want to vaccinate their child but are not empowered to make health-care or financial decisions because of prevalent gender norms. To measure empowerment, the analysis relied on the SWPER (survey-based women's empowerment index) Global Index, an indicator for social independence based on national health surveys in low- and middle-income countries.[4] Of the 74 countries studied, only 33 had empowerment data. In Nigeria, the data showed the greatest gap in vaccination coverage linked to the level of empowerment experienced by mothers. There, the prevalence of zero-dose children among mothers with a low level of empowerment was 53.2 per cent compared with a 10.8 per cent prevalence among mothers with a high level of empowerment *(see Figure 2.4)*.

Figure 2.4. Children whose mothers have little education are less likely to be immunized
Women's education and prevalence of zero-dose children for 74 countries by UNICEF programme region

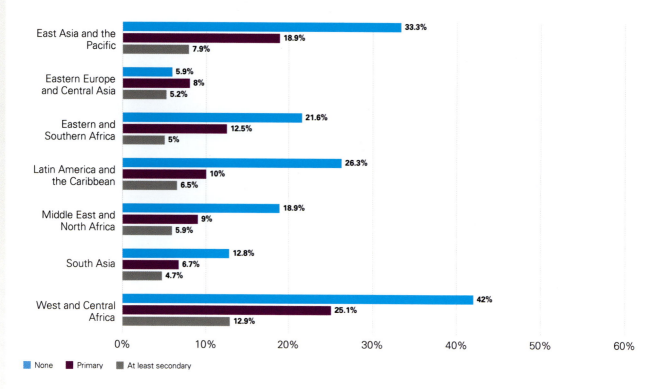

Source: Victora, Cesar, and Aluísio Barros, 'Within-country Inequalities in Zero-dose Prevalence: Background paper for *The State of the World's Children 2023*', International Center for Equity in Health at the Federal University of Pelotas, Brazil, December 2022.

Figure 2.5. Empowered women are more likely to vaccinate their children
Women's empowerment and prevalence of zero-dose children

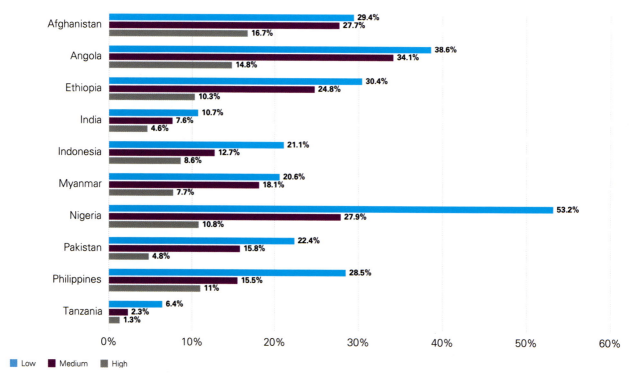

Source: Victora, Cesar, and Aluísio Barros, 'Within-country Inequalities in Zero-dose Prevalence: Background paper for *The State of the World's Children 2023*', International Center for Equity in Health at the Federal University of Pelotas, Brazil, December 2022.

Ethnicity

Disparities in children's health outcomes between different ethnic groups have been the subject of study in high-income countries. However, in low- and middle-income countries, data on inequity between ethnic groups has only recently become available.

The analysis for this report examined data about ethnicity and vaccination coverage from 53 countries. Ethnicity was determined by indicators reported in health surveys such as ethnic affiliation or language. The analysis highlighted high prevalence of zero-dose children in minority ethnic communities in countries such as Afghanistan, Angola, Ethiopia, Nigeria and the Philippines.

The analysis showed that disparities in immunization among minority ethnic groups may offer a way to identify communities with high numbers of zero-dose children.

Crisis

Instability, violence and disruption – the hallmarks of conflict and crisis – can wreak havoc on health systems and hinder children's opportunities to be immunized. In 2018, some 40 per cent of the world's children who had not been immunized lived in fragile or conflict-affected settings.[5]

There are multiple ways in which conflict and crisis interrupt vaccination. They can displace health workers; halt financing; impair supply chains; and cause damage to roads, electricity grids, and water and sanitation systems.[6] In conflict, collateral and purposeful attacks on health-care facilities make accessing health services dangerous.

In addition, crisis compounds economic hardships for families, communities and nations. Travel becomes expensive because of fuel shortages, loss of public transportation, and dangers on the road. Displacement caused by crisis exacerbates already burdened family finances. And outreach activities are hampered by inaccurate data, danger and the dissolution of basic services. Finally, crisis can lead to the erosion of trust and a rise in suspicion of outsiders and authority – prime conditions for misinformation about vaccination to spread.[7]

With periods of crisis in particular, vaccination coverage tends to fall.[8]

Displacement

Conflict and crises can also displace children and families from their homes.[9] Some migrate from their homes to camps for refugees or internally displaced persons; others land in informal settlements or communities.

Displacement can make it difficult to find and estimate the numbers of children who need vaccinations.[10] Sometimes, displaced populations are trying to remain hidden. But displacement can also result in a loss of belonging to a community. It can sever families from the people and services they depend on for health-care interventions such as immunization.

> Instability, violence and disruption – the hallmarks of conflict and crisis – can wreak havoc on health systems and hinder children's opportunities to be immunized.

NIGERIA

A First for Fawaz and Samuel: Reaching zero-dose children in urban slums

On a typical Tuesday morning, Jemlat would have been hard at work hawking bread on the crowded streets of Gengere, a shanty-filled neighbourhood at the end of the popular Mile 12 Market in Lagos.

But one Tuesday, short of money to buy her inventory, Jemlat and her four-year-old son Fawaz took a slow disappointed walk home and happened on a life-saving opportunity: a team of health workers providing vaccines to protect children against potentially lethal diseases.

Jemlat jumped at the opportunity.

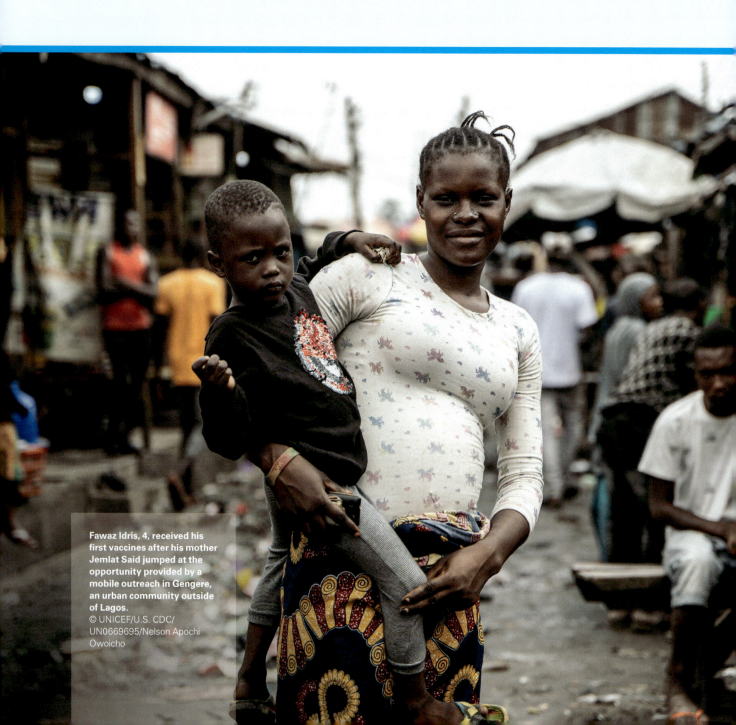

Fawaz Idris, 4, received his first vaccines after his mother Jemlat Said jumped at the opportunity provided by a mobile outreach in Gengere, an urban community outside of Lagos.
© UNICEF/U.S. CDC/UN0669695/Nelson Apochi Owoicho

"My son has never been vaccinated but he has also never been terribly ill," Jemlat said. "He was born in my grandmother's church."

For Fawaz, vaccination was a bit of a shock and he let out a yell. Health workers quickly comforted him with biscuits. With a first set of vaccines, Fawaz was on the way to being protected from life-threatening diseases including measles and polio.

"I want my child to succeed," Jemlat said. "That is my greatest ambition now."

Though Gengere sits on the outskirts of one of the world's greatest financial centres, vaccination services are not easily accessible for a population that faces challenges including poverty, low levels of education, little free time and limited means for reaching even relatively nearby health services.

Once a temporary shelter for wholesalers at the nearby Mile 12 Market, Gengere has mushroomed into a sprawling neighbourhood of noise and garbage. Basic services such as water, sanitation and education are scarce. Crime is plentiful. The nearest primary health care centre is more than 5 kilometres away.

Nigeria is home to the second largest number of zero-dose children in the world, 2.2 million. In Lagos State, the Alimosho Local Government Area (LGA) had over 35,000 zero-dose children in 2021, the highest number of any LGA in Nigeria. The LGA where Jemlat and her son live, Kosofe, had nearly 17,000 zero-dose children in 2021. It also had around 17,162 partially immunized children, the second highest number for an LGA in Lagos State.

The country health officials and partners have long worked to overcome the barriers that prevent mothers from vaccinating their children. However, addressing these barriers requires multiple kinds of outreach efforts, said Elizabeth Unoroh, the state immunization officer for Lagos. One approach is the Routine Immunization Intensification Programme. With support from UNICEF and the United States Government, the programme provides weekly integrated immunization outreach aimed specifically at reducing the number of zero-dose children in the State.

However, in Gengere, where much of the population is in constant transition, reaching children on the move demands daily outreach, increased funding and more neighbourhood-level primary health care, Unoroh said.

On the day Fawaz received his first vaccines, the mobile outreach team was deployed as part of a daily effort to reach zero-dose children and vaccinate them against vaccine-preventable diseases including measles and polio, and their caregivers against COVID-19. The team also provided vitamin A supplements.

Another resident, Esther Sunday, was among the first mothers to get in line to take advantage of the services in Gengere.

Esther gave birth to her son Samuel in 2021 in a Lagos hospital, where he received a dose of Bacille Calmette–Guérin (BCG), the vaccine that protects against tuberculosis. But since then, Samuel had not received any vaccines. At the Gengere health post, Samuel was immunized with all diphtheria, tetanus and pertussis-containing (DTP) vaccines – the backlog of vaccine doses he had missed.

As a single mother of three children, Esther makes her living washing laundry for residents of a nearby residential estate. She started working at about age 10 when her parents sent her to work as an apprentice for a food vendor in the rural area where they lived. Like Samuel, the majority of zero-dose children in Nigeria are born to poor struggling families. To get by, many caregivers keep multiple low-paying jobs in communities where health-care facilities are not available. For these families, access to routine immunization services means paying for transport – a further stretch of their already lean financial resources.

In Gengere, Esther pays about US$1.50 a day for her lodging and about US$0.50 a day for water and the use of a toilet. The outreach was her main opportunity to secure vaccinations for Samuel because taking Samuel to the nearest health centre would cost about half her daily income.

"I would be homeless if I didn't work for one day," she said. ■

Availability, accessibility and affordability

The barriers to immunization caused by poverty, location, marginalization and crisis can also be seen as issues of availability, access and affordability.

The barriers to immunization caused by poverty, location, marginalization and crisis can also be seen as issues of availability, access and affordability. Whether vaccines are available is determined by whether they can be delivered to health centres or outreach campaigns. Issues of accessibility are about whether the vaccines and services are located in a place and offered at a time when children and families can get to them. Affordability can be a question of financial resources to pay for the health service. But it is also about whether families have money for bus fare or the capacity to lose a day's pay to get to the health centre.

Availability, accessibility and affordability issues differ in rural, urban and crisis settings, which suggests that reaching these children will require context-specific interventions.

Remote rural

Vaccination services – and vaccines – are not always available in remote rural areas. These areas are often characterized by small settlements, low population density and few available services. Families live far away from health-care facilities.

In these areas, supply chain limitations, financing bottlenecks, shortages of health workers, and a lack of electricity, water and sanitation are significant barriers to the availability of vaccines. These barriers also get in the way during outreach campaigns aimed at increasing vaccination coverage.

When vaccines are available, they are not always affordable or accessible. Whether parents and caregivers have time and money for immunization can depend on the vagaries of agricultural incomes and the fluctuations of food prices, climate shocks and the weather.

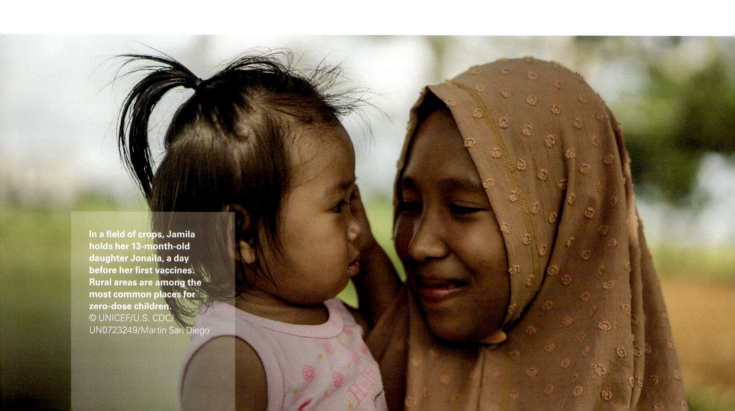

In a field of crops, Jamila holds her 13-month-old daughter Jonaila, a day before her first vaccines. Rural areas are among the most common places for zero-dose children.
© UNICEF/U.S. CDC/UN0723249/Martin San Diego

Urban

In urban slums and informal settlements, geography does not present the same problems. However, the availability of vaccines can be hindered by a patchwork primary health care system ill-equipped to meet the needs of large and growing populations. Far too often, the needs are not even fully understood because data are hard to collect in rapidly changing urban settlements, many of which attract displaced families and migrant populations. In addition, the political will to provide services is often tempered by an interest in discouraging the growth of informal settlements and slums.

Affordability is also a barrier for poor urban households. For parents and caregivers who juggle multiple jobs and responsibilities, clinic hours can be inconvenient and accessing vaccination and other health services means setting priorities that have an impact on a family's financial bottom line.

Crisis

Availability, access and affordability are also critical in crisis contexts, where vaccination services are usually delivered in outreach activities. But outreach activities are not always able to deliver when health-care facilities are damaged, when health workers are not available, and when supplies are hard to find. Availability is hurt because of inaccurate administrative data when people are on the move. In addition, security concerns can limit health workers' outreach activities and their safe access to children.

Affordability often suffers because of economic fallout from crisis. Fuel shortages, limited transportation, and damage to roads and services can also put vaccination out of financial reach for governments and individuals.

Solutions

Removing availability, accessibility and affordability barriers is critical for reaching the children whose lives are impacted by multiple social and economic determinants of health.

Put another way, reaching zero-dose and under-vaccinated children means making vaccination as available, convenient and inexpensive as possible. Achieving this goal requires interventions that take account of availability, accessibility and affordability barriers. Examples of such interventions include incentives that address the concerns of poor families.[11] In some settings, incentives have included food, goods, monetary support or certificates of recognition.

Combining vaccination reminders with incentives has also been effective. In Kenya, for example, a randomized trial found that a short SMS reminder led to marginal increases in immunization rates. However, when parents received an SMS and a small monetary incentive, the number of fully immunized children grew significantly.[12]

Prompts and reminders can also be effective particularly if they are linked to vaccination records. In Pakistan, for example, reminder interventions were shown to be effective in securing DTP3 vaccination, the third dose of the vaccines that protect against diphtheria, tetanus and pertussis.[13]

> Reaching zero-dose and under-vaccinated children means making vaccination as available, convenient and inexpensive as possible. Achieving this goal requires interventions that take account of availability, accessibility and affordability barriers.

FOR EVERY CHILD, VACCINATION

Why it matters

> Vaccination fuelled the child survival revolution of the twentieth and twenty-first centuries, sparing countless children the suffering of disease and death.

Overcoming barriers of availability, accessibility and affordability is critical to overcoming inequity in immunization and reaching zero-dose and under-vaccinated children. Ultimately, overcoming these barriers will save lives.

Indeed, immunization saves about 4.4 million lives a year. If the world reaches 2030 global goals for immunization to reach zero-dose and under-vaccinated children, the number of lives saved could climb to 5.8 million.[14]

But immunization does more than just save lives: It improves the health and wealth of individuals and communities. It helps children survive and thrive.

Survive and thrive

Vaccination is regarded as one of humanity's greatest public health achievements.[15]

Vaccination fuelled the child survival revolution of the twentieth and twenty-first centuries, sparing countless children the suffering of disease and death. Vaccination is the first line of defence against measles;[16] it can protect against pneumonia, which kills more than 700,000 children a year;[17] and can prevent diarrhoea, which kills more than 484,000 a year.[18] In addition, vaccines can prevent diphtheria, tetanus, whooping cough (pertussis), tuberculosis (TB), hepatitis, flu, polio, yellow fever, dengue and cervical cancer.

Excitingly, new vaccines hold the promise of protecting children against even more diseases. In the fight against malaria, for example, a new vaccine, RTS,S,[19] along with other preventive measures, hold the promise of preventing a vector-borne disease that killed 416,000 children under age 5 in 2019.[20] In addition, new vaccines for dengue and Ebola, and a next-generation polio vaccine, are in use. And new vaccines against TB and all influenza strains are in the pipeline.[21]

The value of vaccination

Immunization can bolster family finances, gender equity, education and community health.[22] And it does all this while also being good value for the money.

Poverty
In addition to the emotional strain, caring for a sick child can drain household savings and force parents and caregivers to miss work and pay.[23] For some families, these disruptions lead to impoverishment – and it is usually the poorest families at greatest risk.[24] A study in Nigeria, for example, showed that a third of families – and more than half of the poorest families – faced catastrophic costs after a child fell ill with pneumonia or a related disease.[25]

Gender equity
As the COVID-19 pandemic reminded us, women remain the main caregivers for children,[26] carrying out as much as three quarters of the unpaid work in the

home.[27] By preventing childhood illness, immunization plays an important role in reducing the time that parents and caregivers have to take off work to care for sick children.[28] Given the outsized role that mothers play in protecting children's health, these gains are likely to be strongest for women.

Education

Immunization also allows children to participate in education without extended absences for vaccine-preventable illnesses. Evidence from a number of countries shows that immunization can prevent absences from school and help them achieve in the classroom. In India, a study indicated that being fully vaccinated was associated with a 6–12 per cent improvement in basic reading, writing and mathematics skills among 8- to 11-year-old children.[29] Research in Ethiopia, India and Viet Nam has also shown that immunizing children against measles early in life is linked to improved learning outcomes.[30]

Health

When a child is vaccinated, the entire community benefits. With herd immunity, newborns and vulnerable populations who cannot get vaccinated can be protected because their friends and neighbours have been immunized.[31]

In addition, immunization against childhood disease can limit the spread of antimicrobial resistance by reducing the overuse of antibiotics, thereby curtailing the growth of superbugs – illnesses that do not respond to antibiotics.[32] These superbugs directly cause 1.27 million deaths a year, of which one in five is a child under age 5. Overwhelmingly, these children live in low- and middle-income countries.[33]

Return on investment

Vaccination has long been considered one of the most cost-effective interventions aimed at improving society's health, productivity and economies.[34]

Based on a 'cost-of-illness' approach, every US$1 invested in vaccination delivers a return on investment of US$26.[35] (This figure was calculated for 10 diseases in 24 low- and middle-income countries between 2011 and 2020.)[36] A broader 'value of a statistical life' approach, which captures wider economic benefits, gives an even higher figure for return on investment: around US$52 for every US$1 spent on immunization.[37]

Making the case

In a world where governments face tough choices on spending and a range of competing demands, immunization is a cost-effective method for protecting children, their health and the health of their families and communities.[38] Securing the funding and political will – globally, nationally and locally – is essential to vaccinate every child. Country-specific investment cases are also essential, but they can be complex to calculate. Therefore, developing national capacity to generate these country-specific investment cases would help secure political will and provide an opportunity to show governments, communities and families the immense value of immunization.[39]

> In a world where governments face tough choices on spending and a range of competing demands, immunization is a cost-effective method for protecting children, their health and the health of their families and communities.

NICARAGUA
Community Health Network: Reaching indigenous children at home

On an October morning, three community nurses dressed in white uniforms walked among the traditional *tambo* wood homes in the indigenous Miskito community of Sisin, a tiny town about 50 kilometres from the coast of Nicaragua.

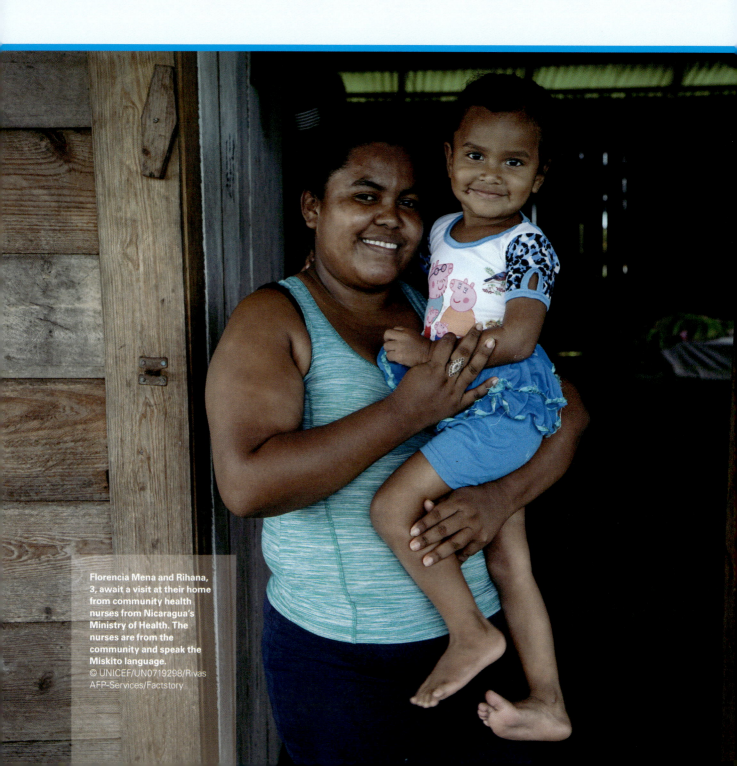

Florencia Mena and Rihana, 3, await a visit at their home from community health nurses from Nicaragua's Ministry of Health. The nurses are from the community and speak the Miskito language.
© UNICEF/UN0719298/Rivas AFP-Services/Factstory

One carried a high-tech thermos for vaccines, another a scale, and the third a bag of vitamins and medicine.

As they climbed the staircase to Florencia Mena's home, the nurses greeted Mena and her three-year-old daughter, Rihana, in the Miskito language. Since before her daughter was born, these nurses from Nicaragua's Ministry of Health have been regular visitors.

"The doctor and the nurses have seen me every month to keep a close eye on my daughter's development," Mena said.

Part of that task has been to keep on top of her daughter's vaccination schedule.

In a remote and poor community in the North Caribbean Coast Autonomous Region, where houses built on pillars protect people from an often punishing climate, the visiting nurses are a vital link between an indigenous community and immunization.

"Children are given routine vaccines according to their schedule, their height and weight," said Reynilda Cramer, one of the regular visitors to Mena and Rihana. "Heights are measured, deworming and vitamins are administered if appropriate. If anyone else in the family has health problems, we also take care of that other person."

Cramer and her colleagues are part of the Community Health Network, a nationwide programme supported by UNICEF in collaboration with the Nicaragua Ministry of Health. The visiting nurses are volunteers elected at community-wide meetings. They are trained by the Ministry of Health to provide routine health care including immunization. As active members of the community, the nurses are a critical link between national primary health care services and populations that traditionally have been hard to reach. They play an important role

in coordinating primary health care activities and encouraging participation. They are at the forefront of an effort to bring services to the most remote areas of Nicaragua.

Success of the Community Health Network can be measured in vaccination rates in North Caribbean Coast Autonomous Region, which includes Sisin, that stayed at 98 per cent in 2020 despite the COVID-19 pandemic and two disastrous hurricanes, Eta and Iota.

The success was also helped when the Community Health Network incorporated the Intercultural Health Care Model, a programme for indigenous communities that involves faith leaders in primary health care efforts.

"This closeness of the health system to the community is one of the reasons for Nicaragua's outstanding vaccination rates," said Dr. Jazmina Umaña, the Ministry of Health's national coordinator of the Expanded Programme on Immunization.

The key is working with nurses like Cramer, a member of the Miskito community, who can closely monitor the health of children from vulnerable communities, Umaña said.

"Everyone plays a key role in promoting vaccines and other health services, because [the community nurses] are trustworthy people for the population," she said.

For Florencia Mena, the Community Health Network helped convince her that vaccination was important for Rihana, she said.

"She received the first vaccine at birth, and although at that time I was afraid that my daughter would get pain and fever, today I see her healthy and full of life," Mena said. "I am proud to have accepted the recommendations of my family and health personnel." ■

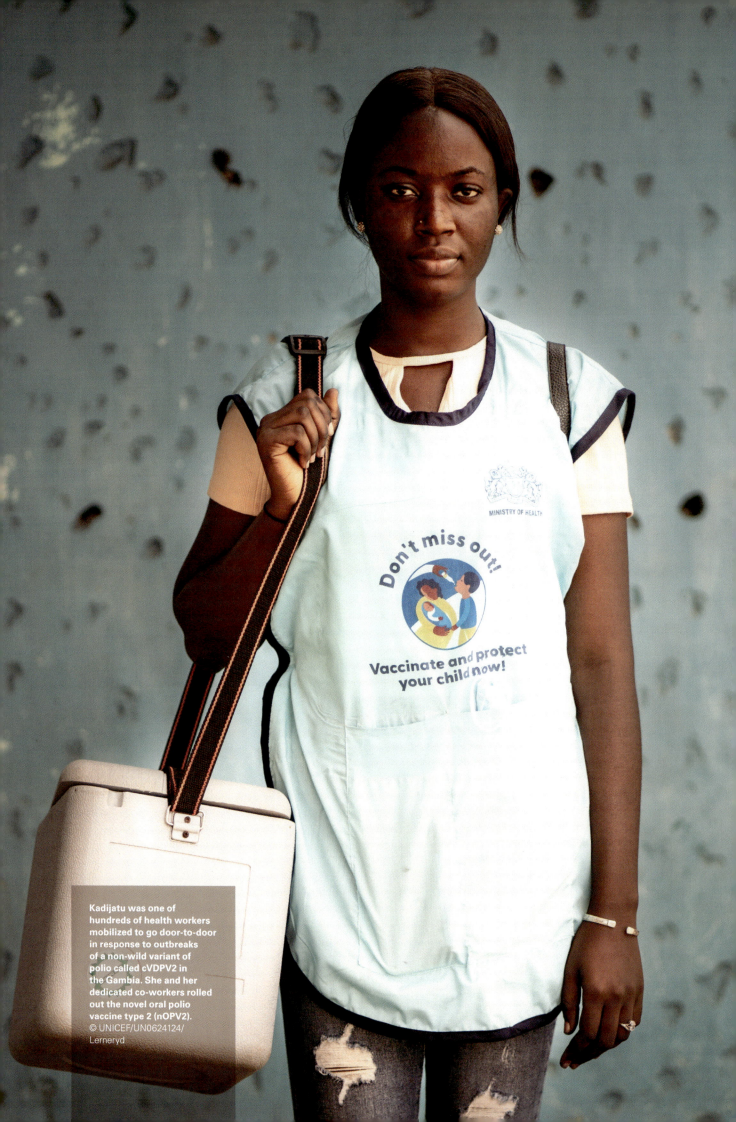

Kadijatu was one of hundreds of health workers mobilized to go door-to-door in response to outbreaks of a non-wild variant of polio called cVDPV2 in the Gambia. She and her dedicated co-workers rolled out the novel oral polio vaccine type 2 (nOPV2).
© UNICEF/UN0624124/Lerneryd

CHAPTER 3

Immunization and primary health care

Stemming a historic backsliding in vaccination – and reaching the children historically left behind – requires an examination of the structures that serve as the backbone for immunization. It requires bolstering primary health care services in facilities, outreach campaigns and humanitarian settings. And it means strengthening the health workforce and encouraging community engagement.

A health-care facility. An outreach campaign. A humanitarian setting.

For the most part, these are the settings where children are immunized, though the details and décor may differ from place to place. Tragically, though, many millions of children never make it to the health-care facility. They are not reached by the campaign. They have no access in a setting where there is a humanitarian crisis. They are left behind.

Structures and challenges

As noted throughout this report, millions of children are left behind. And millions more missed out during the height of the COVID-19 pandemic.

But vaccination, in many ways, has been a remarkable health intervention for decades. It has benefited from well-coordinated global partnerships among governments, communities and donors – partnerships that have helped reach many millions of children in low- and middle-income countries with life-saving vaccines.

In most countries, governments are responsible for service delivery – human resources, transport of supplies and interaction with children and families. Governments have also directed capital investments into health infrastructure. But, especially in low-income countries, donors, international organizations and other partners have provided significant funding and coordination. Globally, donors and partners have also provided normative guidance, policy frameworks and coordinated funding mechanisms.

Weak primary health care

Though the structures and processes vary from country to country, childhood vaccination is most often part of routine maternal and child health services. It is provided by trained health-care professionals in primary health care facilities.

However, in many low- and middle-income countries, and often in poor underserved neighbourhoods of high-income countries, there are limited numbers of reliable, stable and adequately funded primary health care facilities. Where they exist, many operate with limited resources.

In a broad sense, zero-dose children miss out because they live in places without adequate primary health care. In places where primary health care services do exist, failure to reach zero-dose children reflects on the efficacy of services that operate in low-resource settings. Under-vaccinated children have, at some point, come in contact with a health-care structure. However, these health-care providers have lost track of them, missing an opportunity to protect these children from disease.

Box 5
Gavi, the Vaccine Alliance

At the global level, multiple donors and partners are involved in the policy, governance, monitoring, financing and procurement required to immunize children. They include international organizations such as the World Health Organization (WHO) and UNICEF and multiple non-governmental organizations. Founded in 2000, Gavi, the Vaccine Alliance has helped to immunize over 981 million children, contributing to efforts that cut child mortality in half in 73 lower-income countries. As a public–private partnership, Gavi has mobilized more than US\$40 billion to: support routine immunization; strengthen health systems; hold preventive campaigns; build emergency stockpiles; contribute to outbreak response campaigns; and contribute to pandemic response, including the COVAX response to the COVID-19 outbreak. Gavi brings together founding partners WHO, UNICEF, the World Bank and the Bill & Melinda Gates Foundation, governments, the vaccine industry, technical agencies, civil society and other private sector partners.

Outreach campaigns

In communities that lack basic primary health care infrastructure, donor funding has augmented government investment, often with disease-specific interventions aimed at particular communities. Historically, this approach has meant campaigns to reach children in remote rural, urban and crisis settings.

Campaigns also are used to address outbreaks of a vaccine-preventable disease. Indeed, many campaigns have successfully immunized zero-dose children and have increased coverage above what was achieved by routine services.

In places with limited primary health care systems, outreach services are essential for reaching zero-dose and under-vaccinated children. In addition, health centres often deploy regular temporary campaigns aimed at reaching children and families who do not make it to the local facility.

The problem is that, by definition, campaigns are short-term initiatives.

Health workforce

Vaccine programme delivery involves many kinds of health-care professionals, including doctors, nurses, managers, community health workers and data analysts. Increasing the health workforce is a major global development goal, but the task largely falls to national and local governments, which are responsible for training, retaining and incentivizing the health workforce.[2] Many governments struggle to maintain the workforce required to provide health care – including immunization – to children and families. Globally, there are shortages.[3] And, unfortunately, the shortages in the workforce are significant barriers to the access, availability and affordability of health services, including vaccination.

In many ways, the workforce barrier to vaccination is also a gender issue. Women provide most of the work of immunization on the ground.[4] And, in most parts of the world, they face challenges including low pay, informal employment, lack of career opportunities and threats to their security.[5] Indeed, women make up 63.8 per cent of the health sector workforce in low- and middle-income countries and 75.3 per cent in high-income countries.[6] These women earn an average of 20 per cent less than men.

The vast wage inequalities come in part because women are more likely to work in the lower-paid parts of the sector, while men are more represented in the higher-paying jobs.[7] In addition, the gap in pay between women and men widens at higher levels of employment – so, women in top-level positions are much more likely to be paid much less than men in the same jobs.[8]

Box 6
Global Polio Eradication Initiative

The Global Polio Eradication Initiative (GPEI) is an example of a global structure linked with national and local partners.[1]

Founded in 1988, GPEI operates as a public–private partnership led by national governments and six global partners: the World Health Organization (WHO), Rotary International, the United States Centers for Disease Control and Prevention (CDC), UNICEF, Bill & Melinda Gates Foundation and Gavi, the Vaccine Alliance.

Though the incidence of polio has decreased by more than 99.9 per cent since GPEI was founded, the disease is not yet consigned to history. In the effort to eradicate polio, GPEI's strategy uses all opportunities to reach every last child and focuses on increased political will of governments, stronger community partnerships, an enhanced disease surveillance system, application of a gender perspective to programming, and integration with essential immunization and health services, where possible, in polio-priority geographies.

YEMEN
Women's Work: Alleviating suffering motivates a vaccinator and midwife

For Ghada Ali Obaid, vaccinating children is not a job. It's a calling.

On an average day, Ghada dashes through the hallways of Dar Sa'ad Medical Compound counselling mothers about the benefits of immunization and vaccinating their children.

But few of Ghada's days are average.

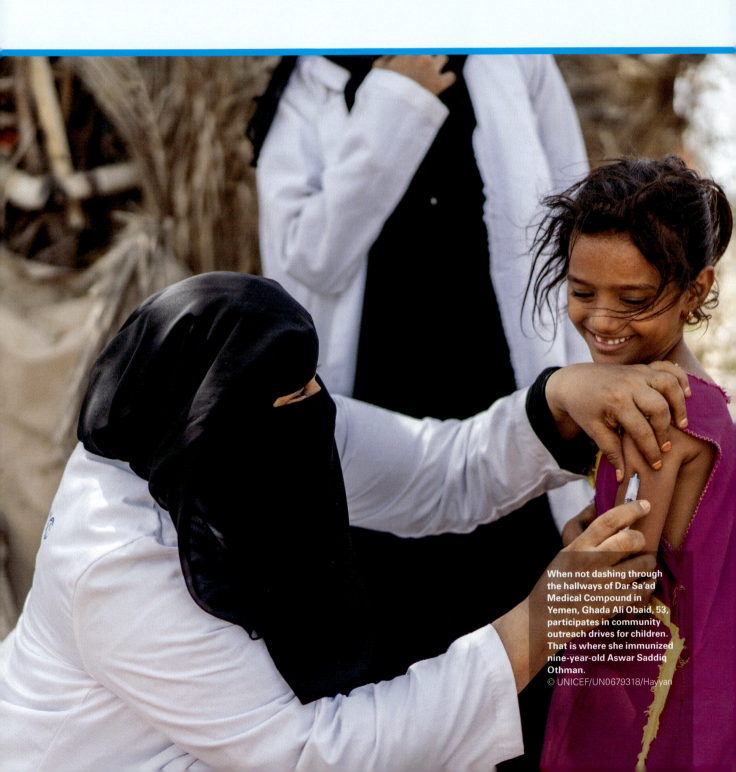

When not dashing through the hallways of Dar Sa'ad Medical Compound in Yemen, Ghada Ali Obaid, 53, participates in community outreach drives for children. That is where she immunized nine-year-old Aswar Saddiq Othman.
© UNICEF/UN0679318/Hayyan

As head of immunization at the health centre in Dar Sa'ad district of Aden, Ghada also takes to the streets to reach out to children who might otherwise miss vaccines against preventable diseases. In June, for example, Ghada was part of a response to a measles outbreak in Yemen. The immunization campaign reached over 1.2 million children between ages 6 months and 10 years with vaccinations against measles and rubella.

"The essence of our work is saving peoples' lives and reducing the suffering of women and children," said Ghada. "Personally, this is the most significant indicator of success in my work and life."

In Yemen, Ghada is part of a corps of women whose life's work is to be the first line of defence against vaccine-preventable diseases. Indeed, women are the backbone of health care in Yemen, a country with more than 4,500 health-care facilities.

According to Saadia Farrukh, UNICEF Yemen Health Manager, all community midwives and health workers are women because it is culturally and socially acceptable for women to provide antenatal check-ups and midwifery services. In rural areas, which are not covered by the national health system, women provide essential maternal and newborn health care in the communities.

"The female community health workers are more accepted by communities and more able to access households to provide the life-saving primary health care services with a focus on children and their mothers, yet not excluding other populations at community level," Saadia said.

As a trained midwife, Ghada witnessed the needless suffering that can occur when children are not immunized.

"One of the worst moments of my life occurred when I met a baby girl who had gone blind from contracting measles," Ghada said. "The fact that it was preventable and was, in part, the result of Yemen's deteriorating health-care system, is what motivated me to become a vaccinator."

At Dar Sa'ad Medical Compound, about 35 children are vaccinated daily, though the number can rise to

as many as 100, said Dr. Jamilah Saeed, immunization supervisor for the district of Dar Sa'ad. Her team at the health centre also provides reproductive health services and education on child health and nutrition.

Though the health centre claims multiple successes, "our organization's most significant intervention, by far, is being able to provide free vaccines regularly, thanks to UNICEF," Dr. Jamilah said.

For Ghada, providing free vaccines means much more than putting needles in arms.

"Over the past 11 years, a big part of my role has been helping Yemenis to understand that many diseases and epidemics could be eliminated, and the mortality and morbidity rates could be reduced," she said.

The work has challenges. The health centre lacks medical staff, especially midwives, an issue she attributes to the lack of job incentives, rewards and promotions. As trained medical staff leave, they are often replaced by volunteers who need training. When going door to door, Ghada must contend with the heat, unreliable electricity sources and distant locations.

Ghada also struggles to find a balance between work and family. She works at the health centre from 8 a.m. to 2 p.m. When involved in a vaccination campaign, she heads to remote locations in the afternoon.

Finding that balance is possible with support from her husband Ehab Faisal.

Ehab takes time off from his job as a taxi driver to take her to remote areas for vaccination campaigns. He has learned to fend for himself and their five-year-old son when Ghada has to work late. But even more than that, he nurtures her desire to help children and families.

"Ghada's job is a calling more than an occupation," Ehab said. "I encourage her to show up every day because she is so passionate about it, and she has my full respect." ■

Missing in leadership

Since the early 2000s, there has been some limited growth in the number of women in the upper echelons of the health workforce. But globally women are still over-represented in lower-paid and lower-skilled jobs – suggesting a gender segregation that puts women at a disadvantage.[9] For example, women are more likely to hold technical jobs in health care – nurse, midwife, lab technician – while men are more likely to hold so-called 'professional' jobs – advanced nursing, doctor, administrator, manager.[10]

According to a 2019 WHO report, 69 per cent of organizations in global health were led by men and only 25 per cent had gender parity in senior leadership, despite women making up 70 per cent of the workforce.[11] As a result, the report declared that global health was delivered by women but led by men.[12]

This lack of women in leadership points to vast inequalities in career advancement. However, it could be interesting to explore a link between female leadership and health or immunization outcomes. It is a link that has been noted in the education sector. For example, some studies have indicated that female leadership in schools is associated with improved learning outcomes, with the suggestion that women leaders adopt practices and behaviours that lead to success for students.[13]

Community health workers

Part of the reason for the inequity in pay in the health sector is that many women serve in unpaid and underpaid roles, typically as community health workers – about 6 million according to Women in Global Health.[14] As a rule, community health workers are tasked with collecting household data, communicating with families and communities, and vaccinating children.[15]

Vaccine services, in particular, rely on female community health workers.[16] In many parts of the world, women community workers are best placed to reach out to other women and children – a population out-of-reach for men because of social, gender and cultural norms.[17] They often work in remote and underserved areas, and serve as a bridge between families and communities and health systems.

However, gender inequalities mean that female community health workers usually work in low-level positions, lack formal recognition as employees, deal with poor working conditions and face threats including gender-based violence, verbal abuse and discrimination.[18] They are most often poorly paid and struggle with the pressures of childcare and household responsibilities.[19]

> In many parts of the world, women community workers are best placed to reach out to other women and children – a population out-of-reach for men because of social, gender and cultural norms.

Solutions

Reaching children who historically have missed out on all or most vaccinations will be more expensive than business as usual. It will require solutions tailored to the complex contexts where these children live – human-centred solutions established and embraced by their communities. It will demand strong primary health care systems and data that allow health workers to keep in touch with families, especially those who live mobile and complicated lives.

Ultimately, securing vaccination access for all children will require coordinated efforts by governments, donors, partners and communities. It will mean strengthening family-centred primary health care systems, so that children have better and sustained access to care, while also bolstering targeted outreach initiatives to zero-dose and under-vaccinated populations.

Strengthen primary health care

For at least the past 45 years, efforts to promote global health have focused on the importance of primary health care.[20] With the adoption of the Sustainable Development Goals, universal health care became a core objective of the current global development agenda, and primary health care was acknowledged as a key component to achieving this global goal.[21] With the Astana Declaration of 2018, government leaders and ministers of health committed to high-quality, assessable, available and affordable primary health care for all.[22]

Primary health care focuses on meeting people's needs throughout the life course with integrated services that prevent, promote, cure, rehabilitate and provide palliative care.[23] Primary health care also addresses the social determinants of health including poverty, crisis, and maternal education and empowerment. And it aims to galvanize individuals, families and communities so they can advocate for effective policies that promote and protect health.

To strengthen primary health care, it is essential to renew efforts in: service delivery; access to medical products, vaccines and technologies; and health information systems. In addition, it will be essential to have financing backed by strong political commitment and strengthened human resources – especially community-based services. To succeed, these efforts will need to be backed by increased community engagement in the design and delivery of primary health care.

Integrate immunization in primary health care

The link between primary health care and immunization is critical. For the most part, zero-dose children and under-vaccinated children experience multiple other health deprivations.[24] Indeed, zero-dose children often have mothers who had no or few antenatal care visits and did not deliver the baby in a health-care facility. Their mothers were less likely to seek care for a sick baby and fewer had hand-washing facilities. For example, mothers of zero-dose children were 46 per cent

> The link between primary health care and immunization is critical.

less likely to have had four or more antenatal care visits, 43 per cent less likely to have delivered their baby in a health-care facility and 36 per cent less likely to have hand-washing facilities. Conversely, fully vaccinated children were more likely to have mothers who had received other important interventions.[25]

Immunization can play a vital role in primary health care. Indeed, the *Immunization Agenda 2030* emphasizes the importance of embedding national immunization services within primary health care as the basis for achieving both high vaccination coverage and universal health care.[26]

As a well-established point of contact with children, families and communities, vaccination services can be an entry-point for the delivery of more essential services and contribute to improvements in access.[27] The converse is also true: Primary health care systems can contribute to efforts to halt the backsliding in vaccination coverage and reach those left behind.

> The UNICEF synthesis of research indicated that there was no one model of integration that provided greater results than another. Indeed, success of integration was highly context specific.

Integrating vaccination into primary health care and other services is part of the seven strategic priorities set out in the *Immunization Agenda 2030*.[28] This integration offers a cost-effective avenue to reach the children and mothers who have missed out on immunization and other basic services.[29] And integrating immunization and primary health care with other services is also critical in communities experiencing malnutrition.

A UNICEF synthesis of the evidence on integration of services identified two main pathways for integration: primary health care services integrated into immunization initiatives and immunization integrated into other primary health care services. For the most part, this integration occurred in the health-care facility, as part of outreach programmes and as part of community-based platforms.

In general, facility-based integration of family planning services with high-performing immunization services increased coverage for family planning without a negative impact on the immunization coverage. An effort in South Sudan to integrate immunization into a nutrition service increased compliance with full vaccination schedules.

Mobile outreach services are also an effective way to integrate services. For example, services that combined maternal, newborn and child health (MNCH) services with immunization improved vaccination coverage in various settings, including in northern Nigeria and parts of Afghanistan.

Mothers and children in humanitarian settings also benefit from the integration of vaccination services with MNCH initiatives. Research shows that these initiatives are most effective if they are sustained – repeated in one location for one or two days and repeated every two months. In Afghanistan, for instance, a mobile health team was able to increase the proportion of women who received antenatal care visits from 61 per cent in places without the integrated services to 84 per cent in places with the service.[30]

Ultimately, the UNICEF synthesis of research indicated that there was no one model of integration that provided greater results than another. Indeed, success of integration was highly context specific.

Optimize outreach campaigns

As noted in the research on integration of services, mobile clinics and targeted outreach campaigns can be effective tools for vaccinating children, especially zero-dose children – even on their own. In many instances, these tools have been able to increase vaccination coverage. In Kenya and Uganda, for example, house-to-house visits by community health workers contributed to an increase in immunization coverage and a decrease in the number of children who did not receive follow-up doses of vaccines against measles and diphtheria, tetanus and pertussis.

However, integration efforts do not come cheap – at least not at first. Global donors and national and local partners need to recognize that these services will be expensive. And that they will need to be repeated – sustained – to achieve the goal of reducing the numbers of zero-dose and under-vaccinated children in the world.

Community engagement

In addition to its focus on integrating immunization in primary health care systems, the *Immunization Agenda 2030* places significant emphasis on engagement with communities.[31] With reason.

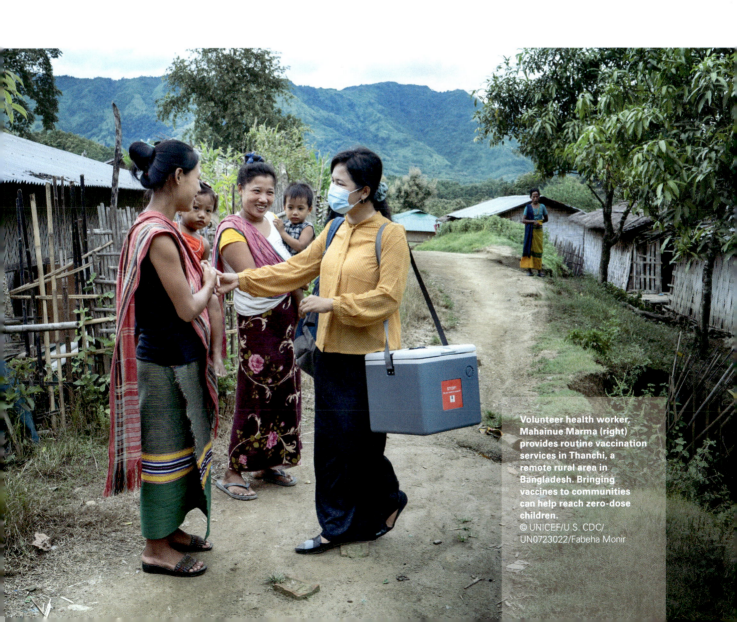

Volunteer health worker, Mahainue Marma (right) provides routine vaccination services in Thanchi, a remote rural area in Bangladesh. Bringing vaccines to communities can help reach zero-dose children.
© UNICEF/U.S. CDC/UN0723022/Fabeha Monir

PAKISTAN

Earned Trust: Integrated service delivery changes minds about polio vaccines

There was a time when Halima would have set the dog on any polio worker who arrived at her door with vaccines for her grandchildren.

But Saima Gul was not any polio worker.

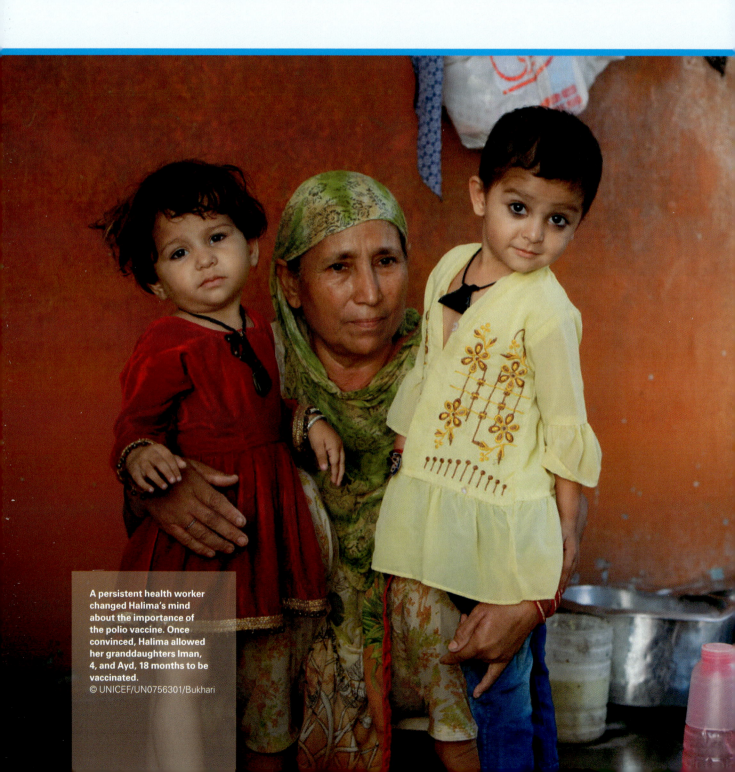

A persistent health worker changed Halima's mind about the importance of the polio vaccine. Once convinced, Halima allowed her granddaughters Iman, 4, and Ayd, 18 months to be vaccinated.
© UNICEF/UN0756301/Bukhari

For two years, Saima visited Halima's home in Gujro, on the outskirts of Karachi. She brought medicines and mosquito nets as gifts. She spoke to Halima in Pashto, the language of many families in Gujro.

On one visit, Saima noticed that Halima had a skin allergy, and she took the 50-year-old grandmother to the nearby Jannat Gul health centre. At the health centre, Halima received help with her skin and treatment for her troublesome knees. The care convinced Halima to trust Saima and the health centre – trust them enough to allow polio vaccinations for her granddaughters, Iman, 4, and Ayd, 18 months.

"Only iron can tackle iron," Halima said. "We don't let outsiders come here … Saima is Pathan (Pashtun). And so a Pathan will be straightened out by another Pathan."

As a polio front-line worker for the government locality – the Union Council – Saima is part of an Integrated Service Delivery (ISD) initiative that links polio vaccination to multiple services including health care, nutrition, water, sanitation, hygiene and birth registration.

The initiative was developed in response to feedback from parents and caregivers in poor communities whose demands for improved water, sanitation or basic health services were too often ignored. However, it also stemmed from a recognition that polio cases were more likely to arise in communities that faced multiple deprivations.

In Pakistan, the Polio Eradication Programme delivers integrated services in 43 Union Councils that face the greatest risk of polio. Gujro, a neighbourhood of about 650,000 residents in Karachi, Sindh Province, was chosen to be part of the initiative because of its history of political, religious and cultural resistance to vaccination against polio – a disease that once instilled fear around the world, but now lingers on the brink of eradication.

In Gujro, the ISD initiative has significantly contributed to a dramatic decline in the number of people who refused to have their children vaccinated against polio: from 4,254 refusals in 2019 to 1,209 in 2022 – a 72 per cent drop. In addition, Gujro and the Karachi area have stayed polio-free even as the disease has re-emerged in Pakistan after 15 months. From April to December 2022, there were 20 polio cases reported in Pakistan.

ISD at the Mother and Child Health Centre (MCHC) Jannat Gul Town started in 2019, with the support of the Bill & Melinda Gates Foundation, Rotary International, UNICEF and World Health Organization. It now includes services such as paediatrics, nutrition, family planning, antenatal services, newborn delivery, kangaroo mother care for babies born with low birthweight, birth registration and essential vaccines. In addition, the initiative includes six dispensaries, water filtration plants and provides off-site health camps linked to polio campaigns.

"When we started, the [outpatient department] had 25 patients a day," said Dr. Quratulain Janjua, the paediatrician who is part of the ISD initiative. "It has gone up to 500 to 600 a day now. We held community awareness sessions and, as awareness grew among people, the number went up, the patient flow increased."

Gulmina, a mother who came to the area from Afghanistan, said she had refused to have her eldest child vaccinated against polio. But a polio worker convinced her to come to the health centre, where she gave birth to her fourth child. Since then, Gulmina has taken all her children to the health centre for check-ups and has had all her children vaccinated against polio and all other vaccine-preventable diseases. She has also told her family members about the MCHC Jannat Gul Town.

"I am happy with the treatment," Gulmina said. "My sister-in-law and other women from our families also gave birth here." ■

> **Significant evidence indicates that vaccination interventions designed, delivered and evaluated by members of the communities they serve can increase equity and efficacy.**

Significant evidence indicates that vaccination interventions designed, delivered and evaluated by members of the communities they serve can increase equity and efficacy.[32] Engagement with community and religious leaders can provide inside information on location-specific barriers to immunization and help ensure that services are culturally appropriate.[33] This engagement can also help stem the influence of rumour and misinformation and bolster widespread support for immunization.

Community health workers and other local volunteers also play a critical role as a link between immunization service providers and children and families.[34] This is a role that can be supported. For example, systematizing community health workers' efforts could provide inside information on the location of hard-to-reach children.[35] And low-cost technologies such as mobile phones would help them communicate with children, families and other health workers.

Support for health workers

In every corner of the globe, it is the health workers who are the key ingredient to the success of vaccination programmes. Indeed, they are the key to the health of children and communities. Supporting them is fundamental to any effort to increase vaccination coverage and strengthen primary health care.

Increasing the health workforce in low- and middle-income countries is a focus of the WHO Workforce 2030 strategy.[36] But bolstering the ranks is only one part of the solution. Training is an important part of this effort. And evidence indicates that training in integrated management of childhood illnesses improves health workers' skills in immunization, nutrition and other areas critical to children's health and well-being.[37]

> **Addressing gender inequities in the health workforce means altering compensation structures with less short-term contracting and ad hoc and intermittent funding, and increasing opportunities for full-time recognized employment.**

Health workers need employment packages that focus on good and regular pay, decent working conditions and opportunities for career advancement. Evidence also indicates that providing clear and supportive supervision and management accountability are critical strategies for bolstering the health workforce in underserved areas of low- and middle-income countries.[38]

Addressing gender inequities in the health workforce means altering compensation structures with less short-term contracting and ad hoc and intermittent funding, and increasing opportunities for full-time recognized employment.[39] It also requires established education pathways that provide career development and training opportunities for female health workers, including community health workers. Eliminating gender inequities in health means empowering women in their work and career development.[40] It will require a deeper understanding of the inequities, investment in education and training opportunities for women that will provide them with access to the top jobs in health care. It also demands transparency about salaries and wages for men and women.[41]

As part of this effort, it will be critical to have a particular focus on the role of community health workers. Despite recognition of their indispensable efforts, community health workers are rarely equipped to deliver to their full potential. Far too often they are unpaid or underpaid and work without the training and protections that come with formal recognition as health workers.[42]

To better rely on community health workers, more information is needed on how many there are, the impact they have on immunization services, and the pay they receive (or do not receive) for their work.[43] Investment in community health programmes has a tenfold return on investment through improved health, deaths averted and increased productivity.[44] However, community health workers need to be recognized and regularized in the systems that deliver immunization and primary health care services. They need to be paid for their work based on their training, their role and the complexity of their tasks.

Next steps

In the past decades, the structures in place for delivering vaccination to children have benefited from strong engagement with national and local governments, and global partners. Vaccination has also benefited from unified goals. These structures have successfully reached many millions of children – protecting them from illness and death. But, historically, too many were missed. And COVID-19 has meant that many more have fallen behind.

Catching up and accelerating progress towards global goals for immunization will require multiple kinds of solutions tailored to the needs of families and communities. Most importantly, immunization efforts need to be deeply integrated into primary health care services. And where those services are limited, immunization efforts need to bolster primary health care.

Success with this task will require immunization and health-care initiatives driven by local knowledge and expertise. Most importantly, it will demand a health workforce – including community health workers – who are paid, professional and prepared to reach children in hard-to-reach communities.

INDIA
To the Mountain Top: Health workers brave challenging terrain to deliver vaccines

In the eastern mountains of Northeast India, where the sun rises early, Dematso Khamblai's day of delivering vaccines starts well before dawn. He is a member of the area's Alternative Vaccine Delivery System.

At 3:30 a.m., Dematso leaves his home and heads to the local health centre. There, he stocks up on vaccines, packing them into a grey insulated carrier. By 4:30 a.m., he is on the road, bumping along for as far as a motorbike.

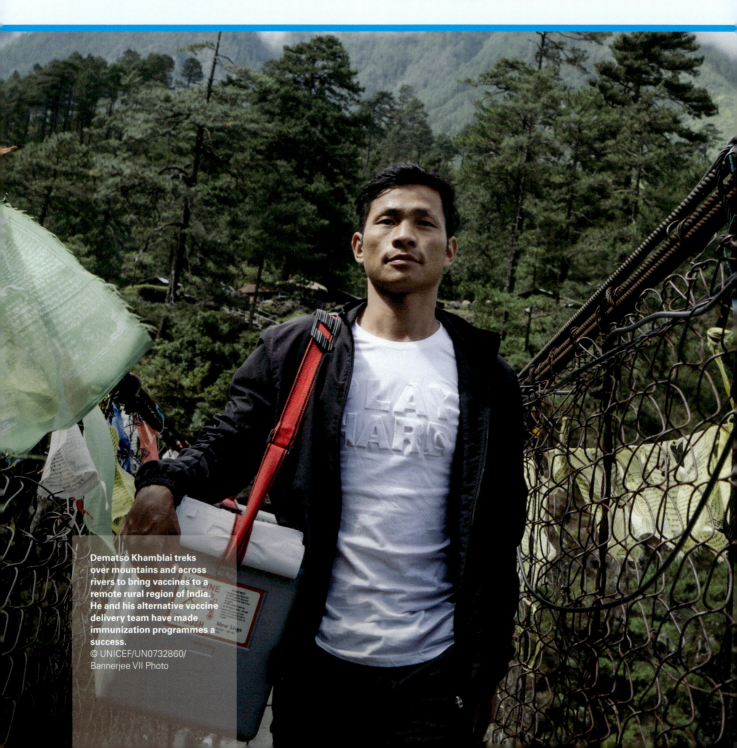

Dematso Khamblai treks over mountains and across rivers to bring vaccines to a remote rural region of India. He and his alternative vaccine delivery team have made immunization programmes a success.
© UNICEF/UN0732860/Bannerjee VII Photo

When the roads end, he begins his trek over hills, through valleys and across rickety suspended bridges. His mission: to deliver vaccines to villages hidden away in the mountains of this north-east corner of India.

"The mountains are steep, and we have to be very careful while hiking," Dematso said. "It becomes dangerous during the monsoon season as rains make the trek slippery. There are also frequent landslides during the monsoon season, which make the trek tough."

Northeast India, known for its natural beauty and rugged terrain, poses a challenge for health workers striving to ensure that all children receive necessary vaccinations. High mountains, deep gorges, and dense forests, combined with unpredictable weather conditions, make the journey to reach vulnerable communities perilous.

The vaccinators who brave the journey need skills, courage, and patience to transport and maintain vaccines at the right temperatures across these winding and treacherous trails.

Dematso is a member of the area's alternative vaccine delivery system, which consists of a corps of health workers who bring vaccines to one of the most remote rural regions in the world. Most of the villages that depend on Dematso's team for immunization, cannot be accessed by road, often having to cross turbulent rivers on suspended wooden bridges

"Earlier there was no health facility available here," said Kheti Meyor, a Gaon Burha (elder). "But now Dematso Khamblai and his team members visit us periodically to immunize the children."

Sushma Meyor credits Dematso and his team with helping her make sure that her eight-month-old son is vaccinated.

"They come to us and explain everything to us," she said. "They also tell us about the date of next vaccine. We don't have to worry at all. The team arrives here at the scheduled time and immunizations are done."

Long distances without roads is not the only challenge to immunizing children in this region.

The remote location means that few children are born in health-care facilities and few families record the birth of the children, said Dr. S. Nayil, a district health officer specializing in reproductive and child health. In addition, limited internet connection makes record-keeping difficult, and lack of accessibility and awareness of vaccines makes micro-planning difficult.

As a result, the alternative vaccine delivery team and health workers are also required to register births in the villages they cover. With this information, district health officials are able to track children's immunization histories and plan vaccination outreach on a micro level. The alternative vaccine delivery team now informs parents and caregivers directly of upcoming vaccination opportunities. The result has been universal vaccination coverage for children in the district, Dr. Nayil said.

During the height of the COVID-19 pandemic, the alternative vaccine delivery (AVD) teams were under extreme stress. Instead of 7 or 8 days in a month of trekking through the remote region, the teams were on foot for at least 20 days a month.

In addition, populations are scattered throughout the steep terrain.

"There are some villages in the region that require a trek of seven to eight hours to reach one village," Dr. Nayil said. "The AVD teams are quite motivated, and it is because of their motivation that we have been able to succeed so far."

Despite the hours of trekking and the dangers of monsoons and landslides, Dematso said he has discovered a sense of purpose in the job.

"Earlier, the duty seemed like instructions to be followed," he said. "But now I feel it as my responsibility."

As the sun sets over the mountains, these health workers return to their homes, exhausted but satisfied with the knowledge that they have made a difference in their communities. Their work may be difficult, but it is also fulfilling and rewarding.

Thanks to their efforts, more children in Northeast India are receiving the vaccines they need to stay healthy and thrive. ■

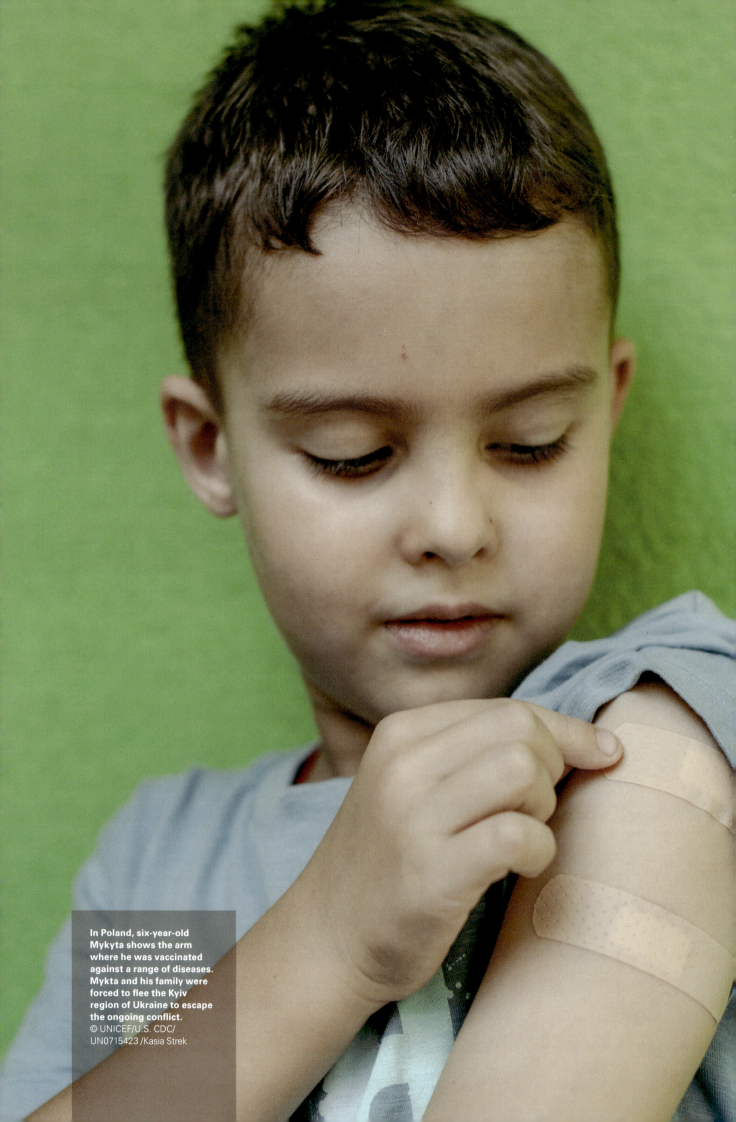

In Poland, six-year-old Mykta shows the arm where he was vaccinated against a range of diseases. Mykta and his family were forced to flee the Kyiv region of Ukraine to escape the ongoing conflict.
© UNICEF/U.S. CDC/ UN0715423 /Kasia Strek

CHAPTER 4

How can we build vaccine confidence?

The decision to vaccinate a child depends in part on trust – a parent's or caregiver's level of faith in government, the health-care system, health workers, vaccine producers and vaccines. Worryingly, there are signs in many countries of declines in vaccine confidence. In response, stronger action is needed to reassure parents and caregivers, including through community engagement and ownership, social listening and pro-vaccine education, and by empowering women and girls.

Numerous factors help to determine whether a child is vaccinated, including whether services are affordable, available and accessible, especially to the most marginalized communities *(see Chapter 2)*. But even if parents and caregivers are able to get a child vaccinated, they may not always be willing to. They must also be motivated. Despite powerful evidence of the benefits of vaccination, fear, ambivalence or outright opposition to vaccines can emerge within families and communities.

Data collected before and after the start of the COVID-19 pandemic suggest that, in many countries, the perception of the importance of vaccines for children has slipped – a worrying sign. If confidence in vaccines has faltered, it may be harder to meet global goals for childhood immunization.

Vaccine confidence can fluctuate depending on factors including rumours and misinformation, what is showing up in social media feeds, and on the state of wider issues, such as experience, trust in government and political polarization.[1] Maintaining and building confidence requires close contact with communities to understand what they are hearing about vaccines and their concerns, and engaging with them to build the kind of trust and confidence parents and caregivers need to vaccinate their children.

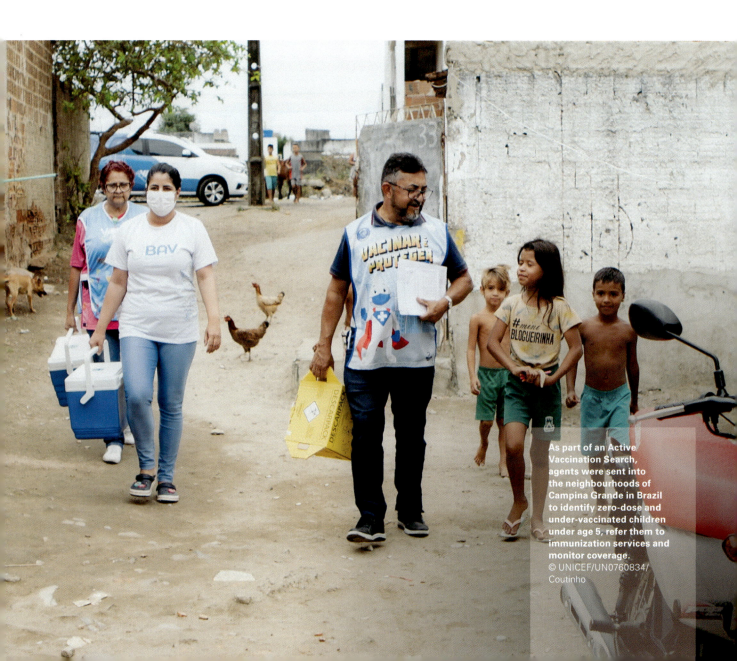

As part of an Active Vaccination Search, agents were sent into the neighbourhoods of Campina Grande in Brazil to identify zero-dose and under-vaccinated children under age 5, refer them to immunization services and monitor coverage.
© UNICEF/UN0760834/Coutinho

Shaken trust

Along with vaccination accessibility, availability and affordability, trust is a critical factor that influences whether parents and caregivers immunize their children. Parents and caregivers must understand the benefits of vaccines so that they feel that immunization is an essential part of caring for a child. Research shows that high confidence in vaccination is significantly associated with vaccine uptake.[2] On the other hand, ambivalence or reluctance around vaccination can prevent children from receiving life-saving vaccines.

A lack of trust in vaccines is as old as the practice of immunization itself.[3] And the reasons for it are multiple and mutable. Vaccine confidence is also notoriously volatile,[4] and any trends are time and location specific.

Nevertheless, there are worrying signs that confidence in vaccines has declined in many countries *(see Figure 4.1)*. Data provided for this report by the Vaccine Confidence Project at the London School of Hygiene & Tropical Medicine indicate that, in all but 3 of 55 countries for which data are available, confidence in the importance of vaccines for children has declined.[5] Conversely, some countries with very large populations, notably China and India, saw increases in the perception of the importance of vaccines for children.

Other indicators of vaccine confidence assessed by the Vaccine Confidence Project – perceptions of vaccine safety and effectiveness *(see Box 7)* – also showed declines, although the declines were not quite as marked as on the question of the importance of vaccines for children.

Across Africa, there were declines in every country for which data were available on all three questions. In South America, the picture was more mixed, with some countries not showing major declines on the questions of vaccine importance for children and vaccine safety. In Europe, there were declines on the question of vaccine importance for children. But there was a more nuanced picture surrounding the questions of vaccine safety and effectiveness, with some countries showing either no change or improvements.

Gender and age differences were also apparent in perceptions of the importance of vaccines for children *(see Figures 4.2 and 4.3)*. For example, declines in the perceptions of the importance of vaccines were more noticeable among people under the age of 35 and among women. Though there was variation across countries, the data underline the need for vaccination initiatives to focus on human behaviour as part of the effort to reach every child.

More broadly, more work and data collection are needed to better monitor confidence in vaccines, including in real time, so that responses can be tailored to respond to the volatile and often highly location-specific nature of changes in confidence.

> Along with vaccination accessibility, availability and affordability, trust is a critical factor that influences whether parents and caregivers immunize their children.

FOR EVERY CHILD, VACCINATION

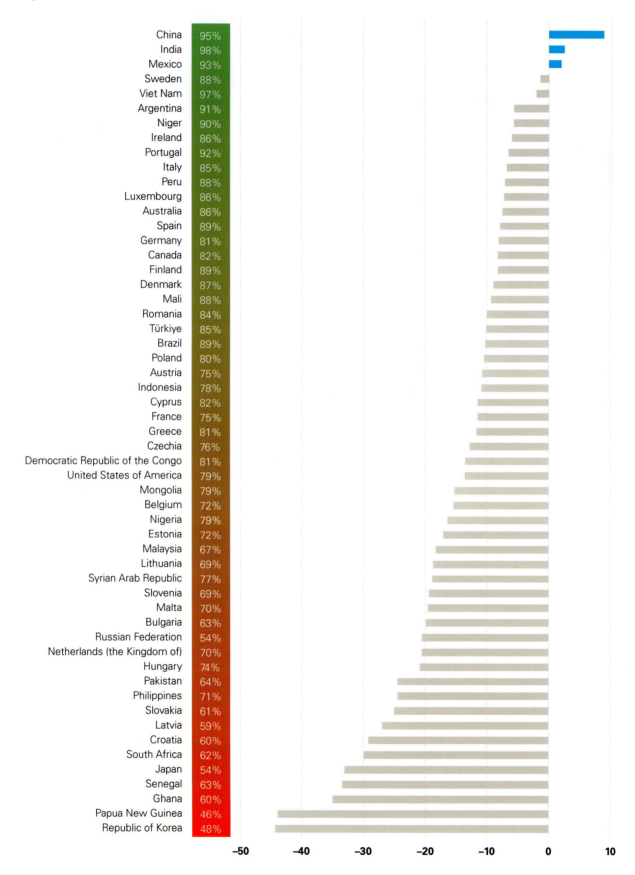

Figure 4.1. Confidence that vaccines are important for children dropped after the start of the pandemic
Percentage point change in perception of the importance of vaccines for children, before and after the start of the pandemic

Source: UNICEF analysis based on data from The Vaccine Confidence Project, London School of Hygiene & Tropical Medicine, 2022.

Figure 4.2. People under age 35 were more likely than people older than 65 to lose confidence in the importance of vaccines for children after the start of the pandemic

Percentage point change in survey respondents who agreed that vaccines were important for children by age group

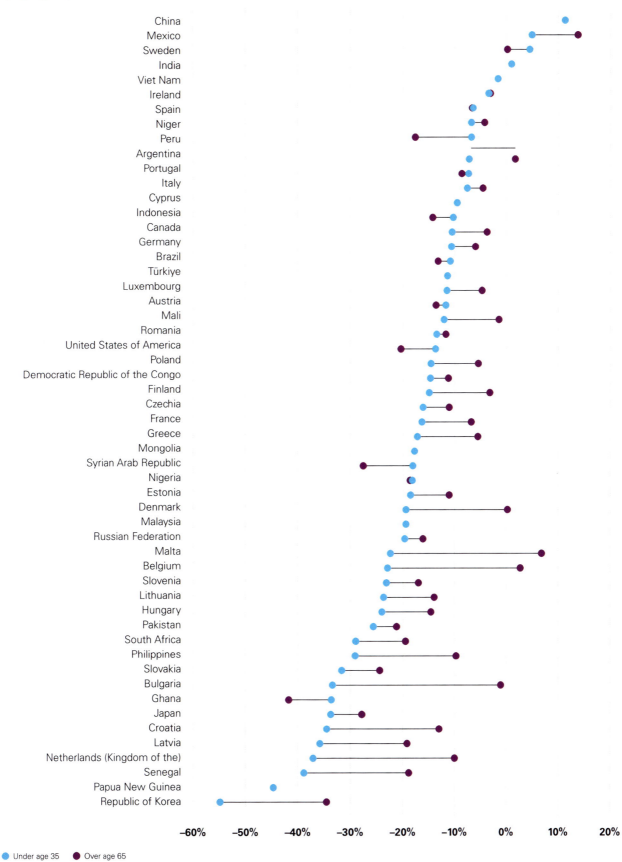

● Under age 35   ● Over age 65

Source: UNICEF analysis based on data from The Vaccine Confidence Project, London School of Hygiene & Tropical Medicine, 2022.

FOR EVERY CHILD, VACCINATION

Figure 4.3. In most countries, women were more likely than men to report less confidence about vaccines for children after the start of the pandemic

Percentage point change in survey respondents who agreed that vaccination was important for children by gender

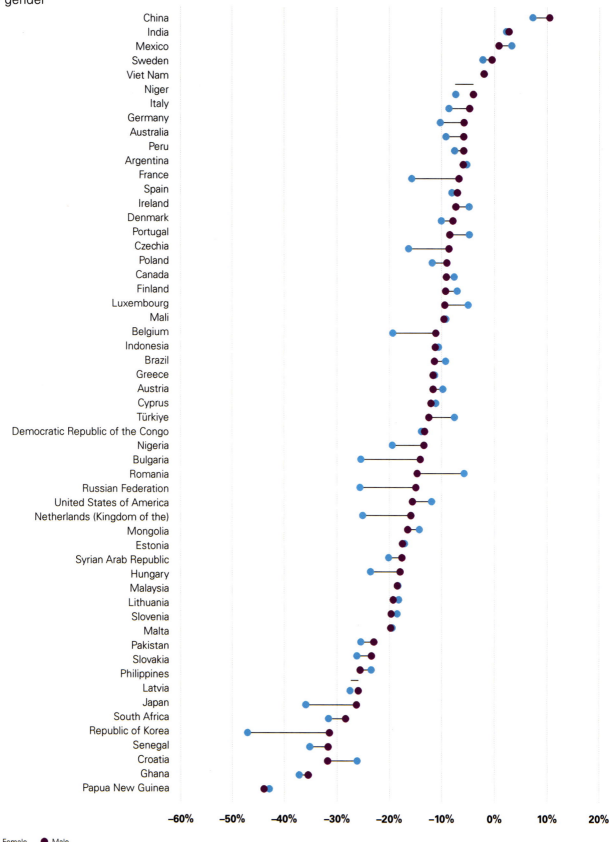

Source: UNICEF analysis based on data from The Vaccine Confidence Project, London School of Hygiene & Tropical Medicine, 2022.

The impact of COVID-19

What caused these declines? Vaccine hesitancy long predated the pandemic and had already been identified by the World Health Organization (WHO) as an issue of concern.[6] But COVID-19 brought new dimensions to the problem at a global scale.

Uncertainty about the course of the pandemic and the global response along with the rapid introduction of new vaccines probably all played a part in denting confidence.[7] Questions around vaccines led many people to search online for information, where scientifically accurate information is often presented alongside a bewildering mix of misinformation and disinformation.[8] Longer term, the increasing political polarization in many societies and declining trust in expertise are also probable factors.[9]

Even as the worst effects of the pandemic appear to be fading in much of the world, the factors undermining confidence in vaccination are unlikely to go away anytime soon. The findings of the Vaccine Confidence Project underline the need to tackle these challenges urgently.

Motivation and hesitancy

Addressing confidence requires an understanding of what motivates and discourages parents and caregivers to make immunization a priority in their lives. Ready access, low cost and low opportunity cost are factors. But a complex set of other elements influences parents' and caregivers' decisions about whether to commit the time and resources to immunizing their children.

Confidence: Trust, or confidence, in the importance, safety and effectiveness of vaccines and the systems that develop, deliver, procure and administer them plays a key role in the decisions parents and caregivers make about immunizing their children.

Awareness and access to information: Misinformation and conspiracy have become a growing challenge to public perceptions of vaccines. Parents and caregivers aware of factual, evidence-based information relevant to their questions and concerns are more likely to be confident in vaccines.

Complacency: Complacency is the tendency to ignore or delay vaccination because the perceived risk of illness or death is low. It is influenced by responsibilities and priorities that take precedence over vaccination. Research shows that complacency about vaccination decreases with a person's recognition of the risk of disease or death.

Benefit–risk calculation: This involves a parent or caregiver deciding whether the benefits of a vaccine outweigh the costs (including travel) or risks of having a child vaccinated.

Box 7

Investigating vaccine confidence

The Vaccine Confidence Project (VCP) at the London School of Tropical Hygiene & Medicine has been monitoring vaccine confidence for over a decade through nationally representative country surveys. Survey collection has been conducted through collaboration with ORB International along with Africa CDC, the European Commission, the Philippines Survey and Research Center, UNICEF, Wellcome Global Monitor and WHO.

Data presented in this report come from a large-scale retrospective study of changes in vaccine confidence between 2015 and November 2019 and since 2021. Vaccine confidence was assessed based on individual perceptions in three main areas – the importance, safety and effectiveness of vaccines – and measured using Likert-scale questionnaires (from "strongly disagree" to "strongly agree"). Only detailed data on the importance measure is presented in this report. Changes in national-level confidence were evaluated for the sampled populations and within demographic subgroups via statistical tests (Wilcoxon–Mann–Whitney tests with p-values adjusted via Bonferroni correction).

The data in this report represent a subset of data gathered by the VCP. To ensure robust analysis of change over time, only 'like-with-like' data were used, leading to the exclusion of some data gathered by the VCP (especially where Likert-scale responses were not directly comparable). Unlike in some other outputs that draw on VCP data, the data presented here was not →

→ modelled. Data also was not weighted. (In Figure 4.1, for example, weighting produces results with an average difference of 0.4 percentage points; for four countries, the difference is between 2 and 4.7 points.) These factors may account for small variations in results between what is reported here and in other reports drawing on VCP data.

Data and findings presented here were provided by the VCP and will shortly appear in a forthcoming paper entitled 'Global Declines in Vaccine Confidence from 2015 to 2022: A large-scale retrospective analysis'.

Convenience: Easy access to vaccination services can also determine whether a child is vaccinated – or not. A 2021 study in Nigeria showed that living more than 30 minutes from a vaccination facility influenced whether a child was fully vaccinated.[10]

Collective responsibility: This denotes the sense of communal orientation, collectivism and empathy that drives an individual to seek vaccines in order to encourage herd immunity and protect others. A lack of collective responsibility is associated with a lower uptake of vaccines.

Constraints: Certain cultural or religious beliefs can act as a barrier to trust in vaccines and decisions about immunizing children, as can language and the ability to navigate health-care systems.

Compliance: Sometimes it is not the vaccine, but the policies about immunization that influence parents' and caregivers' decisions. Some of these policies include the use of mandates in schools, day-care centres and workplaces.

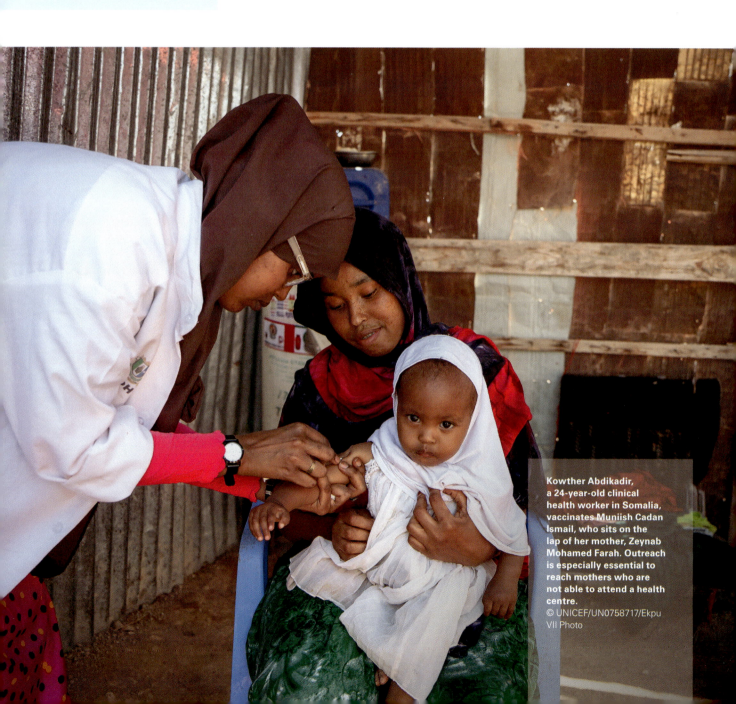

Kowther Abdikadir, a 24-year-old clinical health worker in Somalia, vaccinates Muniish Cadan Ismail, who sits on the lap of her mother, Zeynab Mohamed Farah. Outreach is especially essential to reach mothers who are not able to attend a health centre.
© UNICEF/UN0758717/Ekpu VII Photo

The toll

While the reasons parents or caregivers decide not to immunize a child may be complex, the consequences are straightforward: greater risk of illness and death.[11]

One of the most notorious examples of plummeting vaccine confidence stemmed from a 1998 article that linked the measles, mumps and rubella (MMR) vaccine with autism.[12] The article was debunked and later retracted. But amplification on social media kept the misinformation alive. In the United Kingdom, where the article originated, vaccination was 92 per cent in 1998. By 2003, it had dropped to 79 per cent in England.[13]

In Samoa, a deadly mistake became even more lethal because it eroded trust in measles vaccination. In 2019–2020 a measles epidemic killed 83 people, mostly small children.[14] The epidemic followed the death of two children who were given, by mistake, an MMR vaccine mixed with the wrong diluent. The consequence was a catastrophic drop to 31 per cent of children being immunized against measles.

In the Philippines, a scare involving risks related to a new dengue vaccine led to a precipitous fall in confidence that vaccines were important – from 93 per cent in 2015 to 32 per cent in 2018.[15] As a result, parents and caregivers did not vaccinate their children against any diseases. In 2019, measles cases soared in various parts of the country.[16]

The power of social media in the spread of misinformation was on display in Pakistan in 2019.[17] A staged video claimed that a polio vaccine had hospitalized children and showed staged images of children lying motionless in beds. The fake video drew 24,000 interactions on Twitter within 24 hours, according to a study by First Draft.[18] In Peshawar, an estimated 45,000 children were taken to the hospital by fearful parents within the week that the video hit social media. In the same week, a mob set fire to a health clinic in Peshawar, killing two police officers and a health worker. Five days after the misinformation first circulated, authorities suspended an anti-polio campaign.[19]

In an age of instant information – and disinformation – trust in vaccination is hard won and easily lost. Certainly, vaccination must be available, accessible and affordable for parents and caregivers to make it a priority in their lives. But, as recent research shows, the very human element of trust – of confidence in vaccines and those who procure, deliver and provide them – may play an ever-increasing role parents' and caregivers' decisions about immunizing their children.

> While the reasons parents or caregivers decide not to immunize a child may be complex, the consequences are straightforward: greater risk of illness and death.

KYRGYZSTAN
Social Influence: Faith leaders, volunteers and health workers build vaccine confidence in rural areas

Though her daughter, Aila, was first vaccinated shortly after birth, Meerim Omurkanova hesitated when it was time for follow-up immunizations.

"I read on the internet that vaccinations could cause cerebral palsy and autism," Omurkanova said. "And because of this, I initially did not want her to receive vaccinations."

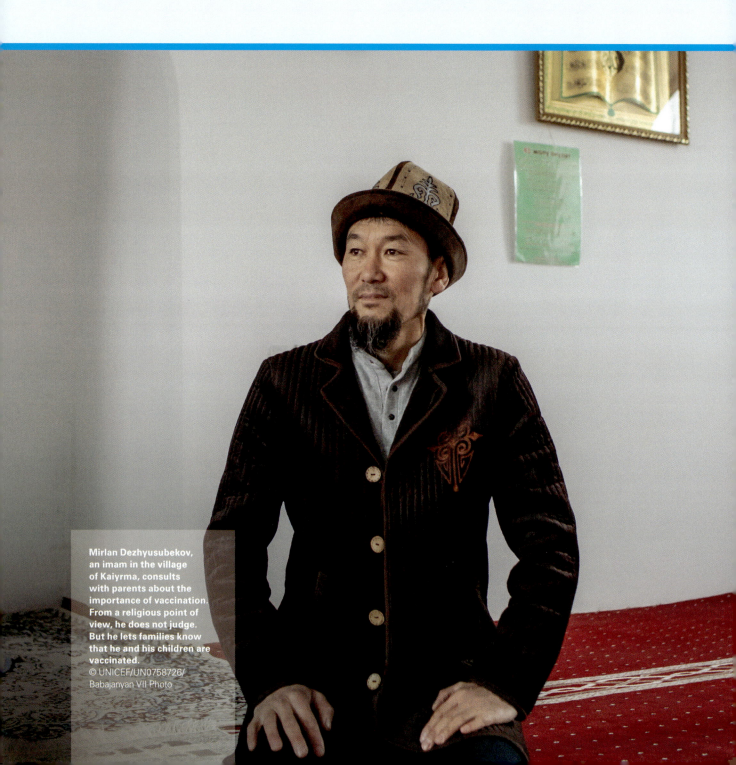

Mirlan Dezhyusubekov, an imam in the village of Kaiyrma, consults with parents about the importance of vaccination. From a religious point of view, he does not judge. But he lets families know that he and his children are vaccinated.
© UNICEF/UN0758726/Babajanyan VII Photo

The internet misinformation – thoroughly disproven – ultimately fell apart under the influence of a much more respected source: Mirlan Dezhyusubekov, the imam of the mosque in Kaiyrma village, where Omurkanova and her family live.

"From a religious point of view, we cannot judge parents' decisions to vaccinate or not to vaccinate their children," Dezhyusubekov said. "But I tell families that I was vaccinated, as well as my children, and we have all been well."

Misunderstanding and a lack of confidence in vaccination has been a concern in Kyrgyzstan, where the Republican Immunoprophylaxis Centre has received a growing number of reports of vaccination refusals since 2016. In 2021, there were more than 10,000 refusals.

In addition, the number of infants in Kyrgyzstan who received a third dose of a vaccine against diphtheria, tetanus and pertussis (DTP3), fell in 2020 to 87 per cent, from 95 per cent in 2019 and 94 per cent in 2018.

To address the rate of vaccination refusal, in 2019 Kyrgyzstan's Republican Health Promotion and Mass Communication Centre, with support from UNICEF and Gavi, the Vaccine Alliance, embarked on an effort to build confidence in vaccines throughout Kyrgyzstan and increase immunization coverage. The initiative focused on equipping volunteer Village Health Committees so they could coordinate with parents, caregivers, health-care professionals and religious leaders.

"When we began communicating with [hesitant parents] about the fact that vaccines protect from 12 types of infections and that immunity grows within a child, protecting them like little soldiers, they began to understand what immunity meant," said Kulyash Beyshenbaeva, a specialist with the Health Promotion Committee in the Jayyl district of northern Kyrgyzstan, which coordinates 31 Village Health Committees including the one in Kaiyrma.

This communication has helped changed minds in communities throughout Kyrgyzstan. In Jayyl district, 164 of the 486 families who refused vaccination in 2022 changed their minds by the end of the year.

In addition, UNICEF social mobilization efforts in four of Kyrgyzstan's seven provinces helped change the minds of thousands of parents and caregivers. In that time, more than 2,000 more children were immunized and were entered into medical and national registries.

As a result of these efforts, Kyrgyzstan has a vibrant model of collaboration between parents, caregivers, medical workers, volunteers and religious leaders at the community level who can work to build and maintain trust in vaccination.

In Kaiyrma, communication about vaccination often begins with Rysbuby Uturova, a nurse and the only health worker in the village of about 90 families. Uturova was trained in interpersonal communication, which includes social mobilization skills. Indeed, nearly a third of medical workers in vaccination services receive similar training.

Uturova's clinic is next to the mosque where Dezhyusubekov is the imam. The closeness is symbolic of their collaboration.

"[Uturova] and I are neighbours, and she sometimes shares issues with me, suggests taking part in solving them, and carrying out informative activities," Dezhyusubekov said.

In addition to the nurse and the imam in Kaiyrma, the Village Health Committee also plays a vital role in building confidence in vaccines. For example, Susar Abdraeva, a volunteer with the committee, reached out to Omurkanova about vaccinating Aila.

"We informed her about the usefulness of vaccines and that illnesses could be prevented through vaccinations," Abdraeva said.

For Omurkanova, the consultations influenced her decision. She immunized her daughter and has followed up faithfully. ■

Building vaccine confidence

The most effective way to promote vaccine confidence is to deploy multiple strategies in a comprehensive approach.

The most effective way to promote vaccine confidence is to deploy multiple strategies in a comprehensive approach.[20] Political will and a national commitment to immunization is a precondition for vaccine acceptability.[21] Once established, understanding what is driving vaccine confidence in each community is critical to designing interventions that work.[22] Officials managing national or local immunization programmes need to understand what factors or mix of factors (e.g., concerns around vaccine safety, questions about effectiveness and/or cost–benefit questions) may be holding people back. The involvement of community representatives, behavioural scientists, programme managers and other stakeholders is key to this understanding, as is collection, analysis and use of behavioural and social data. Health authorities must also assume accountability for the performance of vaccination programmes, as measured by vaccine coverage rates against set targets.

Community engagement, dialogue and ownership

A key principle of the *Immunization Agenda 2030* is ensuring vaccination efforts are people-centred. Considerable evidence indicates that vaccination interventions designed, delivered and evaluated by members of the communities they serve can increase equity and efficacy.[23] Engagement with community and religious leaders can provide inside information on the location-specific barriers to immunization and make sure that services are culturally appropriate.[24] This engagement can also help stem the influence of rumour and misinformation, and bolster widespread support for immunization.

Vaccination interventions informed, designed and implemented by local communities can be powerful. A study based in Remo North, Nigeria is instructive. The project involved the community – community members, front-line health workers, and local government officials – in participatory research to develop immunization interventions.[25] It then brought the stakeholders together for joint planning, implementation and evaluation.[26] The results were dramatic: Full immunization coverage of children older than 9 months increased by 30 percentage points.[27]

Trust is foundational to vaccine confidence – especially faith in vaccines, health-care providers, and institutions such as health authorities and government.

Research shows that informal training of traditional and religious leaders can also empower them to help increase immunization. In one study in Cross River State, Nigeria, traditional and religious leaders were first trained in leadership, effective communication, vaccination and community mobilization.[28] They then provided vaccination education in community meetings, using data summarized by trained health workers. The intervention increased the proportion of children with at least one vaccine, and those who completed pentavalent vaccination.[29]

Trust is foundational to vaccine confidence – especially faith in vaccines, health-care providers, and institutions such as health authorities and government.[30] Dialogue helps foster trust, opening the door for people to share their feelings and concerns about vaccination. It builds the foundation for individuals' and communities' understanding of the importance of life-saving vaccines. Where a lack of knowledge or awareness about vaccines has been observed to be a major hindrance to vaccine uptake, a trusted person discussing the risks and benefits of vaccination with the population has proven effective.[31] Health-care providers are consistently the most trusted voice on vaccines, and a provider recommendation is a strong driver of vaccine acceptance and uptake.[32] That is why motivating and equipping immunization providers – and the community health workers supporting them – to have impactful conversations about vaccination is so important.

Interventions designed around community engagement strategies have been shown to overcome barriers to vaccination in a variety of low- and middle-income country contexts, and in a cost-effective manner. An analysis of 61 studies of community engagement strategies showed that, taken together, these efforts increased the rate of children who were fully vaccinated by 14 percentage points.[33] They did so at modest cost: for every 1 percentage-point increase in absolute immunization coverage across the study populations, the cost for each vaccine dose per child was US$3.68.[34]

Front-line health workers play a critical role in community engagement to increase vaccination, according to a review of interventions in Ethiopia, Myanmar, Nigeria and Pakistan.[35] Interventions successfully obtained community buy-in by centring community members, especially leaders; ensuring their participation in monitoring; and making immunization an agenda item on community platforms.[36]

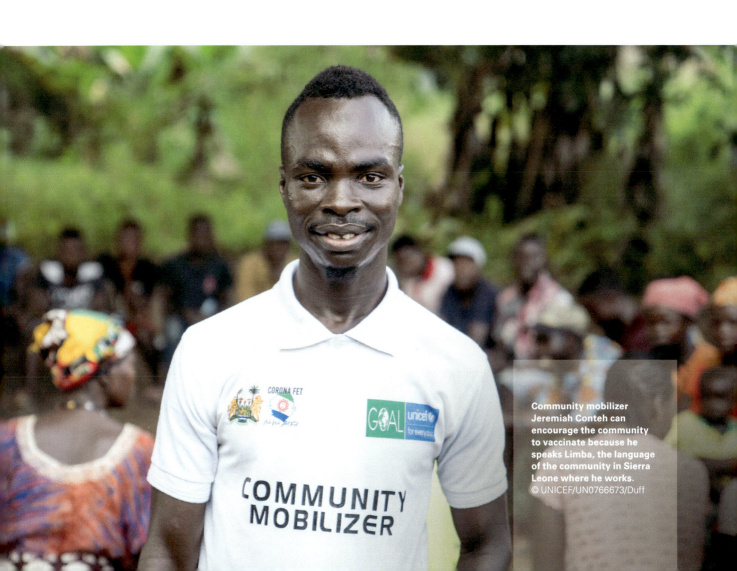

Community mobilizer Jeremiah Conteh can encourage the community to vaccinate because he speaks Limba, the language of the community in Sierra Leone where he works.
© UNICEF/UN0766673/Duff

By engaging communities in a variety of ways, interventions in these four countries sought to tackle vaccine delivery issues and behavioural, social and logistical obstacles caregivers faced. Almost all interventions included a component on health worker sensitization and training and assigned key roles to community leaders in awareness-raising and health system monitoring to improve immunization coverage. Most either leveraged existing community institutions or set up their own platforms to create opportunities for dialogue between service providers and the community. These environments facilitated collective ownership and action.

Another study, in Uttar Pradesh, India, illustrates the impact of community-level engagement. The project used village meetings to provide information on health service entitlements, education service entitlements, and village governance requirements. By the conclusion of the one-year study, infant vaccinations had increased by 25 per cent compared with the control group – with similar results across low-caste and medium-to-high caste households.[37]

Improving the communication skills of providers can help improve trust and rapport between patient and provider. Training equips providers with knowledge and approaches that make them more confident in discussing vaccination with patients. An online training programme being rolled out globally by the International Pediatric Association offers guidance for these vaccine conversations between health-care professionals and patients[38].

Social data and social listening

Investing in understanding people's attitudes to vaccines in real time – that is, social listening – is essential to the success of any vaccination programme. Routine monitoring of vaccine acceptance through regular surveys that include questions about attitudes, intentions and behaviours, would allow programme managers and communications specialists to identify signals of increasing hesitancy around vaccines, tailor strategies to improve confidence, and measure the impact of interventions. Validated tools that measure vaccine acceptance are now available for childhood immunization.[39]

UNICEF has published detailed guidance for establishing or strengthening a national vaccine social listening programme.[40] It helps with the formation of strategic and well-coordinated national action plans to rapidly counter vaccine misinformation and build demand for vaccination that are informed by social listening.

In addition, a dashboard developed by UNICEF, the Public Good Projects and the Yale Institute for Global Health monitors misinformation and equips users to respond to it with effective strategies. The Vaccination Demand Observatory (VDO) dashboard tracks trending vaccine misinformation along with fact checks.[41] It indicates the risk level of emerging misinformation, along with recommendations on when actively debunking it would be effective.[42] The website offers training materials on how to respond to misinformation, and when a country joins the VDO, it receives access its own country-specific dashboard.[43]

Pro-vaccine education and public messaging

Educational interventions have also proven effective in contexts where inadequate information, rumours, parental concerns about safety, and lack of awareness have hindered uptake.[44] When informed by data on a community's attitudes towards vaccines, educational interventions using videos, posters and lectures are shown to have improved vaccine acceptance.[45] Evidence shows that effective public communications campaigns on vaccines should be context-specific, culturally appropriate, and informed by behavioural and local insights.[46]

Filling information gaps with reliable, resonant, relevant information should be central to any public communications strategy.[47] For example, a study conducted using social marketing campaigns in rural areas of North Carolina, the United States of America raised awareness among parents and reduced barriers to accessing the HPV (human papillomavirus) vaccine.[48] HPV vaccination rates increased among 9- to 13-year-old girls within six months of the campaign launch.[49] In northern Nigeria, a relative increase of about 310 per cent in the polio vaccination uptake was observed through an educational intervention with a video containing awareness messages about polio vaccination.[50]

> Filling information gaps with reliable, resonant, relevant information should be central to any public communications strategy.

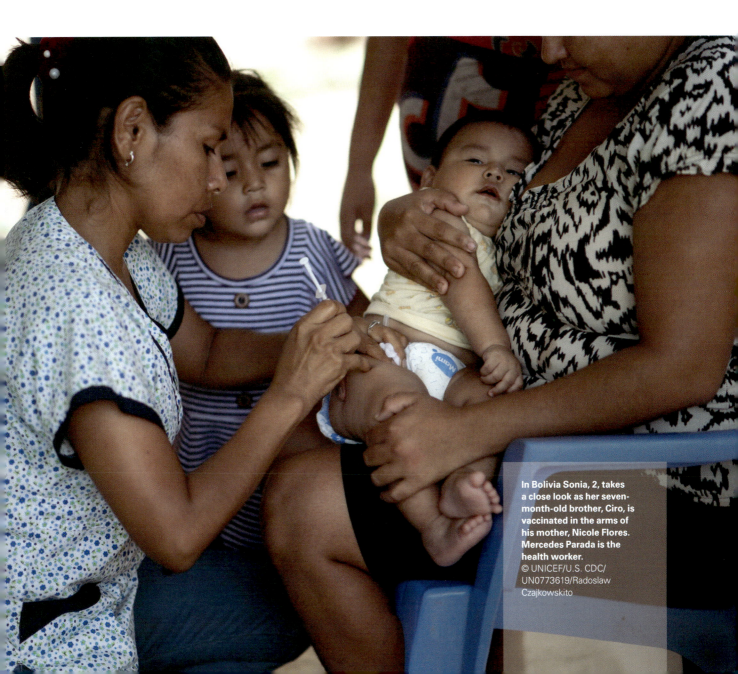

In Bolivia Sonia, 2, takes a close look as her seven-month-old brother, Ciro, is vaccinated in the arms of his mother, Nicole Flores. Mercedes Parada is the health worker.
© UNICEF/U.S. CDC/UN0773619/Radoslaw Czajkowskito

Applying a gender lens

A deeper understanding of how gender impacts vaccine uptake can help greatly with the design of more effective programmes. Women, especially in lower-income and emergency settings, tend to have less access to and control over resources that may influence immunization outcomes (e.g., time, money, information and transportation). This is especially the case for single mothers, and those in low-income households in rural areas.[51] In a study in Nigeria, the most reported barrier to accessing immunization was the lack of financial resources for the costs of transportation or services.[52]

Community-based outreach to women can improve immunization rates, research shows. In Bihar, India, for example, health education was incorporated into women's self-help group meetings, using stories, songs and picture puzzles on a variety of topics including routine immunization.[53] Women who had participated in the sessions were 9 per cent more likely to access age-appropriate immunization for their children.[54] Another study in north-west Ethiopia engaged women-led health development armies to visit households, providing education and appointment reminders, and encouraging vaccination.[55] The project saw increases in pentavalent-3 and measles coverage, and 84 per cent of children who had missed doses during the study were identified and caught up.[56] Research also shows that women conducting outreach and education – known as 'social mobilizers' – have also improved attitudes towards polio vaccination in India and Pakistan.[57]

> Women's decision-making and agency have been strongly associated with children's immunization status. Women's empowerment can improve immunization coverage – while restricting women can hamper it.

Such approaches are also relevant to school-aged girls around HPV vaccination. There is urgent need to establish a sustainable way to reach school-aged children with a broader array of preventive care in ways that are acceptable to them and their parents. For example, mother and daughter communications integrating cervical cancer screenings with discussions about the importance of HPV vaccination provide motivation to complete HPV vaccination.[58] A study in Malawi showed that reading of a magazine targeting girls with HPV vaccine-related messages was associated with greater uptake of the vaccine.[59] Engaging school-aged girls and their families can foster better programme design and uptake.[60]

Empowering women and girls

Women's decision-making and agency have been strongly associated with children's immunization status.[61] Women's empowerment can improve immunization coverage – while restricting women can hamper it, research shows.[62] Greater gender equality, then, enables women to access life-saving services, including vaccines for their children.[63]

For example, a study in Nigeria showed that the greater women's autonomy and decision-making capability, the more likely they were to get their children immunized.[64] Studies throughout South Asia have shown that greater decision-making autonomy for women translates into greater use of maternal and child health services and positive health outcomes.[65]

Further research in Ethiopia revealed that women who had the power to decide about use of financial resources were more likely to have their children partially or fully immunized, compared with women who had no part in such decisions.[66] The study also found that women who made financial decisions together with their husbands were even more likely to have their children vaccinated, compared with women who made financial decisions independently.[67] This finding points to the value of engaging men alongside their partners to improve immunization outcomes.[68]

Religious or cultural norms also affect women's mobility and ability to seek vaccination. For example, in the Nigerian Hausa tradition, unrelated men may not speak to women without permission from their husbands.[69] In polio eradication activities, deploying women front-line workers has increased the effectiveness of immunization delivery, as in many settings only women are allowed to access households and vaccinate children within them.[70] By contrast, a study in three Nigerian states found that all-male vaccinator teams were ineffective – deploying them posed a barrier to polio eradication efforts.[71] A review of polio immunization in Afghanistan over a 16-year period also suggested that mothers' refusals were related to interactions with all-male vaccination teams.[72]

The differing positions that women tend to occupy in societies and families have a bearing on child immunization – so immunization efforts must understand their needs and design programmes around them. Whether through greater logistical support, outreach to men to build vaccine awareness or promoting gender equality, applying a gender lens can improve routine immunization rates.

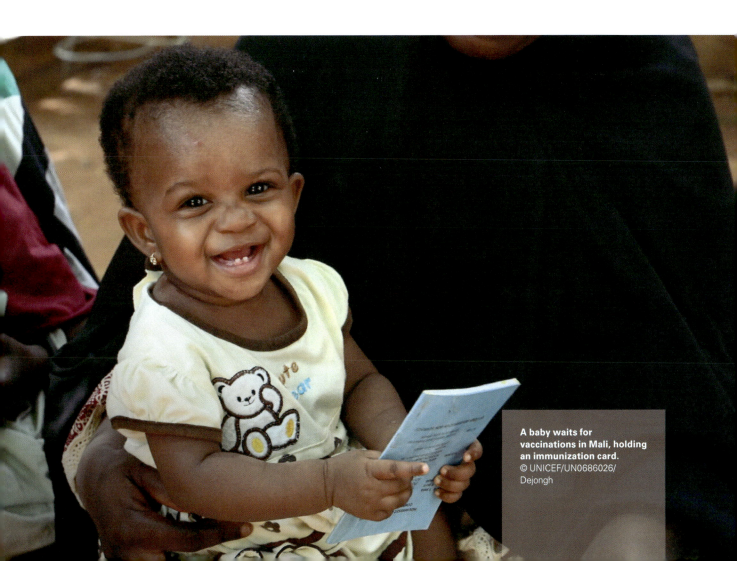

A baby waits for vaccinations in Mali, holding an immunization card.
© UNICEF/UN0686026/Dejongh

ECUADOR
The Power of Community: Volunteers keep watch over children's immunization

After a morning of tending her dairy farm and delivering milk, María Ortencia Catucuago switches gears: She puts on a vest and backpack and begins her daily rounds to neighbourhood homes in her role as a community health volunteer.

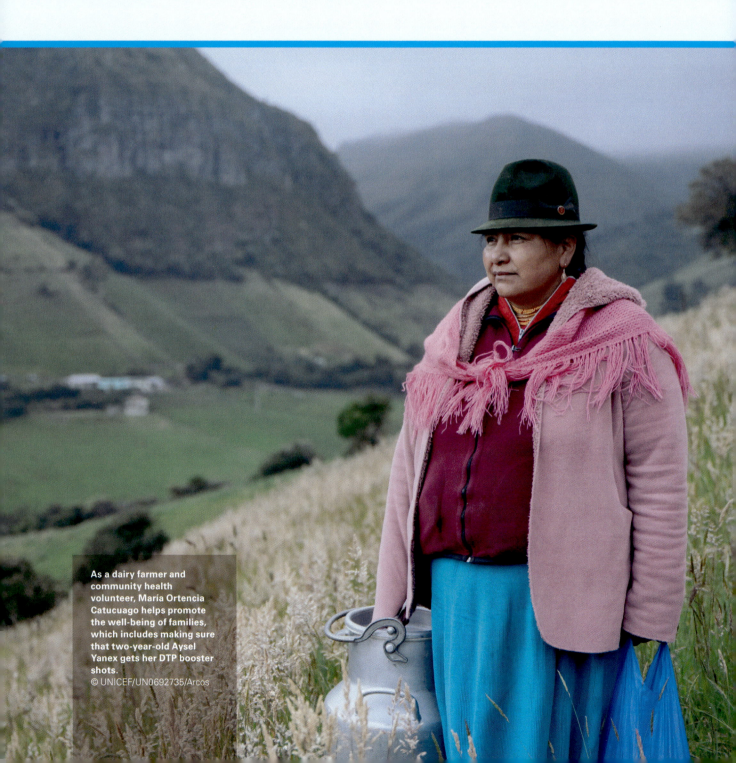

As a dairy farmer and community health volunteer, María Ortencia Catucuago helps promote the well-being of families, which includes making sure that two-year-old Aysel Yanex gets her DTP booster shots.
© UNICEF/UN0692735/Arcos

"I feel passionate about helping others," Catucuago said. "For many years, I have been involved in community activities that promote the well-being and health of families."

Catucuago cares for Turucucho community, which is nestled in the foothills of the north-eastern highlands of Ecuador. She is part of a corps of indigenous members who volunteer to keep watch over the health and well-being of children under the age of 5 and pregnant women.

On a recent morning, Catucuago started rounds as a community health volunteer at the home of Fernanda Valdivieso and her two-year-old daughter, Aysel Yanez. Aysel was born premature and struggled with chronic malnutrition. The little girl had recently missed a diphtheria, tetanus and pertussis (DTP) booster and a check-up on her weight and height.

"One of my responsibilities is reporting to health centre colleagues so they can quickly respond," Catucuago said. "I called the health personnel, then they came and gave her the vaccine she lacked."

For Valdivieso, Catucuago's visit provided a critical reminder.

"Next time, I won't forget her check-up," Valdivieso said.

Catucuago's volunteer work is part of a community health monitoring strategy in 137 communities of indigenous peoples and nationalities in the Imbabura and Pichincha Provinces and in the Monte Sinai part of Guayaquil, Ecuador's largest city. Operated in coordination with the Ministry of Public Health and UNICEF, the community health monitoring strategy was implemented to empower communities to actively prevent the spread of COVID-19. Since it was effective in the pandemic, the strategy was expanded to encourage routine immunization and keep track of the health of pregnant women and children under age 5.

Part of the aim of the community health monitoring strategy is to tackle chronic malnutrition, which affects four out of ten indigenous children under the age of 2. Essential to the effort to curb malnutrition are vaccines including pneumococcal and rotavirus. However, in 2020 and 2021, a vaccine shortage and low attendance at health centres led to a drop in coverage. In 2021, the rates of complete rotavirus vaccination in Ecuador was 60.5 per cent and 62.2 per cent for pneumococcus vaccination. Now that the vaccine shortage has ended, the health ministry aims to achieve coverage over 95 per cent.

The monitoring strategy has allowed the community to alert public health officials where there are difficulties with services, said Pacha Cabascango the technical coordinator of the Community-based Epidemiological Surveillance programme at the Ecuadorian Society for Public Health.

Volunteers such as Catucuago work with an average of 25 families in their communities. The corps of about 500 volunteers have reached about 8,200 children younger than 5 years since the programme began in 2020, and it is one of the country's more successful models of community outreach, Cabascango said.

"Through their work, we have seen that families, especially the new generations, have less resistance to vaccination and recognize its importance in the health and development of children," he said.

Catucuago was invited to become a community health volunteer at a community-wide meeting in 2020.

After a long day of visits, calls and conversations with neighbours in the community, Catucuago returns home to her farm. The work of helping Aysel get a check-up and her DTP vaccine brings her a great sense of purpose, she said.

"I want all the children in my community to grow up healthy, happy and with the same opportunities," Catucuago said. ■

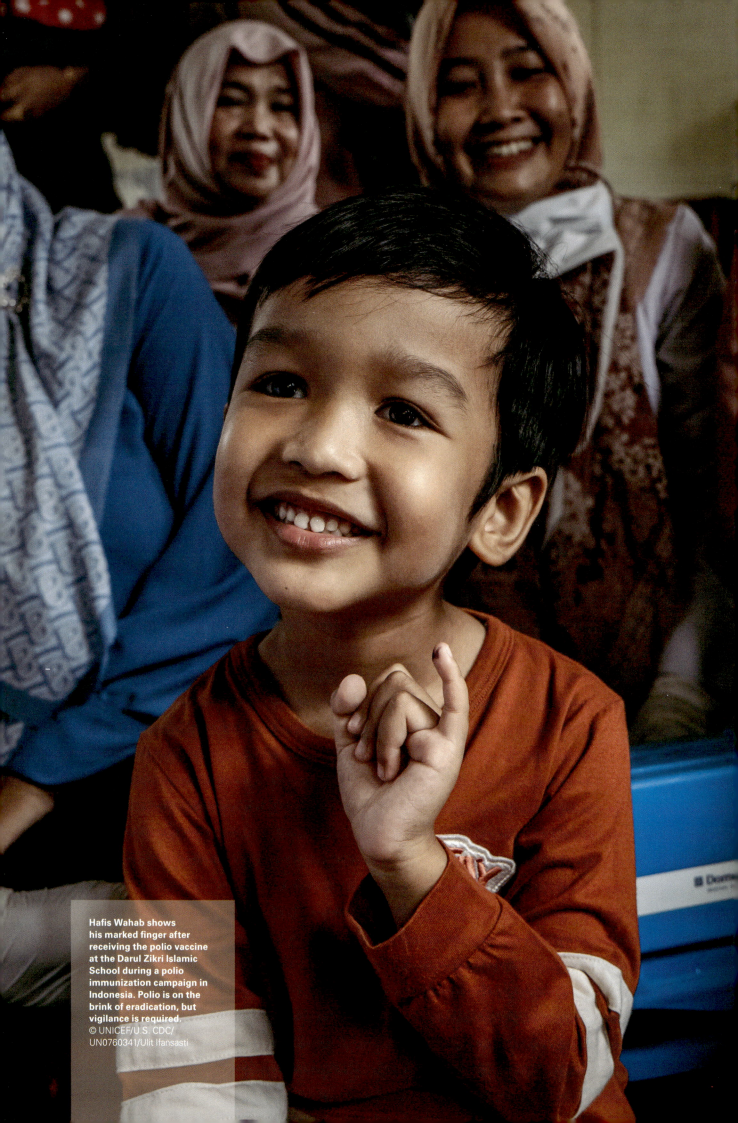

Hafis Wahab shows his marked finger after receiving the polio vaccine at the Darul Zikri Islamic School during a polio immunization campaign in Indonesia. Polio is on the brink of eradication, but vigilance is required.
© UNICEF/U.S. CDC/ UN0760341/Ulit Ifansasti

CHAPTER 5

Funding and innovation for the future

Vaccinating every child means investing in new approaches with the promise of ensuring sustainable, equitable funding and a pipeline of game-changing vaccines and cutting-edge technologies.

The term 'innovation' is most often applied to technology. But its actual definition encompasses not only new devices or products but also new ideas and ways of doing things.

To vaccinate every child, we need to innovate on all fronts – especially in immunization financing, vaccine research, product development and vaccine delivery. Ensuring sustainable, equitable funding and a steady pipeline of vaccine development will strengthen our efforts to reach every child – now and into the future.

Funding: The current situation

The disparities between budget allocation and expenditure highlight an opportunity to strengthen health and finance systems to increase spending on immunization. Prioritizing such investments is all the more important in times of economic turmoil and constrained budgets.

Immunization's success is underpinned by substantial investments. From 2000 to 2017, US$112.4 billion was spent on immunization in low- and middle-income countries.[1] In 2017, about US$40 was spent on immunization for each surviving infant in low-income countries, and US$42 per surviving infant in lower-middle-income countries.

Governments are the largest contributors overall to immunization, with donors providing other essential funds. The funding mix in each country depends on its income level and other factors.[2] In 2017, for example, development assistance provided the largest share of spending on immunization in low-income countries.[3] With many countries facing serious fiscal constraints, such donor assistance for vaccination will remain critical.

Since its inception, Gavi, the Vaccine Alliance, has made significant contributions to vaccine funding in low- and middle-income countries. From 2000 to 2017, Gavi channelled about US$13.3 billion of the estimated US$31.7 billion provided as development assistance in low- and middle-income countries.[4] About US$18.3 billion was dispersed through other development agencies.

Economic instability

The disparities between budget allocation and expenditure highlight an opportunity to strengthen health and finance systems to increase spending on immunization. Prioritizing such investments is all the more important in times of economic turmoil and constrained budgets. In the shadow of the COVID-19 pandemic, global instability and conflict, and a potential global recession, economic insecurity is all but assured.[5] The World Bank estimates that 41 countries will likely not return to pre-COVID levels of government spending until 2027 – essentially a "lost decade" for public investment with consequences for government investment in people's health.[6]

Tragically, these global financial pressures arrive exactly at a time when it is most critical to reclaim lost ground for childhood immunization. Missed immunizations during the pandemic offer a stark reminder that live-saving vaccines must be prioritized. Reaching zero-dose and under-vaccinated children is imperative for the health of those children – and for the health of the world.

Government budgets

Despite great gains in reaching children over many decades, there is significant room to improve the efficiency and effectiveness of planning, budgeting and expenditure procedures in immunization.[7] And as governments and donors seek to prioritize immunization in tight financial circumstances, it will also be critical to find ways to spend more effectively and efficiently.

Governments face multiple challenges when it comes to immunization financing, allocation and spending, especially in low- and middle-income countries. The issues include:

1. Too little funding is allocated for immunization in many countries. Some countries do not even specify a budget line for vaccines.
2. The amount of money a government allocates for health is not always the same as the amount spent.[8]
3. Allocated budget is underspent because of procurement and coordination issues.
4. The funds that are spent are exposed to loss, misuse and inefficiencies.

A study of domestic budgets showed that 22 low- and middle-income countries underspent their budgets by an average of 30 per cent.[9] One country in the study underspent by 76 per cent. Underspending of budgets can lead to inefficiencies and bottlenecks in procuring essential commodities required for vaccination. For example, 20 of the countries studied experienced vaccine shortages and 12 had immunization coverage rates below the global average.[10]

Overall, it is estimated that countries can waste 20–40 per cent of their health resources.[11] This kind of waste can be reduced with sound public financial management that allows for budget transparency. Technical efficiency can be achieved with efficient budget execution practices such as careful consideration of central controls and local autonomy, evaluation of capital expenditures, and standard procedures for workforce engagement.[12] At the programme level, there is an opportunity to increase cost efficiencies with more effective procurement, innovations in service delivery, and use of innovations in vaccine technology and cold-chain equipment.[13]

Much can be achieved with efficiency improvements. However, they can only help optimize expenditures; they are not a substitute for a commitment to investment in immunization and primary health care.[14]

Despite great gains in reaching children over many decades, there is significant room to improve the efficiency and effectiveness of planning, budgeting and expenditure procedures in immunization.

Financing immunization's future

Successfully achieving immunization goals will demand more than just more money. It will require a complex combination of funding, partnerships and political will: a combination of investment and commitment.

Interventions that reach zero-dose and under-vaccinated children – the hardest children to reach – will take significant investment. Tackling that task while also stemming a pandemic-era decline in immunization coverage may take a historic investment.

Certainly, some of this investment will centre on money. But successfully achieving immunization goals will demand more than just more money. It will require a complex combination of funding, partnerships and political will: a combination of investment and commitment. It will mean that governments, donors and partners will need to prioritize investment in immunization and focus on working together to more efficiently and effectively plan, budget and provide services. In addition, donors can harmonize their support to countries, centring their efforts on strengthening primary health care.

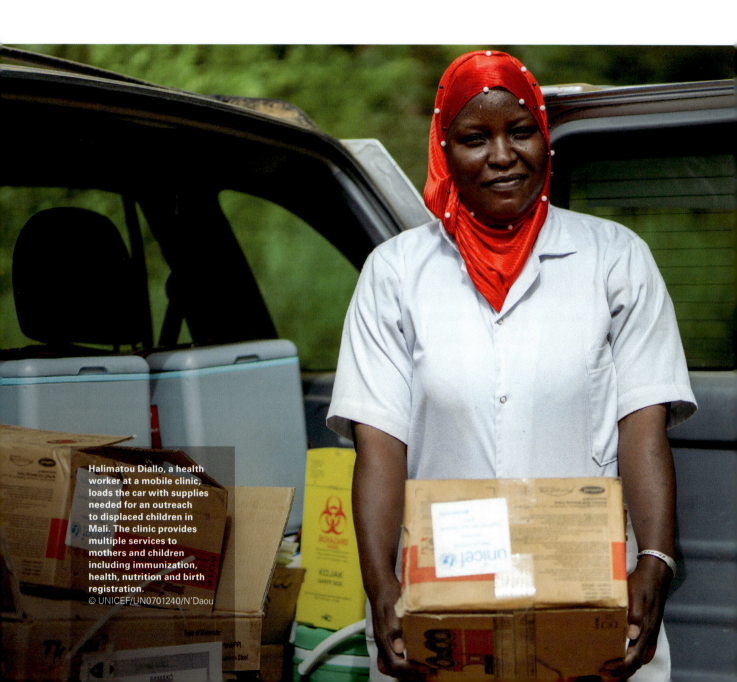

Halimatou Diallo, a health worker at a mobile clinic, loads the car with supplies needed for an outreach to displaced children in Mali. The clinic provides multiple services to mothers and children including immunization, health, nutrition and birth registration.
© UNICEF/UN0701240/N'Daou

Funding

As outlined in the *Immunization Agenda 2030* – and throughout *The State of the World's Children 2023* – planting immunization firmly within primary health care provides benefits for vaccination coverage and the goal of universal health care.[15] However, primary health care is notoriously underfunded – especially in low-income countries. On average, low-income countries spent US$26 per capita on primary health care. In contrast, lower-middle-income countries spend US$61, upper-middle-income countries US$193 and high-income countries US$1,333.[16]

In low- and middle-income countries, nearly half of the money for primary health care comes from private sources, which includes individuals paying for services, private insurance and other domestic private sources.[17] In low-income countries, 18 per cent of funding comes from governments and in lower-middle-income countries, 35 per cent comes from governments.[18]

Partnerships

Though country investment in immunization and primary health care is a foundation for sustainability, donor contributions remain fundamental to the success of immunization efforts – especially in low-income countries.[19] With an economic forecast that predicts economic struggles in the future, it may be unrealistic to rely on more government spending on immunization and primary health care.[20] In a 2022 update to the World Bank's *From Double Shock to Double Recovery – Implications and options for health financing in the time of COVID-19*, the authors state that: "Collaborative efforts now, including increases in development assistance for health and debt relief in countries facing debt distress, can enable countries to heal recent wounds, repair old scars, and jointly create conditions for a healthier, more secure, and more prosperous future."[21]

Challenges

Increasing expenditure on immunization and primary health care is not simple – for donors or governments.[22] Challenges include:[23]

- ✓ Availability of tax revenues
- ✓ Reliability of health insurance contributions in countries that depend on informal workforces
- ✓ Fragmented and declining donor funding
- ✓ Reduced budget allocations to health
- ✓ Difficulty in creating pooled resources – resources collected from multiple sources to pay for services, allowing for reduced individual risk and greater equity.

Solutions

Meeting these challenges requires making investments that are effective and efficient. One of the greatest sources of increased spending comes from economic growth – a challenge in times of economic uncertainty.[24] But there are other strategies for increasing revenue and using it more effectively and efficiently, including the following.

Increase government revenue

- ✔ Debt relief that allows struggling countries to devote more funds to health and immunization.[25]
- ✔ Taxes on products that affect health, such as tobacco, alcohol and sugar-sweetened beverages.[26]
- ✔ Mobilize funds through health insurance schemes, user fees, donations and other means.[27]

Improve efficiency and effectiveness in spending

- ✔ Strong financial management with transparent processes that connect dedicated budget allocation with accurate planning, supply and forecasting practices.[28]
- ✔ Cost efficiencies achieved through more efficient and effective planning, procurement, service delivery.[29]
- ✔ A whole-government approach that includes health and finance ministries, civil society and local communities.[30]
- ✔ Pooled procurement such as that used by UNICEF's Supply Division and the Pan American Health Organization (PAHO) Revolving Fund can save costs.[31]
- ✔ Advanced market commitments, such as one established to secure a market for pneumococcal vaccines, can help shape markets and reduce prices.

Optimize donor funding

- ✔ Strategies tailored to specific country and local needs with donor funding aligned to context-specific plans and goals.
- ✔ Donors that listen closely to the needs of governments and communities and execute funding through government systems.[32]
- ✔ Donor flexibility as countries work towards greater self-reliance.[33]

Commitment

Fundamentally, financing immunization based in primary health care is a matter of commitment; it is a political issue. In a world of competing demands for money, investing in immunization and primary health care needs to be acknowledged as a public good because it provides benefits to children, families, communities and nations.

As the world struggles to recover in the wake of COVID-19, reaching every child with vaccination demands historic investment. But when it comes to immunization, history has delivered great success: it has shown that with global, national and local commitment, vaccination for every child is possible.

> **Fundamentally, financing immunization based in primary health care is a matter of commitment; it is a political issue.**

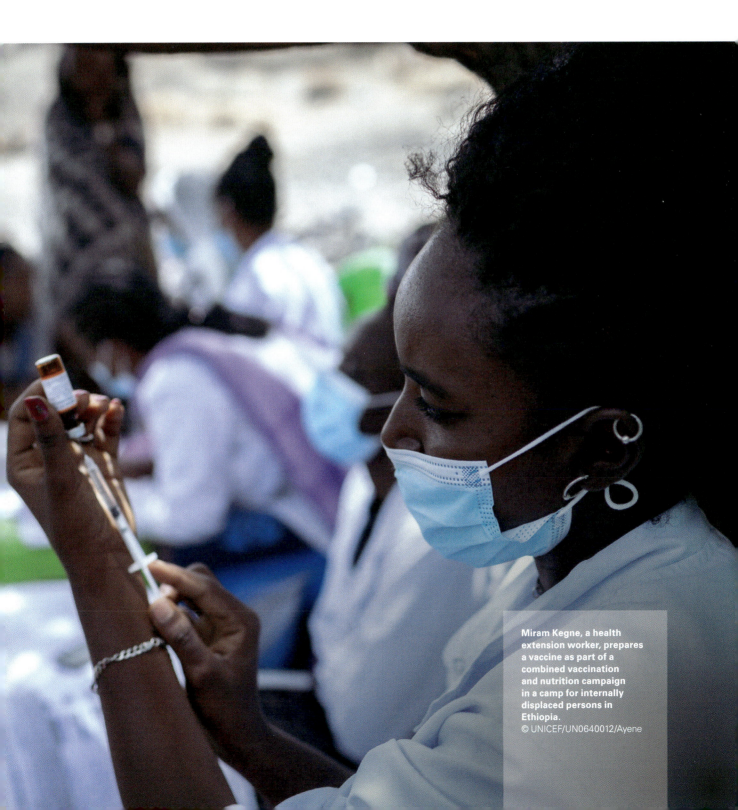

Miram Kegne, a health extension worker, prepares a vaccine as part of a combined vaccination and nutrition campaign in a camp for internally displaced persons in Ethiopia.
© UNICEF/UN0640012/Ayene

UZBEKISTAN
A Shot of Prevention: HPV vaccine is introduced

At age 14, Shakhrizoda Alanazarova knows all too well the benefits of vaccination.

Five years ago, she and her family lived through a stressful time when a close relative was diagnosed with cervical and breast cancer. Despite treatment, Shakhrizoda's relative died at the age of 43.

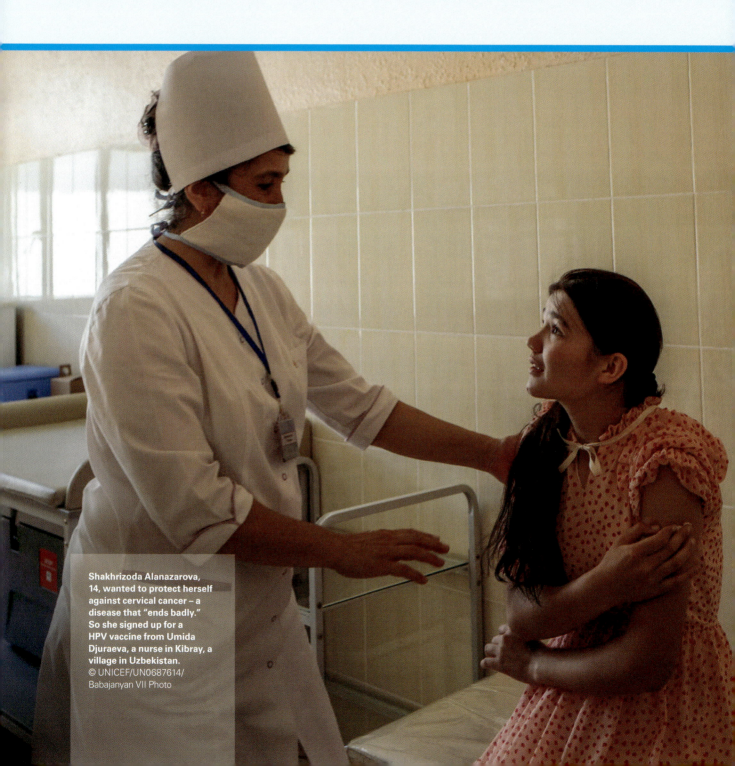

Shakhrizoda Alanazarova, 14, wanted to protect herself against cervical cancer – a disease that "ends badly." So she signed up for a HPV vaccine from Umida Djuraeva, a nurse in Kibray, a village in Uzbekistan.
© UNICEF/UN0687614/ Babajanyan VII Photo

So, when the family health clinic introduced the new vaccine to protect against the virus that causes cervical cancer, Shakhrizoda and her family decided not to miss the opportunity.

"Cancer is a bad illness and ends badly," Shakhrizoda said. "I want to stay healthy. I do not want my mother and father to worry."

As Shakhrizoda and her family know from tragedy, cervical cancer can cause plenty of worry. It has been a concern for the Government of Uzbekistan as well.

Every year, more than 1,600 new cervical cancer cases are diagnosed and about 850 women die of the disease. In response, the Government of Uzbekistan introduced the human papillomavirus (HPV) vaccine in the national immunization calendar in 2015 and began implementation in 2019 with coverage that reached 98.6 per cent of eligible girls. Since the HPV vaccination requires two doses, the second phase landed in the middle of the COVID-19 pandemic lockdowns: a potential challenge for the roll-out of the new vaccine, said Dilorom Tursunova, head of the Immunization Department and Expanded Programme on Immunization (EPI) at the Sanitary and Epidemiological Welfare and Public Health Service of the Ministry of Health.

Despite the concerns, the country persevered, and when the second doses were provided in June 2020, the coverage rate reached 97.8 per cent.

The introduction of the HPV vaccine in Uzbekistan was supported by Gavi, the Vaccine Alliance, UNICEF and the World Health Organization. The organizations offered technical, financial, and monitoring and evaluation support. In addition, they contributed to communication efforts and training for teachers and school health-care providers.

Winning public trust for the vaccine was one of the biggest challenges, Tursunova said. Rumours linked the HPV vaccine with infertility. In response, the ministry and its partners launched a campaign on multiple media platforms that included tailored messages for parents and religious leaders, and endorsements from key influencers.

"We did convince our population, after all," Tursunova said.

In Uzbekistan, only girls aged 9–14 are given the HPV vaccine. Like Shakhrizoda, many girls and their families receive invitations from schools or local clinics.

"Nowadays, people come voluntarily," said Umida Djuraeva, the nurse who administered Shakhrizoda's vaccination at the Central Multidisciplinary Policlinic of Kibray in the Tashkent region. "They have realized the vaccine is safe and tolerated well."

Shakhrizoda's mother, Sabokhat Alanazarova, for one, was convinced that the vaccine was the right step for her daughter.

"It is easier to prevent an illness than to cure it later," she said.

With one dose successfully in her arm, Shakhrizoda said she would be back in six months to complete the vaccination process.

"I am afraid of shots and thought it would be painful," she said. "But it did not hurt. It was fine and I feel good now." ■

New vaccines and products

> **Despite disruptions in earlier phases of the pandemic, vaccines against some of the deadliest infectious diseases – pneumonia, rotavirus, malaria, respiratory syncytial virus (RSV) and polio – made significant progress in recent years.**

Beyond financing, innovation in vaccines and vaccine products is crucial to ensuring every child receives life-saving immunizations. As discussed in Chapter 1, the pandemic shifted the vaccine landscape dramatically – increasing pharmaceutical industry and government investment in research and development (R&D), hastening new vaccine platforms such as messenger RNA (mRNA), and speeding development and regulatory timelines. This changed landscape offers opportunities to advance life-saving vaccine-related innovation.

Despite disruptions in earlier phases of the pandemic, vaccines against some of the deadliest infectious diseases – pneumonia, rotavirus, malaria, respiratory syncytial virus (RSV) and polio – made significant progress in recent years. Broadly protective influenza vaccines, novel oral polio vaccines, and vaccines that can help combat antimicrobial resistance are also in development. Mucosal vaccines in the form of liquid drops, sprays or tablets can enhance immunogenicity, facilitate administration to children and are easier to use in low-resource settings.

The use of non-traditional vaccine platforms such as nucleic acid vaccines (e.g., mRNA vaccines) and material science approaches (e.g., lipid nanoparticles) is expanding, and may offer ways to develop vaccines where traditional approaches have failed. The speed with which COVID-19 vaccines were developed and produced also opened the potential for faster vaccine development and approval.[34] The global community must avail itself of these pandemic outcomes to ensure a strong pipeline for R&D, approval, manufacture and distribution of vaccines against infectious diseases that kill children.

Recent vaccine developments

High prices and limited supply of pneumococcal conjugate vaccines (PCVs) – which protect against the pneumococcus bacterium, the leading cause of deadly childhood pneumonia – have hindered access and uptake, especially in self-financing middle-income countries.[35] Today, pneumonia still kills more children than any other infectious disease, claiming the lives of more than 700,000 children under age 5 each year.[36] In 2019, the availability of a new and more affordable PCV marked a key step in reducing the cost and supply barriers – and reaching the 55 million children who previously lacked access to PCVs.

Several new vaccines are emerging for malaria, which kills half a million children each year.[37] The world's first malaria vaccine, Mosquirix (RTS,S/AS01), was recommended by the World Health Organization (WHO) in 2021 for children at risk in central and southern Africa and other regions with moderate to high transmission of malaria.[38] Gavi has initiated a malaria vaccination programme to support a broader roll-out of the vaccine in Gavi-supported countries, and WHO prequalified the vaccine in 2022. Unfortunately, current production capacity of Mosquirix is limited, severely constraining the number of children who can be protected. A second vaccine candidate, R21, is in advanced clinical trials.[39]

Vaccines for rotavirus, which kills approximately 200,000 children annually,[40] have advanced significantly since 2018. For more than a decade, there were only two live oral rotavirus vaccines (LORVs). Four additional lower-cost rotavirus vaccines are now WHO-prequalified and available with Gavi support.

Next-generation rotavirus vaccines, now in advanced clinical development, are showing further promise. They may be more affordable and offer children better protection against disease than existing LORVs. Another approach is administering LORVs to newborns, which could provide early protection, improve vaccine coverage, and potentially be more effective in areas with the highest rates of rotavirus. One candidate is currently in development.

While no vaccine yet exists for respiratory syncytial virus (RSV) – a significant killer of infants under 6 months old – several are in development. RSV causes 3.2 million hospitalizations and as many as 120,000 deaths per year in children under 5, with most deaths in low- and middle-income countries.[41] Many of these vaccine candidates are administered during pregnancy and protect infants in the early, vulnerable months of life.[42]

The year 2021 also saw the introduction of nOPV2, a next-generation polio vaccine that is less likely to seed new cases of vaccine-derived polio type 2 (cVDPV2) and therefore help stop outbreaks.[43] nOPV2 is showing promising results in the fight against cVDPV2, with 500 million doses administered in 23 countries as of October 2022.[44]

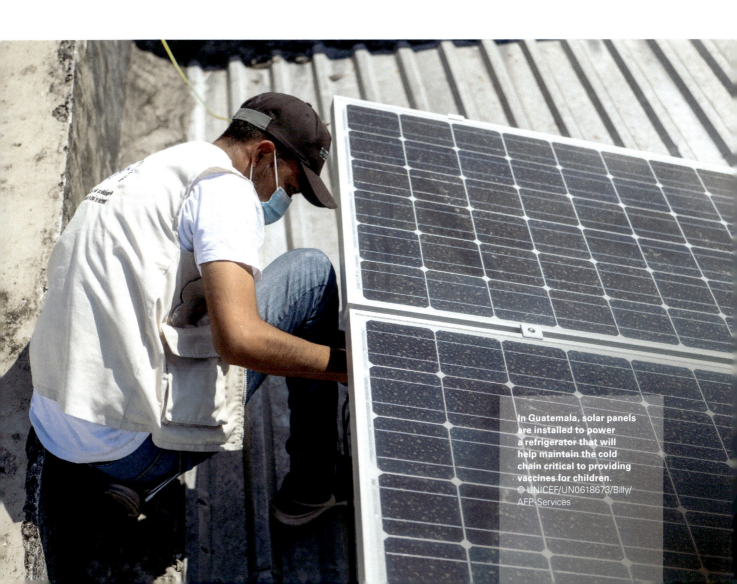

In Guatemala, solar panels are installed to power a refrigerator that will help maintain the cold chain critical to providing vaccines for children.
© UNICEF/UN0618673/Billy/AFP-Services

Vaccine product developments

Vaccine product and formulation innovations are key to maximizing the impact of vaccines themselves. They can simplify logistics, make vaccines easier to administer, improve safety, increase vaccine confidence and facilitate access in hard-to-reach areas.

Vaccine product and formulation innovations are key to maximizing the impact of vaccines themselves. They can simplify logistics, make vaccines easier to administer, improve safety, increase vaccine confidence and facilitate access in hard-to-reach areas. To accelerate the development of vaccine product innovations that better meet the needs of low- and middle-income countries, the Vaccine Innovation Prioritisation Strategy (VIPS) was established in 2017.[45] A partnership of Gavi, WHO, the Bill & Melinda Gates Foundation, UNICEF and PATH, it identifies the most promising innovations and prioritizes them for development. It has selected needle-free technology, systematic use of barcodes and heat-stable vaccines for priority.

- Needle-free MAPs, also referred to as microneedle patches, consist of micron-scale projections that deliver dry vaccine into the skin. MAPs hold promise of increased acceptance among patients and caregivers alike: they are easier to administer and can help avoid reconstitution errors and needlestick injuries.[46] Given their dry-vaccine format, they could also be less susceptible to damage or loss of potency from heat or freezing. The most advanced vaccine MAP products – for seasonal influenza, hepatitis B and measles–rubella vaccines – are in clinical development.

- Barcodes on vaccine packaging – encoding information such as vaccine product number, serial number, supplier data, batch number and expiration date – can be scanned to instantly capture information. Barcodes, which can take multiple forms including QR codes, bring efficiencies to vaccine inventory and supply chain management. They improve both traceability and authentication (i.e., screening for counterfeit products). Barcodes compliant with Global Standards 1 (GS1, an international standard recognized in more than 100 countries) are recommended by WHO and required by Gavi and UNICEF as of 2021. However, barcodes are not typically included on primary packaging, for example on vials themselves, in low- and middle-income countries. Including them could improve tracking of adverse events following immunization. They could also increase data accuracy and save health worker time for service delivery when integrated into electronic immunization records.

- Heat-stable or controlled temperature chain (CTC)-qualified vaccines are sufficiently heat stable to protect against loss of potency and wastage from exposure to high temperatures. Use of heat-stable/CTC-qualified vaccines can foster efficiencies, facilitate vaccine access in hard-to-reach communities, and alleviate cold-chain constraints. Several vaccines, including those against meningitis A, human papillomavirus (HPV), cholera and pneumonia are CTC qualified. A hepatitis B birth dose is also being explored for use in a CTC.

Logistics and supply chain innovations

Innovations in vaccine supply chains over the last five years are coming to market and will result in improved potency and better access to poor and remote areas. One example is vaccine vial monitors (VVMs), small temperature-sensitive indicators on vaccines that allow health workers to monitor vaccines for heat exposure. Newer models, called VVM-TIs (vaccine vial monitor–threshold indicators), signal exposure to temperature above a specific threshold.

Several additional logistics-related innovations are notable. First, a new set of freeze-preventive vaccine carriers can prevent accidental freezing and a loss of potency during transport. Second, drones are being successfully used to deliver health commodities in a number of African countries. This airborne delivery enables access to hard-to-reach areas. Third, solar direct drive (SDD) refrigeration systems have had a significant impact on vaccine delivery. SDDs are able to keep vaccines at the appropriate temperature without the need for batteries or electricity from a national grid.[47] Since 2017, UNICEF and partners have delivered over 140,000 refrigerators to 113 countries, of which 46 per cent were Solar Direct Drive.

Digital tools

The shift to digital technology in the health sector over the past decade emerged with a focus on improving the quality and timeliness of data. Digital tools were first introduced in immunization programmes with systems such as electronic immunization registries (EIRs), which can replace paper-based record-keeping. EIRs are confidential, population-based information systems that can record data on vaccine doses delivered. They can ensure the right person receives the right vaccination at the right time by enabling client identification, recording vaccine histories and tracking clients who have missed a vaccine.

> Digital tools were first introduced in immunization programmes with systems such as electronic immunization registries (EIRs), which can replace paper-based record-keeping.

A growing number of countries have implemented EIRs to improve data quality and programme performance. In Latin America, EIRs have been in use for more than three decades, beginning with Mexico in 1987. Momentum has built since the early 2010s, with more EIRs implemented in Africa and Asia; today, 50 low- and middle-income countries are using EIRs. EIRs in the United Republic of Tanzania and Zambia reported significant improvements in data accuracy, the ability to identify areas with low vaccine coverage, and the ability to identify children who have missed vaccines. In the Gambia, they produce high-quality, timely and consistent data.[48] EIRs have also proven to be efficient and cost-effective: they reduce time on immunization reporting and management and eliminate the costs of printing.[49]

'Big data' derived from EIRs can be a powerful tool to monitor immunization activities in real time and ensure that communities in need are identified, as a study in Pakistan demonstrates.[50] Following the digital registration of vaccinators who tracked their work with an Android phone-based system, the average number of daily doses of the measles vaccine and the third pentavalent dose administered in high-risk areas increased significantly.[51] Geographic information systems (GIS) mapping tools, which allow the production of maps to analyse and present information, are also now in use to help locate children in need of immunization. These tools are assisting both in routine immunization[52] and in the fight against polio.[53] GIS-enabled planning was more cost-effective than standard methods in a study in northern Nigeria.[54] Another study in Nigeria found that GIS enabled more accurate population targeting for measles vaccination, and improved coverage.[55]

Another important digital tool is civil registration and vital statistics (CRVS) and national identification (ID) systems. These systems capture vital events in an individual's life, such as birth, death and cause of death, and help identify support services needed for individuals. Integrating these systems with EIRs helps track vaccinations for all children and assists with vaccination resource allocation. Other digital systems, including electronic logistics management information systems (eLMIS), can reduce vaccine shortages, improve supply chain efficiency, and increase the availability of vaccines.

Still other digital platforms have shown success. In Indonesia, the RapidPro platform was used to digitally track vaccination progress in the national measles–rubella campaign. The technology enabled vaccinators to send text message reports of the number of children vaccinated each day; that information was automatically uploaded to a database and then represented on an online dashboard.[56] Not only was higher coverage linked with higher utilization of the platform, but full immunization targets were also reached more quickly. The effects were even stronger in districts identified as having increased vaccine hesitancy. In India, the digital health platform TeCHO+ (Technology Enabled Community Health Operations) and the electronic vaccine intelligence network (eVIN) increased vaccination coverage while enhancing case management and data entry efficiency.[57]

Initiatives involving mobile phones (known as mHealth) including text message reminders have been shown to improve vaccine coverage and timelines in a variety of low- and middle-income country settings. For example, an analysis of six studies in low- and middle-income countries revealed that pregnant women were 63 per cent more likely to receive tetanus immunization when they received mobile phone-related interventions.[58] Digital interventions have also been used to improve the vaccine supply chain in India,[59] Kenya[60] and Zambia.[61] The eVIN network in India, which monitored the temperature of cold-chain equipment, was linked to the improvement of vaccination coverage and the availability of doses.[62]

> **Another important digital tool is civil registration and vital statistics (CRVS) and national identification (ID) systems. These systems capture vital events in an individual's life, such as birth, death and cause of death, and help identify support services needed for individuals.**

Strengthening local manufacturing

High-income countries quickly developed, procured and distributed COVID-19 vaccines in the early stages of the pandemic, while low- and middle-income countries were forced to wait. This inequity accelerated a movement to increase low- and middle-income countries' capacities to research and manufacture vaccines themselves. Less than 1 per cent of all vaccines used on the African continent are locally produced, for example, underscoring the region's intense vulnerability and overdependence on foreign supplies. The African Union has set a goal to develop, produce and supply more than 60 per cent of the vaccine doses required on the continent by 2040. It has called on Gavi and other international partners to support this agenda. The goal is for well-managed, regional manufacturing diversification to support equitable access during pandemics, while sustaining affordable prices for, and expanding access to, routine vaccination.[63]

The pandemic sparked other, related initiatives. First, the Developing Countries Vaccine Manufacturers Network, established in 2000, aims to help low- and middle-income countries advance towards greater vaccine self-sufficiency. It is an international alliance of manufacturers that coordinate to provide a sustainable supply of vaccines at affordable prices to developing countries while encouraging increased R&D in those countries. Second, mRNA plants are currently being planned in Africa, Asia and Latin America, with the capacity to produce both COVID-19 vaccines and future mRNA vaccines combating other diseases.[64]

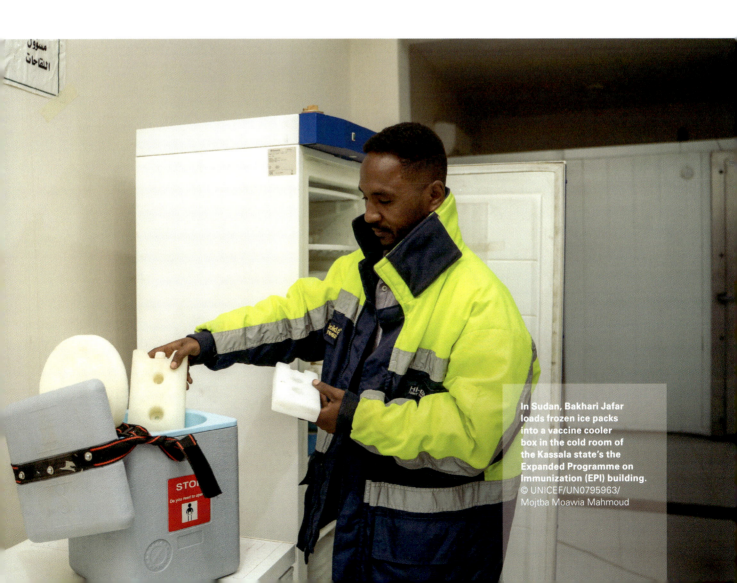

In Sudan, Bakhari Jafar loads frozen ice packs into a vaccine cooler box in the cold room of the Kassala state's the Expanded Programme on Immunization (EPI) building.
© UNICEF/UN0795963/ Mojtba Moawia Mahmoud

HAITI
Solar Solutions: Preserving vaccines, protecting children's health

Every time six-month-old Jamesly needs a vaccine, his mother Rosemirlande makes a 6-kilometre journey from her village to the Sacré Coeur Health Centre.

On one visit, the 27-year-old shopkeeper patiently took a seat in the waiting room, joined by about 20 mothers and caregivers who also held children on their laps. All were eagerly waiting for essential vaccines that will protect their children from diphtheria, diarrhoea, tuberculosis and pneumonia.

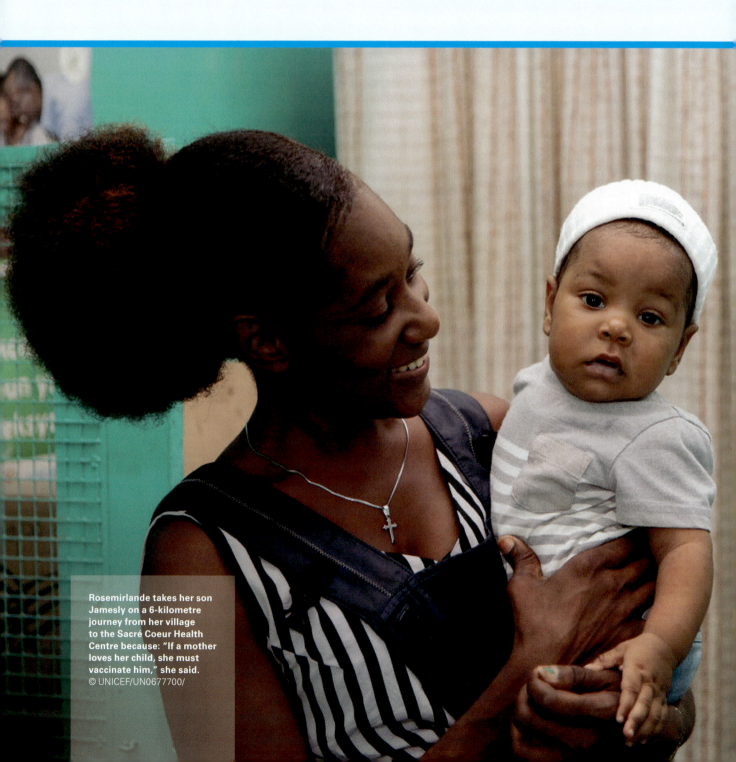

Rosemirlande takes her son Jamesly on a 6-kilometre journey from her village to the Sacré Coeur Health Centre because: "If a mother loves her child, she must vaccinate him," she said.
© UNICEF/UN0677700/

For Rosemirlande, it was worth the effort and the wait.

"If a mother loves her child, she must vaccinate him," she said.

Rosemirlande can put her love into action thanks, in part, to the installation of solar power that has allowed the Sacré Coeur Health Centre in Sud department to overcome persistent electricity shortages.

Over recent years, UNICEF and the Ministry of Public Health and Population have invested in solar energy for health centres. In the tropical country, refrigeration is essential for maintaining perishable health supplies, especially vaccines.

"In the past, we used propane gas canisters, but there were always shortages, putting the cold chain and quality of vaccines at risk," said Mona Yvrose Jean Claude, who has worked as a nurse at Sacré Coeur Health Centre for more than 10 years. "Now ... there are fewer cases of measles, polio, flu or diarrhoea."

"Solar energy is a blessing," she added.

Throughout Haiti, 96 per cent of health-care facilities rely on solar power. The country has over 960 solar refrigerators and two cold rooms – a large warehouse for vaccines. Sud department has more than 150 solar refrigerators.

Despite experiencing a deterioration in immunization coverage because of COVID-19, Sud department managed a coverage of 88 per cent for children protected with the Pentavalent 3 vaccine.

"The electricity problem is solved with solar panels for refrigerators," said Pierre Jean Gardy, cold chain technician at the Sud department Input Supply Centre. "Now, health institutions are continuously well equipped to receive vaccines for children."

But challenges remain.

Rosemirlande was able to walk to the health centre, but for some families the distance is too far. When possible, Mona and her colleagues provide mobile clinics. In some communities, they have encountered adolescents who have never been vaccinated.

"Some people have never had the chance to visit a health centre, so it is our duty to bring the services to them," Mona said.

Sacré Coeur Health Centre offers multiple services, including a robust clinic for HIV. Improvements to the antenatal clinic have increased the number of visits for childhood vaccinations.

"There were few children who came to receive BCG vaccine [for tuberculosis]," Mona said. "So, thanks to the efforts that have been made in our antenatal clinic, we have recorded an increase in the number of visits for vaccination."

The COVID-19 pandemic caused a drop in attendance, especially among pregnant women. However, multi-skilled community health workers (Agent de Santé Communautaire Polyvalent) were trained and deployed in communities.

But maintaining these outreach activities is a financial challenge, especially for an ageing workforce. Continuing with a more versatile community health workforce and establishing assembly stations would allow Mona and her colleagues to continue the effort and reach more children, Mona said.

On the day Rosemirlande brought Jamesly for his vaccinations, nurses were also advising the adults on the importance of food and hygiene in preventing infections.

"For me, it is not the salary but rather the patient's feelings," Mona said. "... Every morning, I know that I will help someone in their physical or psychological suffering. This is what drives me to get up every day and come to work." ■

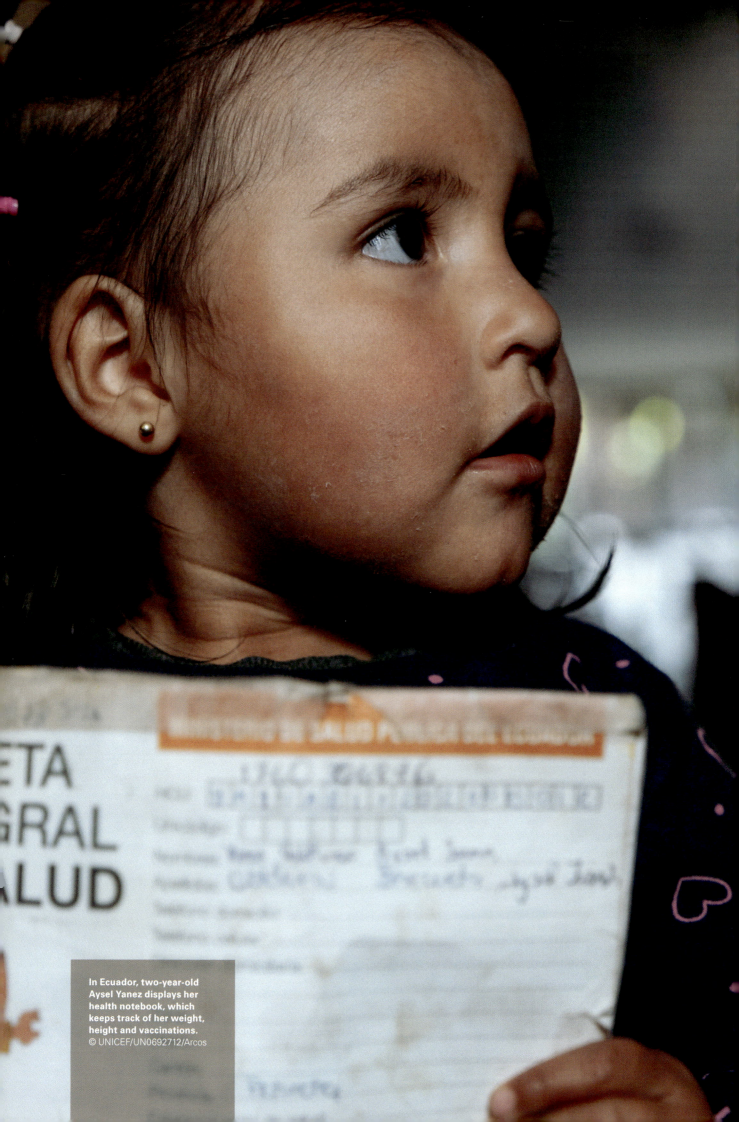

In Ecuador, two-year-old Aysel Yanez displays her health notebook, which keeps track of her weight, height and vaccinations.
© UNICEF/UN0692712/Arcos

CHAPTER 6

For every child, vaccination: An equity agenda

Immunization saves lives. It is central in protecting children's health and well-being and supporting our shared development goals. Scaling up vaccination coverage is a matter of life and death. This chapter proposes a framework for action with key recommendations that global stakeholders should prioritize to reach every child with life-saving vaccination.

Introduction

Despite undeniable progress over many decades, we continue to face critical challenges in immunization. Immunization coverage has fallen back, or stagnated, in too many places. We are persistently missing about one in five children with life-saving vaccines, especially the socially marginalized and poorest children, and the situation has only deteriorated during the COVID-19 pandemic. The failure of health systems to reach every child with vaccines reflects domestic underinvestment in primary health care, inadequate human resources for health, and leadership gaps across different levels and areas of government.

The decline in immunization throughout the pandemic should sound an alarm bell. Routine immunization must be a priority in the coming years. We must take concerted action to catch up on children who missed out on being vaccinated during the pandemic, rebuild systems and tackle major gaps in health systems. Failure to act will devastate the lives of today's children and adolescents – tomorrow's adults – and further set back progress towards reaching the Sustainable Development Goals.

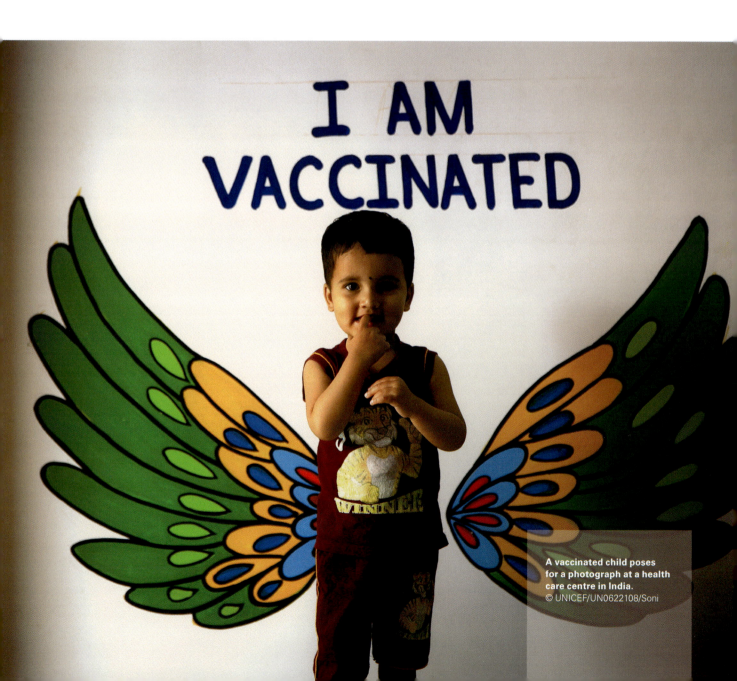

A vaccinated child poses for a photograph at a health care centre in India.
© UNICEF/UN0622108/Soni

For every child, vaccination: An equity agenda

Over the last few years, stakeholders including global governance institutions, development agencies and academics have called for accelerated action in immunization services.

Building on the global strategies outlined in the *Immunization Agenda 2030* and the Gavi Strategy 5.0 to promote equity and sustainably scale up immunization coverage, this report presents an agenda to put childhood vaccination first – a set of concrete and actionable recommendations to reach every child with vaccines and ensure that immunization and primary health care systems are ready to meet future challenges.

Enacting this agenda will require strong political will from governments and other major stakeholders in the immunization landscape. The COVID-19 pandemic has shown the centrality of collective and concerted action to ensure that vaccines reach everyone. We are constantly reminded that "vaccines don't save lives, vaccination saves lives". For vaccination to happen, political will must be a number one priority across countries.

1. Vaccinate every child, everywhere

Equity means this: Vaccines must reach every child, no matter where they were born, who they are or where they are living.[1] That means reaching the children who missed out on vaccination during the pandemic and who are now slipping past the age when they would normally be vaccinated. It means reaching children in the three areas identified as facing particular obstacles to immunization – remote rural villages, informal urban settlements and conflict areas. It also means reaching zero-dose children living in places where barriers to vaccination may not be obvious, often no more than an hour from the nearest health centre.[2]

Key priorities

✓ **Catch up on the vaccination of children missed during the pandemic:** The COVID-19 pandemic response generated enormous momentum for immunization, which can now be used to focus on the needs of children who were not vaccinated during the pandemic. Tailored responses are needed in the countries most affected, backed by financial and other support from key donors and international partners.

✓ **Identify zero-dose and under-vaccinated children and address key inequities:** Use high-quality and fit-for-purpose data to identify zero-dose and under-vaccinated children and inform and guide action, and invest in new technologies and approaches to make data timelier and more granular. Develop an individual child health record system to monitor outcomes, including a community's vaccine status, and monitor progress and needs with publicly accessible dashboards.

Design immunization services to be responsive to addressing key socioeconomic inequities and barriers to accessing immunization.

✔ **Identify children in urban areas, access children in rural areas:** In urban areas, strengthen community engagement to encourage people to engage with health services, improve security for parents and health workers, and offer flexibly timed vaccine services. In rural areas, focus on motivating and retaining health workers with salary top-ups and other incentives, consider using private operators to lower the high marginal cost of delivering vaccine services, and better integrate health services across sectors.

✔ **Meet the challenges in emergency and fragile settings:** Invest in preparedness to ensure countries are equipped to respond, including by creating contingency stocks, building resilience and engaging civil society. Support children and families on the move, ensuring vaccines and health services are available and accessible. Prioritize and invest in innovative solutions, such as using mobile money and digital systems to pay health workers and developing vaccines with longer shelf-lives.

2. Strengthen demand for – and confidence in – vaccination

Many factors affect families' readiness to vaccinate children, and these vary considerably depending on local contexts, culture and societal norms. Questions around the safety and effectiveness of vaccines can be important, as can perceptions of the benefits and costs of vaccination *(see Chapter 4)*. Communities' relationships and experiences with health and government officials can also shape wider attitudes towards the use of immunization and health services. Understanding all these issues with effective social listening is critical to help identify and develop tailored interventions and strategies that can help promote vaccine demand.

Key priorities

✔ **Talk to communities:** Strengthen engagement with communities to better understand their attitudes towards the safety of vaccines and the value of vaccination; their experiences – both good and bad – with health systems and government officials; and the support they need if they are to take the time to vaccinate their children.

✔ **Tackle gender barriers:** Use innovative approaches to inform and educate caregivers, especially mothers; involve and engage fathers and men; and tailor services to meet the needs of time-pressed caregivers.

✔ **Equip health workers to address concerns:** Health workers enjoy high levels of trust. They should be supported to be powerful allies to persuade parents to vaccinate children, counter misinformation in the community, and inform the design of responses that meet families' needs.

✔ **Rethink accountability in health systems to boost trust:** Governments should consider setting up well-designed governance bodies, such as health-care facility committees, to give community leaders a formal mechanism for voicing concerns and tackling issues related to immunization and primary health care services in their area.

3. Spend more and spend better on immunization and health

The COVID-19 pandemic showed that, despite significant global investment in immunization and health systems strengthening over the last decade, health systems in many countries remain fragile. Many suffer from underinvestment and a lack of predictable funding – a particular issue for countries heavily reliant on external donors. With many countries facing the prospect of a lost decade for public investment, it has never been more important to ensure that money is well spent and efficiently targeted. To promote equity, national and subnational governments need to prioritize funding for immunization services and primary health care. They should also look to further strengthen leadership and accountability to oversee efficient and effective spending. For their part, international donors need to do more to harmonize their support and centre it on strengthening primary health care.

Key priorities

- ✓ **Invest in primary health care at the national level:** Governments should prioritize funding for primary health care to ensure it does more to meet the needs of its users and ensures equitable access, especially to underserved communities.
- ✓ **Better align donor support:** Donors should work to integrate their support into national priorities and national systems, shifting from disease-specific initiatives to system strengthening. Better harmonization of support can help to reduce fragmentation and eliminate wasteful overlaps, including the duplication of, among others, infrastructure, service delivery and information platforms.
- ✓ **Strengthen leadership capacity and promote accountability:** Improve mechanisms for social accountability to ensure transparency, adequate budget allocations, quality of service, and community engagement. Such approaches should be part of an overall push to maximize returns on current investment by improving planning and budgeting, identifying budget challenges, improving public financing management systems, and strengthening coordination among national-level ministries and between government at national and subnational levels.
- ✓ **Explore innovative financing:** Stakeholders at all levels need to build on recent successes and explore how innovative financing mechanisms can maximize returns on current investment and tap into new sources of funding. Such approaches need to be informed by a clear understanding of the potential risks involved and the need for governance and oversight.

4. Build resilient systems and shockproof them for the future

Every community has a right to person-centred primary health care with immunization as an integral part of service provision. In turn, immunization can be an entry-point to strengthening primary health care and to improving service delivery, especially in challenging settings. Primary health care should prioritize equity, focusing on those most in need, and should be people-centred, rather than disease-centred. Health workers, and community health workers, are at the heart of primary health: Strengthening their presence, skills and motivation is essential. Resilient systems are able to respond to outbreaks, epidemics or pandemics, while continuing to provide essential services. Building these systems also means providing quality primary health care with a motivated and skilled workforce close to communities; developing data and information systems to monitor immunization needs; and strengthening surveillance, especially of disease outbreaks. It is also essential to secure reliable supplies of vaccines and to make best use of innovations that can help health workers reach the most remote children.

Key priorities

- **Focus on health workers, especially women:** Improve pay and working conditions to motivate and retain health workers, especially the many women working in health systems. They need to be better represented in leadership, offered access to training and professional advancement, protected from discrimination and gender-based violence in the workplace, and provided with flexible working arrangements to help them better manage their family and professional commitments.
- **Improve data collection and disease surveillance:** Within broader information systems for primary health care, it is essential to improve data collection on immunization and ensure it is actionable. Countries also need to build and strengthen comprehensive surveillance systems for vaccine-preventable diseases as part of a national system for public health surveillance, all supported by strong and reliable laboratory networks.
- **Secure vaccine and other supplies:** Ensure a secure supply of high-quality vaccines and related commodities. Making better use of pooled procurement processes and strategies can ensure affordable prices and support strategic stockpiles. The potential of expanded regional manufacturing to speed and diversify vaccine supplies also needs to be fully explored and supported.
- **Develop and promote worthwhile innovations:** Invest in novel delivery technologies, such as solar-powered cold chains, heat-resistant vaccines, and micro-array patches, to ensure access to vaccines for communities in the most challenging settings.

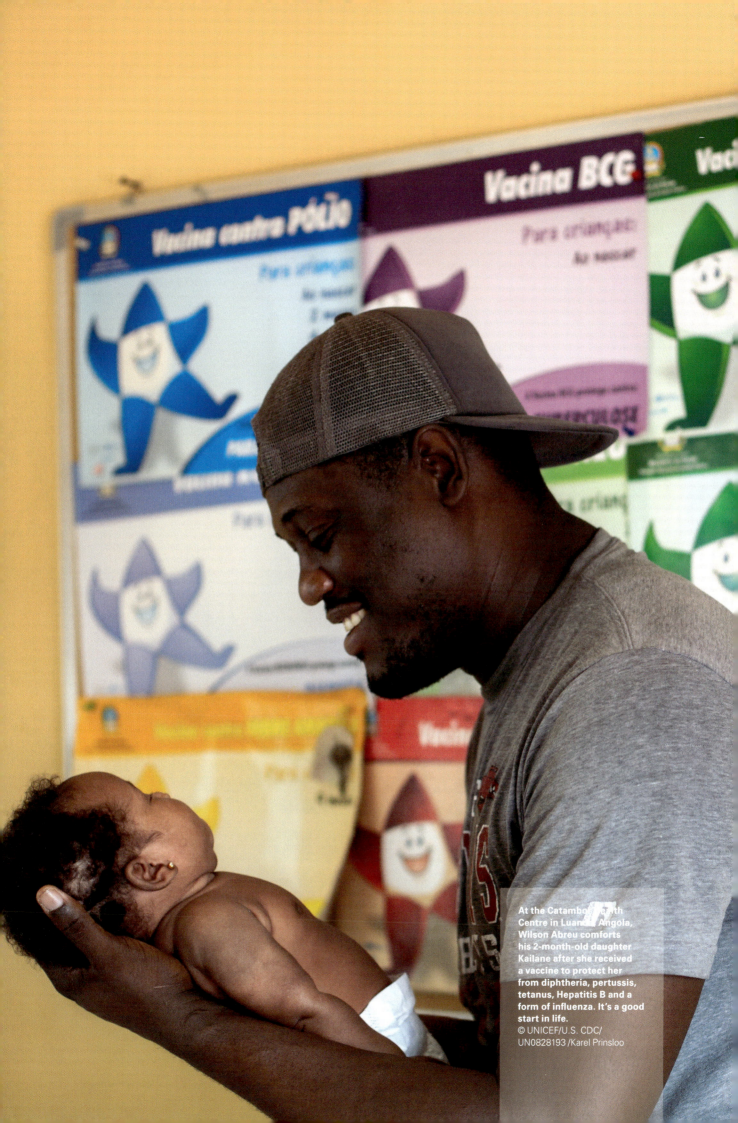

At the Catambor Health Centre in Luanda, Angola, Wilson Abreu comforts his 2-month-old daughter Kailane after she received a vaccine to protect her from diphtheria, pertussis, tetanus, Hepatitis B and a form of influenza. It's a good start in life.
© UNICEF/U.S. CDC/ UN0828193 /Karel Prinsloo

Endnotes

Introduction

1 UN News, 'Nearly 40 Million Children Susceptible to Measles Due to COVID-19 Disruptions', 23 November 2022, <https://news.un.org/en/story/2022/11/1131002>, accessed 23 February 2023.
Centers for Disease Control and Prevention, 'Global Measles and Rubella', 23 November 2022, <www.cdc.gov/globalhealth/measles/index.html>, accessed 23 February 2023.

2 Centers for Disease Control and Prevention, 'Complications of Measles', 5 November 2020, <www.cdc.gov/measles/symptoms/complications.html>, accessed 27 February 2023.
Leal, I., et al. (2015), 'An Old "New" Friend: Postmeasles blindness in the 21st century', BMJ Case Reports, 2015, art. bcr2015211766, <http://dx.doi.org/10.1136/bcr-2015-211766>.
World Health Organization, 'Measles', 5 December 2019, <www.who.int/news-room/fact-sheets/detail/measles>, accessed 27 February 2023.

3 Semba, Richard D., and Martin W. Bloem, 'Measles Blindness', *Public Health and the Eye*, vol. 49, no. 2, March 2004, pp. 243–255, <https://doi.org/10.1016/j.survophthal.2003.12.005>.
'Measles'.

4 Dixon, Meredith G., et al., 'Progress Toward Regional Measles Elimination – Worldwide, 2000–2020', *Morbidity and Mortality Weekly Report*, vol. 70, no. 45, 10 November 2021, pp. 1563–1569, <https://doi.org/10.15585/mmwr.mm7045a1>.

5 World Health Organization and United Nations Children's Fund, *Progress and Challenges with Achieving Universal Immunization Coverage: 2021 WHO/UNICEF estimates of national immunization coverage (WUENIC)*, 15 July 2022, <https://data.unicef.org/wp-content/uploads/2016/07/progress-challenges_wuenic2021.pdf>, accessed 26 July 2022.

6 Ibid.

7 Ibid.

8 *Immunization Agenda 2030: A global strategy to leave no one behind (IA2030)*, n.d., <https://cdn.who.int/media/docs/default-source/immunization/strategy/ia2030/ia2030-draft-4-wha_b8850379-1fce-4847-bfd1-5d2c9d9e32f8.pdf?sfvrsn=5389656e_69&download=true>, accessed 27 February 2023.

9 Henderson, Donald A., 'The Eradication of Smallpox – An overview of the past, present, and future', *Vaccine*, vol. 29, suppl. 4, 2011, pp. D7–D9, <www.sciencedirect.com/science/article/pii/S0264410X11009546>, accessed 27 February 2023.

10 Global Polio Eradication Initiative, *Investment Case 2022-2026: Investing in the promise of a polio-free world*, World Health Organization, Geneva, 2022, p. v, <https://polioeradication.org/wp-content/uploads/2022/04/GPEI-Investment-Case-2022-2026-Web-EN.pdf>, accessed 27 February 2023.

11 World Health Organization, 'Global Excess Deaths Associated with COVID-19, January 2020 – December 2021', May 2022, <www.who.int/data/stories/global-excess-deaths-associated-with-covid-19-january-2020-december-2021>, accessed 27 February 2023.

12 Mattieu, E., et al., 'Coronavirus Pandemic (COVID-19) Vaccinations', Our World in Data, 2020, <https://ourworldindata.org/covid-vaccinations>, accessed on 26 July 2022.

13 Watson, Oliver J., et al., 'Global Impact of the First Year of COVID-19 Vaccination: A mathematical modelling study', *The Lancet Infectious Diseases*, vol. 22, no. 9, September 2022, pp. 1293–1302, <https://doi.org/10.1016/S1473-3099(22)00320-6>.

14 Solis-Moreira, Jocelyn, 'How Did We Develop a COVID-19 Vaccine So Quickly?', MedicalNewsToday, 13 November 2021, <www.medicalnewstoday.com/articles/how-did-we-develop-a-covid-19-vaccine-so-quickly>, accessed 27 February 2023.

15 Watson, et al., 'Global Impact of the First Year of COVID-19 Vaccination'.

16 World Health Organization, *Implementing the Immunization Agenda 2030: A framework for action through coordinated planning, monitoring & evaluation, ownership & accountability, and communications & advocacy*, WHO, Geneva, 2021, <www.who.int/teams/immunization-vaccines-and-biologicals/strategies/ia2030>, accessed 27 February 2023.

17 Strategic Advisory Group of Experts on Immunization, The Global Vaccine Action Plan 2011-2020. *Review and lessons learned*, WHO/IVB/19.07, World Health Organization, Geneva, 2019, <https://apps.who.int/iris/bitstream/handle/10665/329097/WHO-IVB-19.07-eng.pdf>, accessed 27 February 2023.

18 United Nations Children's Fund and World Health Organization, *Immunization Coverage: Are we losing ground?*, WHO and UNICEF, Geneva and New York, July 2020, <https://data.unicef.org/resources/immunization-coverage-are-we-losing-ground/>, accessed 6 July 2022.

19 WHO/UNICEF national immunization coverage estimates, 2021. <https://unicef.shinyapps.io/wuenic-analytics-2022/>, accessed 28 February 2023.

20 *Implementing the Immunization Agenda 2030*.

21 Lindstrand, Ann, et al., 'The World of Immunization: Achievements, challenges, and strategic vision for the next decade', *The Journal of Infectious Diseases*, vol. 224, suppl. 4, 1 October 2021, pp. S452–S467, <https://doi.org/10.1093/infdis/jiab284>.

22 Larson, Heidi J., Emmanuela Gakidou and Christopher J.L. Murray, 'The Vaccine-Hesitant Moment', *New England Journal of Medicine*, vol. 387, no. 1, 2022, pp. 58–65, <https://doi.org/10.1056/NEJMra2106441>.

23 World Health Organization, 'Ten Threats to Global Health in 2019', n.d., <www.who.int/news-room/spotlight/ten-threats-to-global-health-in-2019>, accessed 27 February 2023.

24 Larson, et al., 'The Vaccine-Hesitant Moment'.

25 World Health Organisation, 'Measles and Rubella Global Update January 2023', WHO, Geneva, <www.who.int/teams/immunization-vaccines-and-biologicals/immunization-analysis-and-insights/surveillance/monitoring/provisional-monthly-measles-and-rubella-data>, accessed on 23 January 2023

26 Clarke, Ed, and Beate Kampmann, 'No One is Safe Until Everyone is Safe – From polio too', *BMJ*, vol. 377, 2022, art. o1625, <https://doi.org/10.1136/bmj.o1625>.

27 United Nations Children's Fund, *The Climate Crisis is a Child Rights Crisis: Introducing the Children's Climate Risk Index*, UNICEF, New York, August 2021, <www.unicef.org/reports/climate-crisis-child-rights-crisis>, accessed 28 February 2023.

28 *Immunization Agenda 2030*.

29 United Nations, Convention on the Rights of the Child, United Nations, New York, 20 November 1989, Art. 24, <www.ohchr.org/en/instruments-mechanisms/instruments/convention-rights-child>.

30 *Immunization Agenda 2030*.

31 United Nations Children's Fund, *Costs of Vaccinating a Child*, UNICEF, New York, August 2020.

32 Immunization Economics Community of Practice, 'Return on Investment', 2019, <https://immunizationeconomics.org/dove-roi>, accessed 27 February 2023.

33 Kurowski, Christoph, et al., *From Double Shock to Double Recovery: Implications and options for health financing in the time of COVID-19. Technical update: Old scars, new wounds*, The World Bank, Washington, D.C., September 2022, <https://openknowledge.worldbank.org/bitstream/handle/10986/35298/September%202022.pdf>, accessed 27 February 2023.

34 Kurowski, Christoph, et al., 'From Double Shock to Double Recovery: Implications and options for health financing in the time of COVID-19', Health, Nutrition and Population Discussion Paper, The World Bank, Washington, D.C., March 2021, pp. 45–46, <https://openknowledge.worldbank.org/handle/10986/35298>, accessed 6 March 2023.

Chapter 1

1 MacMillan, Carrie, 'Herd Immunity: Will we ever get there?', Yale Medicine, 21 May 2021, <www.yalemedicine.org/news/herd-immunity>, accessed 28 February 2023

2 World Health Organization, 'Immunization Analysis and Insights', <www.who.int/teams/immunization-vaccines-and-biologicals/immunization-analysis-and-insights/surveillance/monitoring/provisional-monthly-measles-and-rubella-data>, accessed 7 February 2023.

3 WHO Africa, 'Vaccine-Preventable Disease Outbreaks on the Rise in Africa', 28 April 2022, <www.afro.who.int/news/vaccine-preventable-disease-outbreaks-rise-africa>, accessed 3 May 2022.
World Health Organization and UNICEF, 'UNICEF and WHO Warn of "Perfect Storm" of Conditions for Measles Outbreaks, Affecting Children', "Press release", 27 April 2022, <www.unicef.org/press-releases/unicef-and-who-warn-perfect-storm-conditions-measles-outbreaks-affecting-children>, accessed 3 May 2022.

4   Jerving, Sara, 'Is a Measles Spike a Bellwether for Other Vaccine-Preventable Outbreaks?', DEVEX, Inside Development, Global Health, 5 May 2022, <www.devex.com/news/is-a-measles-spike-a-bellwether-for-other-vaccine-preventable-outbreaks-103147>, accessed 6 May 2022.

5   United Nations Children's Fund, *Severe Wasting: An overlooked child survival emergency*, UNICEF Child Alert, May 2022, p. 5, <www.unicef.org/media/120346/file/Wasting%20child%20alert.pdf>, accessed 26 October 2022.

6   FAO, et al., *The State of Food Security and Nutrition in the World 2022: Repurposing food and agricultural policies to make healthy diets more affordable*, Food and Agriculture Organization of the United Nations, Rome, 2022, p. 10, <https://doi.org/10.4060/cc0639en>.

7   Toh, Zheng Quan, et al., 'Human Papillomavirus Vaccination After COVID-19', *JNCI Cancer Spectrum*, vol. 5, no. 2, 2 March 2021, art. pkab011, p. 5, <https://doi.org/10.1093/jncics/pkab011>.

8   Bray, Freddie, et al., 'Global Cancer Statistics 2018: GLOBOCAN estimates of incidence and mortality worldwide for 36 cancers in 185 countries', *CA: A Cancer Journal for Clinicians*, vol. 68, no. 6, 12 September 2018, pp. 394–424, p. 401, <https://doi.org/10.3322/caac.21492>. Erratum in: *CA: A Cancer Journal for Clinicians*, vol. 70, no. 4, July 2020, p. 313.

9   World Health Organization and United Nations Children's Fund, *Progress and Challenges with Achieving Universal Immunization Coverage: 2021 WHO/UNICEF estimates of national immunization coverage (WUENIC)*, 15 July 2022, p. 23, <https://data.unicef.org/wp-content/uploads/2016/07/progress-challenges_wuenic2021.pdf>, accessed 26 July 2022.

10 Ibid., p. 21.

11 Masresha, Balcha Girma, et al., 'The Performance of Routine Immunization in Selected African Countries During the First Six Months of the COVID-19 Pandemic', *Pan African Medical Journal*, vol. 37, suppl. 1, 18 September 2020, art. 12.
Grundy, John, and Beverley-Ann Biggs, 'The Impact of Conflict on Immunization Coverage in 16 Countries', *International Journal of Health Policy and Management*, vol. 8, no. 4, April 2019, pp. 211–221, <https://doi.org/10.15171/ijhpm.2018.127>.

12 Nelson, Roxanne, 'COVID-19 Disrupts Vaccine Delivery', *The Lancet Infectious Diseases*, vol. 20, no. 5, 17 April 2020, p. 546, <https://doi.org/10.1016/S1473-3099(20)30304-2>.
Kurowski, Christoph, et al., 'From Double Shock to Double Recovery: Implications and options for health financing in the time of COVID-19', Health, Nutrition and Population Discussion Paper, The World Bank, Washington, D.C., March 2021, <https://openknowledge.worldbank.org/handle/10986/35298>, accessed 6 March 2023.

13 World Health Organization, *Third Round of the Global Pulse Survey on Continuity of Essential Health Services During the COVID-19 Pandemic: November–December 2021 Interim report*, WHO, Geneva, 7 February 2022, p. 16, <www.who.int/publications/i/item/WHO-2019-nCoV-EHS_continuity-survey-2022.1>, accessed 23 February 2023.

14 Lee Ho, et al., 'Impact of the SARS-CoV-2 Pandemic on Vaccine-Preventable Disease Campaigns', *International Journal of Infectious Diseases*, vol. 119, June 2022, pp. 201–209, <https://doi.org/10.1016/j.ijid.2022.04.005>.

15 World Health Organization, 'Wild Poliovirus Type 1 (WPV1) – Malawi', News item, 3 March 2022, <www.who.int/emergencies/disease-outbreak-news/item/wild-poliovirus-type-1-(WPV1)-malawi>, accessed 11 January 2023.

16 Zeitouny, Seraphine, et al., 'Mapping Global Trends in Vaccine Sales Before and During the First Wave of the COVID-19 Pandemic: A cross-sectional time-series analysis', *BMJ Global Health*, vol. 6, no. 12, 2 December 2022, art. e006874, p. 7, <https://gh.bmj.com/content/6/12/e006874#block-system-main>, accessed 23 February 2023.

17 Ibid., p 1.

18 Dubé, Eve, and Noni E. MacDonald, 'How Can a Global Pandemic Affect Vaccine Hesitancy?', *Expert Review of Vaccines*, vol. 19, no. 10, 18 September 2020, pp. 899–901, <https://doi.org/10.1080/14760584.2020.1825944>.

19 Ota, Martin O.C., et al., 'Impact of COVID-19 Pandemic on Routine Immunization', *Annals of Medicine*, vol. 53, no. 1, 2 December 2021, pp. 2286–2297, <https://doi.org/10.1080/07853890.2021.2009128>.

20 United Nations Children's Fund, 'COVID-19 Market Dashboard', <https://www.unicef.org/supply/covid-19-market-dashboard>, accessed 20 December 2022.

21 Kurowski, Christoph, et al., *From Double Shock to Double Recovery: Implications and options for health financing in the time of COVID-19. Technical update: Old scars, new wounds*, The World Bank, Washington, D.C., September 2022, p. 13, <https://openknowledge.worldbank.org/bitstream/handle/10986/35298/September%202022.pdf>, accessed 27 February 2023.

22 Ibid., p. 48.

23 World Health Organization, *Health Workforce Policy and Management in the Context of the COVID-19 Pandemic Response: Interim guidance*, WHO, Geneva, 3 December, 2020, <www.who.int/publications/i/item/WHO-2019-nCoV-health_workforce-2020.1>, accessed 23 February 2023.

24 Ibid.

25 Gavi, the Vaccine Alliance, 'Evaluation Studies', 20 December 2021, <www.gavi.org/programmes-impact/our-impact/evaluation-studies>, accessed 23 February 2023.

Chapter 2

1   Cesar Victora and Aluísio Barros of the International Center for Equity in Health at the Federal University of Pelotas, Brazil conducted an analysis for *The State of the World's Children 2023* report of nationally representative surveys carried out from 2015 to 2020, covering 74 countries. The surveys included the Demographic and Health Surveys (DHS) and Multiple Indicator Cluster Surveys (MICS). The outcome variable was lack of any doses of the DTP (diphtheria, tetanus and pertussis) vaccine, referred to as no-DTP prevalence, which is a proxy measurement for zero-dose. The analyses included 161,922 children aged 12–23 months who constitute the target group for measuring immunization coverage. Nine stratification variables were studied: wealth quintiles and deciles (derived from household asset indices), urban or rural residence, double stratification by wealth and residence, sex of the child, maternal education and empowerment (using the SWPER or survey-based women's empowerment index), ethnic group and subnational area. All analyses took into account the survey sample design. Pooled estimates were provided by region of the world and country income groups using as weights the child populations in each country.

2   Feletto, Marta, et al., 'A Gender Lens to Advance Equity in Immunization', Discussion Paper 05, Equity Reference Group for Immunization, December 2018, p. 4.

3   Ibid., p. 4.

4   Ewerling, Fernanda, et al., 'SWPER Global: A survey-based women's empowerment index expanded from Africa to all low- and middle-income countries', *Journal of Global Health*, vol. 10, no. 2, December 2022, art. 020434, <https://doi.org/10.7189/jogh.10.020434>.

5   Okwo-Bele, Jean-Marie, et al., 'Tackling Inequities in Immunization Outcomes in Conflict Contexts', Discussion Paper 06, Equity Reference Group for Immunization, December 2018, p. vi.

6   Ibid., p. 4.

7   Ibid.

8   Ibid., p. 2.

9   Ibid., p. 4.

10 Ibid.

11 Singh et al., 'Strategies to Overcome Vaccine Hesitancy: A systematic review', *Systematic Reviews*, vol. 11, art. 78, April 2022, <https://doi.org/10.1186/s13643-022-01941-4>.

12 Gibson, Dustin G., et al., 'Mobile Phone-delivered Reminders and Incentives to Improve Childhood Immunization Coverage and Timeliness in Kenya (M-SIMU): A cluster randomised controlled trial', *The Lancet Global Health*, vol. 5, no. 4, April 2017, pp. E428–E438, <https://doi.org/10.1016/S2214-109X(17)30072-4>.

13 Jarrett, Caitlin, et al., 'Strategies for Addressing Vaccine Hesitancy – A systematic review', *Vaccine*, vol. 33, no. 34, 2015, pp. 4180–4190, <https://doi.org/10.1016/j.vaccine.2015.04.040>.

14 Carter, Austin, et al., 'Modeling the Impact of Vaccination for the Immunization Agenda 2030: Deaths averted due to vaccination against 14 pathogens in 194 countries from 2021–2030', *SSRN*, 26 April 2021, <http://dx.doi.org/10.2139/ssrn.3830781>.

15 Piot, Peter, et al., 'Immunization: Vital progress, unfinished agenda', *Nature*, vol. 575, 6 November 2019, pp. 119–129, <https://doi.org/10.1038/s41586-019-1656-7>.

16 United Nations, 'Nearly 40 Million Children Susceptible to Measles Due to COVID-19 Disruptions', UN News, 23 November 2022, <https://news.un.org/en/story/2022/11/1131002>, accessed 10 December 2022.

17 United Nations Children's Fund, 'Pneumonia', December 2022, <https://data.unicef.org/topic/child-health/pneumonia/>, accessed 7 February 2023.

18 United Nations Children's Fund, 'Diarrhoea', December 2022, <https://data.unicef.org/topic/child-health/diarrhoeal-disease/>, accessed 7 February 2023.

19 *Immunization Agenda 2030: A global strategy to leave no one behind (IA2030)*, n.d., <https://cdn.who.int/media/docs/default-source/immunization/strategy/ia2030/ia2030-draft-4-wha_b8850379-1fce-4847-bfd1-5d2c9d9e32f8.pdf>, accessed 27 February 2023.

World Health Organization, 'WHO Recommends Groundbreaking Malaria Vaccine for Children at Risk', News release, 6 October 2021, <www.who.int/news/item/06-10-2021-who-recommends-groundbreaking-malaria-vaccine-for-children-at-risk>, accessed 7 February 2023.

20 The Lancet, 'Malaria Vaccine Approval: A step change for global health', Editorial, *The Lancet*, vol. 398, no. 10309, p. 1381, <https://doi.org/10.1016/S0140-6736(21)02235-2>.

21 *Immunization Agenda 2030*, p. 6.
Global Polio Eradication Initiative, 'cVDPV2 Outbreaks and the Type 2 Novel Oral Polio Vaccine (nOPV2)', Factsheet, GPEI, Geneva, October 2022, <https://polioeradication.org/wp-content/uploads/2022/10/GPEI-nOPV2-Factsheet-EN-20221011.pdf>, accessed 14 February 2023.

22 Rodrigues, Charlene M.C., and Stanley A. Plotkin, 'Impact of Vaccines; Health, Economic and Social Perspectives', *Frontiers in Microbiology*, vol 11, no. 1526, July 2020, p.1, <https://doi.org/10.3389/fmicb.2020.01526>.

23 Riumallo-Herl, Carlos, et al., 'Poverty Reduction and Equity Benefits of Introducing or Scaling up Measles, Rotavirus, and Pneumococcal Vaccines in Low-income and Middle-income Countries: A modelling study', *BMJ Global Health*, vol. 3, no. 2, March 2018, art. e000613, <https://doi.org/10.1136/bmjgh-2017-000613>.
Johansson, Kjell Arne, et al., 'Health Gains and Financial Protection from Pneumococcal Vaccination and Pneumonia Treatment in Ethiopia: Results from an extended cost-effectiveness analysis', *PLoS ONE*, vol 10, no. 12, December 2015, <https://doi.org/10.1371/journal.pone.0142691>.
de Broucker, Gastien, et al., 'Cost of Nine Pediatric Infectious Illnesses in Low- and Middle-Income Countries: A systematic review of cost-of-illness studies', *PharmacoEconomics*, vol. 38, August 2020, pp. 1071–1094, <https://doi.org/10.1007/s40273-020-00940-4>.
Chang, Angela, Y., et al., 'The Equity Impact Vaccines May Have on Averting Deaths and Medical Impoverishment in Developing Countries', *Health Affairs*, vol. 37, no. 2, February 2018, pp. 316–324, <https://doi.org/10.1377/hlthaff.2017.0861>.

24 Riumallo-Herl, et al., 'Poverty Reduction and Equity Benefits of Introducing or Scaling up Measles, Rotavirus, and Pneumococcal Vaccines in Low-income and Middle-income Countries'.
Johansson, et al., 'Health Gains and Financial Protection from Pneumococcal Vaccination and Pneumonia Treatment in Ethiopia'.
Chang, et al., 'The Equity Impact Vaccines May Have on Averting Deaths and Medical Impoverishment in Developing Countries'.

25 Adamu, Aishatu Lawal, et al., 'The Cost of Illness for Childhood Clinical Pneumonia and Invasive Pneumococcal Disease in Nigeria', *BMJ Global Health*, vol. 7, no. 1, January 2022, art. e007080, <http://dx.doi.org/10.1136/bmjgh-2021-007080>.

26 Power, Kate, 'The COVID-19 Pandemic Has Increased the Care Burden of Women and Families', *Sustainability: Science, Practice and Policy*, vol. 16, no. 1, 21 June 2020, pp. 67–73, <https://doi.org/10.1080/15487733.2020.1776561>.
da Silva, Jorge Moreira, 'Why You Should Care about Unpaid Care Work', OECD Development Matters, 18 March 2019, <https://oecd-development-matters.org/2019/03/18/why-you-should-care-about-unpaid-care-work/>, accessed 10 December 2022.

27 Power, 'The COVID-19 Pandemic has Increased the Care Burden of Women and Families'.
da Silva, 'Why You Should Care about Unpaid Care Work'.

28 Postma, Maarten J., Stuart Carroll and Alexandra Brandão, 'The Societal Role of Lifelong Vaccination', *Journal of Market Access & Health Policy*, vol. 3, no. 1, art. 26962, 12 August 2015, p. 1, <https://doi.org/10.3402/jmahp.v3.26962>.

29 Arsenault, Catherine, Sam Harper and Arijit Nandi, 'Effect of Vaccination on Children's Learning Achievements: Findings from the India Human Development Survey', *Journal of Epidemiology and Community Health*, vol. 74, no. 10, June 2020, pp. 778–784, <http://dx.doi.org/10.1136/jech-2019-213483>.

30 Nandi, Arindam, et al., 'Anthropometric, Cognitive, and Schooling Benefits of Measles Vaccination: Longitudinal cohort analysis in Ethiopia, India, and Vietnam', *Vaccine*, vol. 37, no. 31, June 2019, pp. 4336–4343, <https://doi.org/10.1016/j.vaccine.2019.06.025>.

31 Andre, F.E., et al., 'Vaccination Greatly Reduces Disease, Disability, Death and Inequity Worldwide', *Bulletin of the World Health Organization*, vol. 86, no. 2, 27 November 2007, pp. 140–106, <https://doi.org/10.2471/blt.07.040089>.
Rodrigues and Plotkin, 'Impact of Vaccines; Health, Economic and Social Perspectives'.

32 World Health Organization, *Bacterial Vaccines in Clinical and Preclinical Development 2001: An overview and analysis*, WHO, Geneva, 2022, p. 1, <www.who.int/publications/i/item/9789240052451>, accessed 14 February 2023.

33 Murray, Christopher J.L., et al., 'Global Burden of Bacterial Antimicrobial Resistance in 2019: A systematic analysis', *The Lancet*, vol. 399, no. 10325, 12 February 2022, pp. 629–655, <https://doi.org/10.1016/S0140-6736(21)02724-0>.
McDonnell, Anthony, and Katherine Klemperer, 'Drug-resistant Infections are One of the World's Biggest Killers, Especially for Children in Poorer Countries. We must act now', Center for Global Development, 20 January 2022, <www.cgdev.org/blog/drug-resistant-infections-are-one-worlds-biggest-killers-especially-children-poorer-countries#:~:text=Particularly%20striking%20from%20the%20new,AMR%20nearly%20every%20two%20minutes>, accessed 11 December 2022.

34 Decade of Vaccine Economics, 'Return on Investment', DOVE/ThinkWell, <https://immunizationeconomics.org/dove-roi>, accessed 11 December 2022.

35 Sim, So Yoon, et al., 'Return on Investment from Immunization against 10 Pathogens in 94 Low- and Middle-Income Countries, 2011–30', *Health Affairs*, vol. 39, no. 8, August 2020, pp. 1343–1353, <https://doi.org/10.1377/hlthaff.2020.00103>.

36 Ibid.

37 Decade of Vaccine Economics, 'Return on Investment'.

38 Bärnighausen, Till, et al., 'Valuing Vaccination', *PNAS*, vol. 111, no. 34, 18 August 2014, pp. 12313–12319, <https://doi.org/10.1073/pnas.1400475111>.

39 Based on contributions from participants at 'For every child, vaccines: UNICEF Convening Event on Immunization', UNICEF Innocenti – Global Office of Research and Foresight, Florence, 9–10 June 2022.

Chapter 3

1 Global Polio Eradication Initiative, 'Who We Are' n.d., <https://polioeradication.org/who-we-are/>, accessed 7 February 2023.

2 Micah, Angela E., et al., 'Development Assistance for Human Resources for Health, 1990–2020', *Human Resources for Health*, vol. 20, art. 51, 10 June 2022, p. 2, <https://doi.org/10.1186/s12960-022-00744-x>.

3 GDB 2019 Human Resources for Health Collaborators, 'Measuring the Availability of Human Resources for Health and Its Relationship to Universal Health Coverage for 204 Countries and Territories from 1990 to 2019: A systematic analysis for the Global Burden of Disease Study 2019', *The Lancet*, vol. 399, no. 10341, June 2022, pp. 2129–2154, <https://doi.org/10.1016/S0140-6736(22)00532-3>.

4 Bliss, Katherine E., and Alicia Carbaugh, 'Gender Equity to Improve Immunization Services', CSIS Brief, Center for Strategic & International Studies, Washington, D.C., September 2022, <www.csis.org/analysis/gender-equity-improve-immunization-services>, accessed 8 March 2023.

5 Ibid.

6 World Health Organization and International Labour Organization, *The Gender Pay Gap in the Health and Care Sector: A global analysis in the time of COVID-19*, WHO and ILO, Geneva, 2022, p. viii, <www.who.int/publications/i/item/9789240052895>, accessed 8 March 2023.

7 Ibid.

8 Ibid., p. x.

9 Ibid.

10 Ibid., p. 36.

11 World Health Organization, *Delivered by Women, Led by Men: A gender and equity analysis of the global health and social workforce*, Human Resources for Health Observer Series No. 24, WHO, Geneva, 14 March 2019, <www.who.int/publications/i/item/978-92-4-151546-7>, accessed 8 March 2023.

12 Ibid.

13 Bergmann, Jessica, Maria Carolina Alban Conto and Mattheiu Brossard, 'Increasing Women's Representation in School Leadership: A promising path towards improving learning', Innocenti Research Brief', UNICEF Innocenti – Global Office of Research and Foresight, Florence, 2022, <www.unicef-irc.org/publications/1399-increasing-womens-representation-in-school-leadership-a-promising-path-towards-improving-learning.html>, accessed 15 February 2023.

14 Women in Global Health, 'Subsidizing Global Health: Women's unpaid work in global health systems', Policy Brief, WGH, Washington, D.C., June 2022, <https://womeningh.org/our-advocacy/paywomen/>, accessed 15 February 2023.

15 Bliss and Carbaugh, 'Gender Equity to Improve Immunization Services'.

16 Ibid.

17 Ibid.
'Subsidizing Global Health'.
18 Bliss and Carbaugh, 'Gender Equity to Improve Immunization Services'.
19 Ibid.
20 International Conference on Primary Health Care, 'Declaration of Alma-Ata', September 1978, <https://cdn.who.int/media/docs/default-source/documents/almaata-declaration-en.pdf>, accessed 15 February 2023.
21 World Health Organization, 'Primary Health Care', Fact sheet, 1 April 2021, <www.who.int/news-room/fact-sheets/detail/primary-health-care>, accessed 14 December 2022.
22 Global Conference on Primary Health Care, *Declaration of Astana*, Astana, 26 October 2018, <www.who.int/publications/i/item/WHO-HIS-SDS-2018.61>, accessed 8 March 2023.
23 World Health Organization and UNICEF, A Vision for Primary Health Care in the 21st Century: Towards UHC and the SDGs, WHO, UNICEF, Geneva and New York, 2018, pp. xvii.
'Primary Health Care'.
24 Santos, Thiago M., et al., 'Assessing the Overlap between Immunisation and Other Essential Health Interventions in 92 Low- and Middle-income Countries Using Household Surveys: Opportunities for expanding immunization and primary health care', *The Lancet*, vol. 42, art 101196, December 2021, <https://doi.org/10.1016/j.eclinm.2021.101196>.
25 Ibid.
26 *Immunization Agenda 2030: A global strategy to leave no one behind (IA2030)*, n.d., <https://cdn.who.int/media/docs/default-source/immunization/strategy/ia2030/ia2030-draft-4-wha_b8850379-1fce-4847-bfd1-5d2c9d9e32f8.pdf>, accessed 27 February 2023.
27 Ibid., p. 12.
28 Ibid., p. 30.
29 World Health Organization, *Working Together: An integration resource guide for immunization services throughout the life course*, WHO, Geneva, 2018, pp. 33–39, <https://apps.who.int/iris/handle/10665/276546>, accessed 8 March 2023.
30 Edmond, Karen, et al., 'Mobile Outreach Health Services for Mothers and Children in Conflict-affected and Remote Areas: A population based study', *Archives of Disease in Childhood*, vol. 105, no. 1, 2020, pp. 18–25, quoted in Crocker-Buque, Tim, et al., 'Immunization, Urbanization and Slums: A systematic review of factors and interventions, *BMC Public Health*, vol. 17, art. 556, June 2017, p. 7, <https://doi.org/10.1186/s12889-017-4473-7>.
31 *Immunization Agenda 2030*, p. 22.
32 Crocker-Buque, Tim, et al., 'Immunization, Urbanization and Slums – A systematic review of factors and interventions', *BMC Public Health*, vol. 17, art. 556, June 2017, <https://doi.org/10.1186/s12889-017-4473-7>.
33 Ibid.
34 World Health Organization, *WHO Guideline on Health Policy and System Support to Optimize Community Health Worker Programmes*, WHO, Geneva, 2018, pp. 25, 92–93, <https://apps.who.int/iris/handle/10665/275474>, accessed 8 March 2023.
35 Ibid., pp. 63, 92–93.
36 World Health Organization, *Global Strategy on Human Resources for Health: Workforce 2030*, WHO, Geneva, 2016, <https://apps.who.int/iris/bitstream/handle/10665/250368/9789241511131-eng.pdf>, accessed 8 March 2023.
37 Nguyen, Duen Thi Kim, et al., 'Does Integrated Management of Childhood Illnesses (IMCI) Training Improve the Skills of Health Workers? A systematic review and meta-analysis', *PLoS ONE*, vol. 8, no. 6, 12 June 2013, <https://doi.org/10.1371/journal.pone.0066030>.
38 Equity Reference Group for Immunization, 'Brief on Published Evidence on Human Resources for Health Strategies in Underserved Areas of Low- and Middle-income Countries', Meeting Brief, October 2022.
39 Bliss and Carbaugh, 'Gender Equity to Improve Immunization Services'.
40 Ibid.
41 *The Gender Pay Gap in the Health and Care Sector: A global analysis in the time of COVID-19*, p. 125.
42 Bliss and Carbaugh, 'Gender Equity to Improve Immunization Services'.
43 Ibid.
44 Masis, Lizah, et al., 'Community Health Workers at the Dawn of a New Era: 4. Programme financing', *Health Research Policy and Systems*, vol. 19, suppl. 3, 12 October 2021, art. 107, <https://doi.org/10.1186/s12961-021-00751-9>.

Chapter 4

1 Larson, Heidi J., Emmanuela Gakidou and Christopher J.L. Murray, 'The Vaccine-Hesitant Moment', *New England Journal of Medicine*, vol. 387, 2022, pp. 58–65, <https://doi.org/10.1056/NEJMra2106441>.
2 de Figueiredo, Alexandre, et al., 'Mapping Global Trends in Vaccine Confidence and Investigating Barriers to Vaccine Uptake: A large-scale retrospective temporal modelling study', *The Lancet*, vol. 396, no. 10255, 26 September 2020, pp. 898–908, <https://doi.org/10.1016/S0140-6736(20)31558-0> (see abstract and p. 905).
3 Larson, Heidi J., and David A. Broniatowski, 'Volatility of Vaccine Confidence', *Science*, vol. 371, no. 6356, 26 March 2021, p. 1289, <https://doi.org/10.1126/science.abi6488>.
4 Ibid.
5 The Vaccine Confidence Project carried out a large-scale retrospective modelling study to investigate the extent to which vaccine confidence changed across 54 countries between 2015 and November 2019 (pre-pandemic) and in 2021 and 2022 (post-pandemic). The study collated data from nationally representative surveys comprising over 100,000 individuals. Data collected in 2020 were omitted to ensure a relatively clear distinction between pre- and post-pandemic groups. Vaccine confidence was measured via a four-item Likert-scale questionnaire probing individual perceptions of the importance, safety and effectiveness of vaccines. Changes in national-level confidence were evaluated for the sampled populations and within demographic subgroups via Wilcoxon–Mann–Whitney tests with p values adjusted via Bonferroni correction to account for multiple hypotheses.
6 World Health Organization, 'Ten Threats to Global Health in 2019', n.d., <www.who.int/news-room/spotlight/ten-threats-to-global-health-in-2019>, accessed 15 February 2023.
7 Larson, et al., 'The Vaccine-Hesitant Moment'.
8 Ibid.
9 Ibid.
10 Eze, Paul, et al., 'Factors Associated with Incomplete Immunization in Children Aged 12–23 Months at Subnational Level, Nigeria: A cross-sectional study', *BMJ Open*, vol 11, no. 6, art. e047445, 2021, <https://doi.org/10.1136/bmjopen-2020-047445>.
11 Larson, Heidi J., Leesa Lin and Rob Goble, 'Vaccines and the Social Amplification of Risk', *Risk Analysis*, vol. 42, 14 May 2022, pp. 1409–1422, <https://doi.org/10.1111/risa.13942> (see MMR example, p. 1413).
12 Ibid.
Elliman, David, and Helen Bedford, 'MMR: Where are we now?', *Archives of Diseases in Children*, vol. 92, no. 2, pp. 1055–1057, <http://dx.doi.org/10.1136/adc.2006.103531>.
13 Ibid., p. 1055. Original source specifies England.
14 The Sabin-Aspen Vaccine Science & Policy Group, *Meeting the Challenge of Vaccination Hesitancy*, The Aspen Institute, Sabin Vaccine Institute, Washington, D.C., May 2020, p. 16, <www.sabin.org/resources/meeting-the-challenge-of-vaccination-hesitancy/>, accessed 8 March 2023.
15 Larson, Heidi J., Kenneth Hartigan-Go and Alexandre de Figueiredo, 'Vaccine Confidence Plummets in Philippines Following a Dengue Vaccine Scare: Why it matters to pandemic preparedness', *Human Vaccines & Immunotherapeutics*, vol. 15, no. 3, 12 October 2018, pp. 625–627, <https://doi.org/10.1080/21645515.2018.1522468.
Mendoza, Ronald U., Sheena A. Valenzuela and Manuel M. Dayrit, 'A Crisis of Confidence: The case of Dengvaxia in the Philippines', Working Paper, Ateneo School of Government, Quezon City, January 2020, p. 17.
16 Mendoza, Valenzuela and Dayrit, 'A Crisis of Confidence: The case of Dengvaxia in the Philippines', p. 17.
17 United Nations Children's Fund, et al., *Vaccine Misinformation Management Field Guide: Guidance for addressing a global infodemic and fostering demand for immunization*, UNICEF, New York, December 2020, p. 35, <https://vaccinemisinformation.guide/>, accessed 21 February 2023.
18 Sarika Bhattacharjee and Carlotta Dotto, 'Vaccine Case Study: Understanding the impact of polio vaccine disinformation in Pakistan', First Draft, 19 February 2020, https://firstdraftnews.org/long-form-article/first-draft-case-study-understanding-the-impact-of-polio-vaccine-disinformation-in-pakistan/, accessed, 7 March 2023.
19 United Nations Children's Fund, et al., *Vaccine Misinformation Management Field Guide*, p. 35.
20 Jarrett, Caitlin, et al., 'Strategies For Addressing Vaccine Hesitancy – A systematic review', *Vaccine*, vol. 33, no. 34, 14 August 2015, pp. 4180–4190, <https://doi.org/10.1016/j.vaccine.2015.04.040>.
21 Tripathi Stuti, et al., 'Designing Appropriate, Acceptable and Feasible Community-Engagement Approaches to Improve Routine Immunisation Outcomes in Low- and Middle-Income Countries: A synthesis of 3ie-supported formative evaluations', *PLoS ONE*, vol. 17, no. 10, art. e0275278, 2022, p. 11, <https://doi.org/10.1371/journal.pone.0275278>.

22 Jarrett, et al., 'Strategies For Addressing Vaccine Hesitancy – A systematic review', p. 4185.

23 Crocker-Buque, Tim, et al., 'Immunization, Urbanization and Slums: A systematic review of factors and interventions', *BMC Public Health*, vol. 17, art. 556, June 2017, p. 12, <https://doi.org/10.1186/s12889-017-4473-7>.

24 Ibid., p. 6.

25 Akwataghibe, Ngozi N., et al., 'Using Participatory Action Research to Improve Immunization Utilization in Areas with Pockets of Unimmunized Children in Nigeria', *Health Research Policy and Systems*, vol. 19, suppl. 2, art. 88, 11 August 2021, <https://doi.org/10.1186/s12961-021-00719-9>.

26 Ibid., pp. 1, 8, 12.

27 Ibid., pp. 1, 8, 12.

28 Oyo-Ita, A., et al., 'Effects of Engaging Communities in Decision-Making and Action Through Traditional and Religious Leaders on Vaccination Coverage in Cross River State, Nigeria: A cluster-randomised control trial', *PLoS ONE*, vol. 16, no. 4, 16 April 2021, art. e0248236, <https://doi.org/10.1371/journal.pone.0248236>.

29 Ibid.

30 Larson, Heidi J., et al., 'Measuring Trust in Vaccination: A systematic review', *Human Vaccines & Immunotherapeutics*, vol. 14, no. 7, 10 May 2018, pp. 1599–1609, <https://doi.org/10.1080/21645515.2018.1459252>.

31 Singh, Prem, et al., 'Strategies to Overcome Vaccine Hesitancy: A systematic review', *Systematic Reviews*, vol. 11, art. 78, 26 April 2022, p. 10, <https://doi.org/10.1186/s13643-022-01941-4>.

32 Tuckerman, Jane, Jessica Kaufman and Margie Danchin, 'Effective Approaches to Combat Vaccine Hesitancy', *The Pediatric Infectious Disease Journal*, vol. 41, no. 5, May 2022, pp. e243–e245, <htpps://doi.org/10.1097/INF.0000000000003499>.

33 Jain, Monica., et al., 'Use of Community Engagement Interventions to Improve Child Immunisation in Low- and Middle-Income Countries: A systematic review and meta-analysis', *Campbell Systematic Reviews*, vol. 18, no. 3, 2022, art. e1253.

34 Ibid., p. 13.

35 Tripathi, et al., 'Designing Appropriate, Acceptable and Feasible Community-Engagement Approaches to Improve Routine Immunisation Outcomes in Low- and Middle-Income Countries: A synthesis of 3ie-supported formative evaluations', p. 1.

36 Ibid., p. 1.

37 Pandey, P., et al., 'Informing Resource-Poor Populations and the Delivery of Entitled Health and Social Services in Rural India: A cluster randomized controlled trial', *JAMA*, vol. 298, no. 16, 24 October 2007, art. 1872, <https://doi.org/10.1001/jama.298.16.1867>.

38 See the International Pediatrics Association's Vaccine Trust Project, <www.ipa-world.org/ipa-vaccine-trust-project.php>, accessed 8 March 2023.

39 Opel, Douglas J., et al., 'The Relationship Between Parent Attitudes About Childhood Vaccines Survey Scores and Future Child Immunization Status: A validation study', *JAMA Pediatrics*, vol. 167, November 2013, pp. 1065–1071, <https://doi.org/10.1001/jamapediatrics.2013.2483>.
World Health Organization, *Behavioural and Social Drivers of Vaccination: Tools and practical guidance for achieving high uptake*, WHO, Geneva, 2022, <https://apps.who.int/iris/handle/10665/354459>.

40 See *Vaccine Misinformation Management Field Guide*.

41 United Nations Children's Fund, The Public Good Projects and Yale Institute for Global Health, 'Introducing the VDO Dashboard', Vaccine Demand Observatory, <https://www.thevdo.org/>, accessed 21 February 2023.

42 Ibid.

43 Ibid.

44 Singh, et al., 'Strategies to Overcome Vaccine Hesitancy: A systematic review'.

45 Ahlers-Schmidt, Carolyn R., et al., 'Text Messaging Immunization Reminders: Feasibility of implementation with low-income parents', *Preventive Medicine*, vol. 50, no. 5–6, May–June 2010, pp. 306–307, <https://doi.org/10.1016/j.ypmed.2010.02.008>. Cates, Joan R., et al., 'Evaluating a County-Sponsored Social Marketing Campaign to Increase Mothers' Initiation of HPV Vaccine for Their Preteen Daughters in a Primarily Rural Area', *Social Marketing Quarterly*, vol. 17, no. 1, 2011, pp. 4–26, <https://doi.org/10.1080/15245004.2010.546943>.
Pandey, Deeksha, et al., 'Awareness and Attitude Towards Human Papillomavirus (HPV) Vaccine Among Medical Students in a Premier Medical School in India', *PLoS ONE*, vol. 7, no. 7, July 2012, art. e40619, <https://doi.org/10.1371/journal.pone.0040619>.
Nasiru, Sani-Gwarzo, et al., 'Breaking Community Barriers to Polio Vaccination in Northern Nigeria: The impact of a grass roots mobilization campaign (Majigi)', *Pathogens and Global Health*, vol. 106, no. 3, 2012, pp. 166–171, <https://doi.org/10.1179/2047773212Y.0000000018>.

46 Thomson, Angus, Gaëllee Vallée-Tourangeau and L. Suzanne Suggs, 'Strategies to Increase Vaccine Acceptance and Uptake: From behavioral insights to context-specific, culturally-appropriate, evidence-based communications and interventions', *Vaccine*, vol. 36, no. 44, 22 October 2018, pp. 6457–6458, <https://doi.org/10.1016/j.vaccine.2018.08.031>.

47 *Vaccine Misinformation Management Field Guide*.

48 Cates, et al., 'Evaluating a County-Sponsored Social Marketing Campaign to Increase Mothers' Initiation of HPV Vaccine for Their Preteen Daughters in a Primarily Rural Area'.

49 Ibid., p. 9.

50 Nasiru, et al., 'Breaking Community Barriers to Polio Vaccination in Northern Nigeria: The impact of a grass roots mobilization campaign (Majigi)'.

51 Feletto, M., et al., 'A Gender Lens to Advance Equity in Immunization', ERG Discussion Paper 05, Equity Reference Group for Immunization, New York, 2018.

52 Olorunsaiye, Comfort Z., and Hannah Degge, 'Variations in the Uptake of Routine Immunization in Nigeria: Examining determinants of inequitable access', *Global Health Communication*, vol. 2, no. 1, 22 July 2016, pp. 19–29, <http://dx.doi.org/10.1080/23762004.2016.1206780>.

53 Saggurti, Niranjan, et al., 'Effect of Health Intervention Integration Within Women's Self-Help Groups on Collectivization and Healthy Practices Around Reproductive, Maternal, Neonatal and Child Health in Rural India', *PLoS ONE*, vol. 13, no. 8, 23 August 2018, art. e0202562, <https://doi.org/10.1371/journal.pone.0202562>.

54 Ibid.

55 Demissie, Shiferaw Dechasa, et al., 'Community Engagement Strategy for Increased Uptake of Routine Immunization and Select Perinatal Services in North-West Ethiopia: A descriptive analysis', *PLoS ONE*, vol. 15, no. 10, 29 October 2020, art. e0237319, p. 1, <https://doi.org/10.1371/journal.pone.0237319>.

56 Ibid.

57 Global Polio Eradication Initiative, *Gender Equality Strategy 2019–2023*, World Health Organization, Geneva, 2019.
Global Polio Eradication Initiative, *Technical Brief: Gender*, World Health Organization, Geneva, 2018, p. 12.

58 World Health Organization, *Why Gender Matters: Immunization Agenda 2030*, WHO, Geneva, 2021, p. 35, <www.gavi.org/sites/default/files/2021-12/why-gender-matters-ia2030.pdf>, accessed 21 February 2023.

59 Jones, Amy, and Natalie Kawesa-Newell, 'Using Branded Behaviour Change Communication to Create Demand for the HPV Vaccine Among Girls in Malawi: An evaluation of Girl Effect's Zathu mini magazine', *Vaccine*, vol. 40, suppl. 1, 31 March 2022, pp. A107–A115, <https://doi.org/10.1016/j.vaccine.2021.07.011>, pp. A110, A112.

60 Fisher, Harriet, et al., 'Young Women's Autonomy and Information Needs in the Schools-Based HPV Vaccination Programme: A qualitative study', *BMC Public Health*, vol. 20, art. 1680, 2020, <https://doi.org/10.1186/s12889-020-09815-x>.
Feletto, et al., 'A Gender Lens to Advance Equity in Immunization', pp. 6–11, 15.

61 *Why Gender Matters: Immunization Agenda 2030*, p. 17.

62 Goodman, Tracey, et al., 'Why Does Gender Matter for Immunization?', *Vaccine*, 10 December 2022, p. 4, <https://doi.org/10.1016/j.vaccine.2022.11.071>.
Why Gender Matters: Immunization Agenda 2030, p. 18.

63 Singh, Kavita, Erica Haney and Comfort Olorunsaiye, 'Maternal Autonomy and Attitudes Towards Gender Norms: Associations with Childhood Immunization In Nigeria', *Maternal and Child Health Journal*, vol. 17, no. 5, July 2013, pp. 837–841, <https://doi.org/10.17615/ah06-0141>, pp. 4–5.

64 *Why Gender Matters: Immunization Agenda 2030*, p. 17.
Antai, Diddy, 'Gender Inequities, Relationship Power, and Childhood Immunization Uptake in Nigeria: A population-based cross-sectional study', *International Journal of Infectious Diseases*, vol. 16, no. 2, February 2012, pp. E140–E143, <https://doi.org/10.1016/j.ijid.2011.11.004>.

65 Muralidharan, Arundati, et al., 'Transforming Gender Norms, Roles, and Power Dynamics for Better Health: Evidence from a systematic review of gender-integrated health programs in low- and middle-income countries, 'Futures Group, Health Policy Project, Washington, D.C., September 2015, p. 2, <www.healthpolicyproject.com/pubs/381_GPMIndiaSummaryReport.pdf>, accessed 8 March 2023.

66 Ebot, J.O., '"Girl Power!": The relationship between women's autonomy and children's immunization coverage in Ethiopia', *Journal of Health, Population and Nutrition*, vol. 33, 2015, art. 18, p. 6, <https://doi.org/10.1186/s41043-015-0028-7>.

67 Ibid.

68 *Why Gender Matters: Immunization Agenda 2030*, pp. 18, 35.

69 *Gender Equality Strategy 2019–2023*, p. 12.

70 *Technical Brief: Gender*, p. 12.

71 Ibid., pp. 12–13.

72 Ibid., p. 13.

Chapter 5

1 Ikilezi, Gloria, et al., 'Estimating Total Spending by Source of Funding on Routine and Supplementary Immunization Activities in Low-income and Middle-income Countries, 2000–17: A financial modelling study', *The Lancet*, vol. 398, no. 10314, November 2021, pp. 1875–1893, <https://doi.org/10.1016/S0140-6736(21)01591-9>.

2 Ibid.

3 Ibid.

4 Ibid.

5 *Immunization Agenda 2030: Sustainable financing for immunization*, September 2020, <www.immunizationagenda2030.org/images/documents/BLS20116_IA_Global_strategy_document_SP_6_001.pdf>, accessed 6 March 2023.

6 Kurowski, Christoph, et al., 'From Double Shock to Double Recovery: Implications and options for health financing in the time of COVID-19', Health, Nutrition and Population Discussion Paper, The World Bank, Washington, D.C., March 2021, <https://openknowledge.worldbank.org/handle/10986/35298>, accessed 6 March 2023.

7 Ibid.

8 Piatti-Fünfkirchen, Moritz, et al., *Budget Execution in Health: Concepts, trends and policy issues*, The World Bank, Washington, D.C., 2021, <https://openknowledge.worldbank.org/bitstream/handle/10986/36583/Budget-Execution-in-Health-Concepts-Trends-and-Policy-Issues.pdf?sequence=5&isAllowed=y>, accessed 16 February 2023.

9 Cho, Chloe, Jason Lakin and Ulla Griffiths, 'Underspent Immunization Budgets: A budget credibility analysis of 22 countries', Budget Brief, International Budget Partnership, Washington, D.C., 17 December 2019, <https://internationalbudget.org/publications/underspent-immunization-budgets-a-budget-credibility-analysis-of-22-countries/>, accessed 16 February 2023.

10 Ibid.

11 Kurowski, et al., 'From Double Shock to Double Recovery'.

12 Ibid.

13 Saxenian, Helen, et al., 'Sustainable Financing for *Immunization Agenda 2030*', *Vaccine*, [advance online publication], 2 December 2022, <https://doi.org/10.1016/j.vaccine.2022.11.037>.

14 Kurowski, et al., 'From Double Shock to Double Recovery'.

15 *Immunization Agenda 2030: Sustainable financing for immunization*, p 1.

16 World Health Organization, *Global Expenditure on Health: Public spending on the rise?*, WHO, Geneva, 2021, p. 18, <www.who.int/publications/i/item/9789240041219>, accessed 6 March 2023.

17 Ibid., p. 2.

18 Ibid., p. 18.

19 Ikilezi, et al., 'Estimating Total Spending by Source of Funding on Routine and Supplementary Immunization Activities in Low-income and Middle-income Countries'.

20 Kurowski, Christoph, et al., *From Double Shock to Double Recovery: Implications and options for health financing in the time of COVID-19. Technical update: Old scars, new wounds*, The World Bank, Washington, D.C., September 2022, <https://openknowledge.worldbank.org/bitstream/handle/10986/35298/September%202022.pdf>, accessed 27 February 2023.

21 Ibid.

22 Saxenian, et al., 'Sustainable Financing for *Immunization Agenda 2030*'.

23 Hanson, Kara, et al., '*The Lancet Global Health* Commission on Financing Primary Health Care: Putting people at the centre', *The Lancet Global Health Commissions*, vol. 10, no. 5, May 2022, <https://doi.org/10.1016/S2214-109X(22)00005-5>.

24 Ibid.

25 Kurowski, et al., 'From Double Shock to Double Recovery – Technical update 2'.

26 Hanson, et al., '*The Lancet Global Health* Commission on Financing Primary Health Care'.

27 Ibid.

28 Saxenian, et al., 'Sustainable Financing for *Immunization Agenda 2030*'.

29 *Immunization Agenda 2030: Sustainable financing for immunization*, p. 4.

30 Hanson, et al., '*The Lancet Global Health* Commission on Financing Primary Health Care'.

31 Saxenian, et al., 'Sustainable Financing for *Immunization Agenda 2030*'.

32 Ibid.

33 Ibid.

34 Saville, Melanie, et al., 'Delivering Pandemic Vaccines in 100 days – What will it take?', *The New England Journal of Medicine*, vol. 387, no. 3, 14 July 2022, art. e3, <https://doi.org/10.1056/NEJMp2202669>.

35 Alderson, Mark R., et al., 'Development Strategy and Lessons Learned for a 10-Valent Pneumococcal Conjugate Vaccine (PNEUMOSIL®)', *Human Vaccines & Immunotherapeutics*, vol. 17, no. 8, 24 February 2021, pp. 2670–2677, <https://doi.org/10.1080/21645515.2021.1874219>.

36 United Nations Children's Fund, 'Pneumonia', December 2022, <https://data.unicef.org/topic/child-health/pneumonia/#:~:text=A%20child%20dies%20of%20pneumonia%20every%2039%20seconds&text=Pneumonia%20kills%20more%20children%20than,of%20these%20deaths%20are%20preventable>, accessed 7 February 2023.

37 Roser, Max, 'Malaria: One of the leading causes of child deaths, but progress is possible and you can contribute to it', Our World in Data, 22 March 2022, <https://ourworldindata.org/malaria-introduction>, accessed 7 February 2023.

38 World Health Organization, 'WHO Recommends Groundbreaking Malaria Vaccine for Children at Risk', News release, 6 October 2021, <www.who.int/news/item/06-10-2021-who-recommends-groundbreaking-malaria-vaccine-for-children-at-risk>, accessed 7 February 2023.

39 Moorthy, Vasee, and Fred Binka, 'R21/Matrix-M: A second malaria vaccine?', *The Lancet*, vol. 397, no. 10287, 15 May 2021, pp. 1782–1783, <https://doi.org/10.1016/S0140-6736(21)01065-5>.

40 Institute for Health Metrics and Evaluation, 'Global Burden of Disease Study 2017 Results', <http://ghdx.healthdata.org/gbd-results-tool>, accessed 20 January 2023.

41 Shi, Ting, et al., 'Global, Regional, and National Disease Burden Estimates of Acute Lower Respiratory Infections Due to Respiratory Syncytial Virus in Young Children in 2015: A systematic review and modelling study', *The Lancet*, vol. 390, no. 10098, 6 July 2017, pp. 946–958, <https://doi.org/10.1016/S0140-6736(17)30938-8>.

42 PATH, 'A Roadmap for Advancing RSV Maternal Immunization', <www.path.org/resources/roadmap-advancing-rsv-maternal-immunization/>, accessed 7 February 2023.

43 Global Polio Eradication Initiative, 'nOPV2', <https://polioeradication.org/nopv2/>, accessed 7 February 2023.

44 Global Polio Eradication Initiative, 'cVDPV2 Outbreaks and the Type 2 Novel Oral Polio Vaccine (nOPV2)', Factsheet, GPEI, Geneva, October 2022, <https://polioeradication.org/wp-content/uploads/2022/10/GPEI-nOPV2-Factsheet-EN-20221011.pdf>, accessed 16 February 2023.

45 Gavi, the Vaccine Alliance, 'The Vaccine Innovation Prioritisation Strategy (VIPS)', <www.gavi.org/our-alliance/market-shaping/vaccine-innovation-prioritisation-strategy>, accessed 16 February 2023.

46 Peyraud, Nicolas, et al., 'Potential Use of Microarray Patches for Vaccine Delivery in Low- and Middle income Countries', *Vaccine*, vol. 37, no. 32, 26 July 2019, pp. 4427–4434, <https://doi.org/10.1016/j.vaccine.2019.03.035>.

47 UNICEF Supply Division, *Cold Chain Support Package: Procurement guidelines – Solar direct drive refrigerators and freezers*, United Nations Children's Fund, Copenhagen, 21 December 2020, <www.unicef.org/supply/media/6276/file/E003-solar-direct-drive-refrigerators-freezers.pdf>, accessed 16 February 2023.

48 Sowe, Aliey, and Maria Isabella Gariboldi, 'An Assessment of the Quality of Vaccination Data Produced Through Smart Paper Technology in The Gambia', *Vaccine*, vol. 38, no. 42, 29 September 2020, pp. 6618–6126, <https://doi.org/10.1016/j.vaccine.2020.07.074>.

49 Bello, Isah Mohammed, et al., 'Real-time Monitoring of a Circulating Vaccine-Derived Poliovirus Outbreak Immunization Campaign Using Digital Health Technologies in South Sudan', *Pan African Medical Journal*, vol. 40, art. 200, 4 December 2021, <https://doi.org/10.11604/pamj.2021.40.200.31525>.
Mvundura, Mercy, et al., 'Assessing the Incremental Costs and Savings of Introducing Electronic Immunization Registries and Stock Management Systems: Evidence from the Better Immunization Data Initiative in Tanzania and Zambia', *Pan African Medical Journal*, vol. 35, no. 1, art. 11, 12 February 2020, <https://doi.org/10.11604/pamj.supp.2020.35.1.17804>.

50 Chandir, Subhash, et al., 'Zindagi Mehfooz (Safe Life) Digital Immunization Registry: Leveraging low-cost technology to improve immunization coverage and timeliness in Pakistan', *Iproceedings*, vol. 4, no. 2, 17 September 2018, art. e11770, <https://doi.org/10.2196/11770>.

51 Ibid.

52 Ali, Disha, et al., 'A Cost-Effectiveness Analysis of Traditional and Geographic Information System-Supported Microplanning Approaches for Routine Immunization Program Management in Northern Nigeria', *Vaccine*, vol. 38, no. 6, 5 February 2020, pp. 1408–1415, <https://doi.org/10.1016/j.vaccine.2019.12.002>.

53 Polio Global Eradication Initiative, 'Innovative Digital Technologies Bridge Gaps in the Polio Response and Beyond', News story, World Health Organization, Geneva, August 2022, <https://polioeradication.org/news-post/innovative-digital-technologies-bridge-gaps-in-the-polio-response-and-beyond/>, accessed 16 February 2023.

54 Ali, et al., 'A Cost-Effectiveness Analysis of Traditional and Geographic Information System-Supported Microplanning Approaches for Routine Immunization Program Management in Northern Nigeria'.

55 Oteri, Joseph, et al., 'Application of the Geographic Information System (GIS) in Immunisation Service Delivery; Its use in the 2017/2018 measles vaccination campaign in Nigeria', *Vaccine*, vol. 39, suppl. 3, 17 November 2021, pp. C29–C37, <https://doi.org/10.1016/j.vaccine.2021.01.021>.

56 Jusril, Hafizah, et al., 'Digital Health for Real-Time Monitoring of a National Immunisation Campaign in Indonesia: A large-scale effectiveness evaluation', *BMJ Open*, vol. 10, no. 12, December 2020, art. e038282, <https://doi.org/10.1136/bmjopen-2020-038282>.

57 Saha, Somen, and Zahiruddin Syed Quazi,, 'Does Digitally Enabling Frontline Health Workers Improve Coverage and Quality of Maternal and Child Health Services? Findings from a mixed methods evaluation of TECHO+ in Gujarat', *Frontiers in Public Health*, vol. 10, 22 July 2022, art. 856561, <https://doi.org/10.3389/fpubh.2022.856561>.

58 Yadav, Poonam, et al., 'The Impact of Mobile Health Interventions on Antenatal and Postnatal Care Utilization in Low- and Middle-Income Countries: A meta-analysis', *Cureus*, vol. 14, no. 1, art. e21256, 14 January 2022, pp. 4, 7, <https://doi.org/10.7759/cureus.21256>.

59 Mahanubhav, Damini S., et al., 'Impact of Electronic Vaccine Intelligence Network Application Used in Immunization Sessions in Pune City', *International Journal of Community Medicine and Public Health*, vol. 9, no. 1, 27 December 2021, art. 130, <https://doi.org/10.18203/2394-6040.ijcmph20214857>.

60 Lutukai, Mercy, et al., 'Using Data to Keep Vaccines Cold in Kenya: Remote temperature monitoring with data review teams for vaccine management', *Global Health: Science and Practice*, vol. 7, no. 4, 23 December 2019, pp. 585–597, <https://doi.org/10.9745/GHSP-D-19-00157>.

61 Lamanna, Camillo, and Lauren Byrne, 'A Pilot Study of a Novel, Incentivised mHealth Technology to Monitor the Vaccine Supply Chain in Rural Zambia', *Pan African Medical Journal*, vol. 33, 2019, art. 50, <https://doi.org/10.11604/pamj.2019.33.50.16318>.

62 Mahanubhav, et al., 'Impact of Electronic Vaccine Intelligence Network Application Used in Immunization Sessions in Pune City'.

63 Gavi, the Vaccine Alliance, 'Gavi Sets Course to Support Sustainable Vaccine Manufacturing in Africa with New Action Plan in Support of the African Union's 2040 Vision', News item, 3 November 2022, <www.gavi.org/news/media-room/gavi-sets-course-support-sustainable-vaccine-manufacturing-africa-new-action-plan>, accessed 16 February 2023.

64 Pan American Health Organization, 'Latin American Manufacturers Complete First Training in mRNA Technology in Bid to Improve Regional Vaccine Production', News item, 24 March 2022, <www.paho.org/en/news/24-3-2022-latin-american-manufacturers-complete-first-training-mrna-technology-bid-improve>, accessed 16 February 2023.
Anon., 'mRNA Made in Africa', News in Brief, *Nature Biotechnology*, vol. 40, art. 284, 16 March 2022, <https://doi.org/10.1038/s41587-022-01268-4>.

Chapter 6

1 Equity Reference Group for Immunization, *ERG: Equity Reference Group for Immunization* [advocacy brief], n.d., <https://drive.google.com/file/d/1VpuVX85RWd_vq6FJ4lcmCnPOYJp1AhuM/view>, accessed 23 February 2023.

2 Wigley, Adelle, et al., 'Estimates of the Number and Distribution of Zero-Dose and Under-Immunised Children Across Remote-Rural, Urban, and Conflict-Affected Settings in Low and Middle-Income Countries', *PLoS Global Public Health*, vol. 2, no. 10, 26 October 2022, art. e0001126, p. 4, <https://doi.org/10.1371/journal.pgph.0001126>.

Statistical tables

The statistical tables in this volume present the most recent key statistics on child survival, development and protection for the world's countries, areas and regions. They support UNICEF's focus on progress and results towards internationally agreed-upon goals and compacts relating to children's and women's rights and development.

General note on the data

Data sources

Data presented in the following statistical tables are derived from UNICEF global databases and are accompanied by definitions, sources and, where necessary, additional footnotes. The indicators data draw on inter-agency estimates and nationally representative household surveys such as Multiple Indicator Cluster Surveys (MICS) and Demographic and Health Surveys (DHS). In addition, data from administrative sources and other United Nations organizations have been used. More detailed information on data sources is provided at the end of each table.

The demographic indicators and many of the population-related indicators in these tables were based on the latest population estimates and projections from *2022 Revision of World Population Prospects* and *World Urbanization Prospects: The 2018 revision,* published by the United Nations Population Division, Department of Economic and Social Affairs. They were adjusted based on the *2022 Revision of World Population Prospects.* Data quality is likely to be adversely affected for countries that have recently suffered disasters or conflicts, especially where basic country infrastructure has been fragmented or where major population movements have occurred.

UNICEF supports countries in collecting and analysing data for monitoring the situation of children and women through MICS, its global household survey programme. Since 1995, as many as 349 surveys have been completed in 118 countries and areas. MICS is the leading data source for measuring the 2030 Sustainable Development Goal (SDG) indicators and for shaping government policies and programmes around the world. More information is available at <mics.unicef.org>.

Regional and global aggregates

Unless otherwise mentioned, regional and global aggregates for indicators were generated as population-weighted averages using data from *2022 Revision of World Population Prospects.* They accord with the relevant age and sex groups for each indicator. For example, the indicator for the total number of live births is based on unweighted population averages and the indicator for females aged 15–49 years with anaemia is based on weighted population averages. Unless otherwise noted, global and regional estimates are only reported for indicators with population-level data coverage of at least 50 per cent.

Data disaggregation

The COVID-19 crisis has underscored the importance of disaggregated data for understanding the differential health and socioeconomic effects of the pandemic on women and children, which have exacerbated long-standing structural disparities and discrimination. Beyond the crisis, high-quality, comparable and timely disaggregated data, as well as data simultaneously disaggregated along more than one dimension, are essential to identifying priority groups for various types of interventions and to fulfil the 2030 Sustainable Development Agenda mandate to leave no one behind.

Different sources of data, including household surveys, vital registrations and administrative records are utilized to compile and analyse disaggregated data. While space constraints do not permit the full presentation of these data in the following statistical tables, efforts have been made to present disaggregated data along key dimensions, including sex, age, residence and wealth status. Given UNICEF's core commitment to gender equality and the empowerment of women and girls, the presentation of sex-disaggregated data, when available, is prioritized in the statistical tables, except when statistically significant differences between boys and girls are not observed in the majority of countries for a given indicator. In these instances, the sex-disaggregated data are available online at <data.unicef.org>. For further information about the disaggregation of individual indicators, please refer to the footnotes below the statistical tables.

Data comparability

Efforts have been made to maximize the comparability of statistics across countries and time. Nevertheless, data used at the country level may differ in terms of the methods used to collect data or arrive at estimates, and in terms of the populations covered. Furthermore, data presented here are subject to evolving methodologies, revisions of time-series data (e.g., immunization and maternal mortality ratios), and changing regional classifications. Also, data comparable from one year to the next are unavailable for some indicators. It is therefore not advisable to compare data from consecutive editions of *The State of the World's Children.*

Further methodological information

Data presented in the following statistical tables generally reflect information compiled and updated from January through July 2022, with a specific cut-off time associated with individual indicators described in the 'main data sources' section underneath each table. The 'last updated' time stamp reflects when the data were compiled and updated as part of country consultation or inter-agency processes that are specific to individual topics.

Interested readers are encouraged to visit <data.unicef.org> for methodological details of the indicators and statistics.

Data presented in the tables are available online at <https://www.unicef.org/reports/state-of-worlds-children> and via <data.unicef.org>. Please refer to these websites for the latest data and for any updates or corrigenda subsequent to printing.

Child mortality estimates

Under-five mortality is used as the principal indicator of progress in child well-being. Here are under-five mortality rates and deaths by UNICEF region.

Under-five mortality rate (deaths per 1,000 live births)

UNICEF Region	1980	1985	1990	1995	2000	2005	2010	2015	2021
East Asia and Pacific	73	62	57	49	39	29	22	17	15
Europe and Central Asia	43	37	31	28	21	16	12	10	8
Eastern Europe and Central Asia	65	54	47	45	35	25	18	14	11
Western Europe	16	13	10	8	6	5	4	4	4
Latin America and Caribbean	85	68	55	43	33	26	23	18	16
Middle East and North Africa	125	87	66	54	43	34	27	25	22
North America	15	12	11	9	8	8	7	7	6
South Asia	173	151	130	112	93	77	62	49	37
Sub-Saharan Africa	201	190	179	170	151	124	102	87	73
Eastern and Southern Africa	187	176	163	154	135	106	81	65	53
West and Central Africa	217	205	197	187	168	142	121	107	91
Least developed countries	213	195	176	158	136	109	89	74	63
World	**118**	**104**	**93**	**87**	**76**	**63**	**51**	**43**	**38**

Under-five deaths (thousands)

UNICEF Region	1980	1985	1990	1995	2000	2005	2010	2015	2021
East Asia and Pacific	2,613	2,372	2,379	1,685	1,228	880	695	544	370
Europe and Central Asia	565	486	394	310	218	159	132	108	78
Eastern Europe and Central Asia	468	413	337	270	188	134	109	89	61
Western Europe	97	73	58	40	30	26	23	20	17
Latin America and Caribbean	957	794	650	507	382	288	244	195	155
Middle East and North Africa	927	725	560	440	340	285	259	265	214
North America	56	50	49	40	36	35	32	29	25
South Asia	5,702	5,384	4,875	4,299	3,667	3,011	2,367	1,794	1,287
Sub-Saharan Africa	3,473	3,734	3,925	4,112	4,032	3,700	3,379	3,136	2,904
Eastern and Southern Africa	1,679	1,822	1,885	1,923	1,827	1,586	1,336	1,135	1,010
West and Central Africa	1,794	1,912	2,040	2,188	2,205	2,114	2,042	2,001	1,894
Least developed countries	3,725	3,787	3,703	3,605	3,345	2,898	2,527	2,251	2,079
World	**14,295**	**13,545**	**12,832**	**11,393**	**9,903**	**8,357**	**7,109**	**6,070**	**5,034**

Regional classifications

Aggregates presented at the end of each of the 18 statistical tables are calculated using data from countries and areas as classified below.

East Asia and the Pacific
Australia; Brunei Darussalam; Cambodia; China; Cook Islands; Democratic People's Republic of Korea; Fiji; Indonesia; Japan; Kiribati; Lao People's Democratic Republic; Malaysia; Marshall Islands; Micronesia (Federated States of); Mongolia; Myanmar; Nauru; New Zealand; Niue; Palau; Papua New Guinea; Philippines; Republic of Korea; Samoa; Singapore; Solomon Islands; Thailand; Timor-Leste; Tokelau; Tonga; Tuvalu; Vanuatu; Viet Nam.

Europe and Central Asia
Eastern Europe and Central Asia; Western Europe.

Eastern Europe and Central Asia
Albania; Armenia; Azerbaijan; Belarus; Bosnia and Herzegovina; Bulgaria; Croatia; Georgia; Kazakhstan; Kyrgyzstan; Montenegro; North Macedonia; Republic of Moldova; Romania; Russian Federation; Serbia; Tajikistan; Türkiye; Turkmenistan; Ukraine; Uzbekistan.

Western Europe
Andorra; Austria; Belgium; Cyprus; Czechia; Denmark; Estonia; Finland; France; Germany; Greece; Holy See; Hungary; Iceland; Ireland; Italy; Latvia; Liechtenstein; Lithuania; Luxembourg; Malta; Monaco; Netherlands (Kingdom of the); Norway; Poland; Portugal; San Marino; Slovakia; Slovenia; Spain; Sweden; Switzerland; United Kingdom.

Latin America and the Caribbean
Anguilla; Antigua and Barbuda; Argentina; Bahamas; Barbados; Belize; Bolivia (Plurinational State of); Brazil; British Virgin Islands; Chile; Colombia; Costa Rica; Cuba; Dominica; Dominican Republic; Ecuador; El Salvador; Grenada; Guatemala; Guyana; Haiti; Honduras; Jamaica; Mexico; Montserrat; Nicaragua; Panama; Paraguay; Peru; Saint Kitts and Nevis; Saint Lucia; Saint Vincent and the Grenadines; Suriname; Trinidad and Tobago; Turks and Caicos Islands; Uruguay; Venezuela (Bolivarian Republic of).

Middle East and North Africa
Algeria; Bahrain; Egypt; Iran (Islamic Republic of); Iraq; Israel; Jordan; Kuwait; Lebanon; Libya; Morocco; Oman; Qatar; Saudi Arabia; State of Palestine; Syrian Arab Republic; Tunisia; United Arab Emirates; Yemen.

North America
Canada; United States of America.

South Asia
Afghanistan; Bangladesh; Bhutan; India; Maldives; Nepal; Pakistan; Sri Lanka.

Sub-Saharan Africa
Eastern and Southern Africa; West and Central Africa.

Eastern and Southern Africa
Angola; Botswana; Burundi; Comoros; Djibouti; Eritrea; Eswatini; Ethiopia; Kenya; Lesotho; Madagascar; Malawi; Mauritius; Mozambique; Namibia; Rwanda; Seychelles; Somalia; South Africa; South Sudan; Sudan; Uganda; United Republic of Tanzania; Zambia; Zimbabwe.

West and Central Africa
Benin; Burkina Faso; Cabo Verde; Cameroon; Central African Republic; Chad; Congo; Côte d'Ivoire; Democratic Republic of the Congo; Equatorial Guinea; Gabon; Gambia; Ghana; Guinea; Guinea-Bissau; Liberia; Mali; Mauritania; Niger; Nigeria; Sao Tome and Principe; Senegal; Sierra Leone; Togo.

Least developed countries/areas
[Classified as such by the United Nations High Representative for the Least Developed Countries, Landlocked Developing Countries and Small Island Developing States (UNOHRLLS)]. Afghanistan; Angola; Bangladesh; Benin; Bhutan; Burkina Faso; Burundi; Cambodia; Central African Republic; Chad; Comoros; Democratic Republic of the Congo; Djibouti; Eritrea; Ethiopia; Gambia; Guinea; Guinea-Bissau; Haiti; Kiribati; Lao People's Democratic Republic; Lesotho; Liberia; Madagascar; Malawi; Mali; Mauritania; Mozambique; Myanmar; Nepal; Niger; Rwanda; Sao Tome and Principe; Senegal; Sierra Leone; Solomon Islands; Somalia; South Sudan; Sudan; Timor-Leste; Togo; Tuvalu; Uganda; United Republic of Tanzania; Yemen; Zambia.

Notes on specific tables

TABLE 1. DEMOGRAPHICS

The demographics table contains selected indicators on some of the most important demographic information of each population, including the total population and the total population broken down by age, as well as annual population growth rates. The annual number of births is a function of both population size and current fertility. The total fertility rate allows for the comparison of fertility levels internationally. A total fertility level of 2.1 is called 'replacement level' and represents a level at which, over the long term, the population would remain the same size. Life expectancy at birth is a measure of the health status and the development of a population and continues to increase in almost all countries. The dependency ratio is the ratio of the not-working-age population (i.e., the economically 'dependent' population) to the working-age population (aged 15–64 years years). This can be divided into a child dependency ratio (ratio of children under 15 years of age to working-age population) and an old-age dependency ratio (ratio of population 65 years and older to working-age population). The total dependency ratio is usually U-shaped over time, reflecting a changing age structure as a result of the demographic transition. This can be understood as the combination of opposing trends in child and old-age dependency ratios. For example, decreasing fertility leads to a decreasing share of children in the population and therefore to a decrease in the child dependency ratio. Increasing life expectancy (as a consequence of decreasing mortality) will lead to a larger share of older people and therefore to an increase in the old-age dependency ratio.

The proportion of the urban population and the annual urban population growth rate describe the status and dynamics of the urbanization process. The net migration rate refers to the difference between the number of immigrants and the number of emigrants; a country/area with more immigrants than emigrants shows a positive value, while a country with fewer immigrants than emigrants shows a negative value. All demographic indicators are based on *2022 Revision of World Population Prospects*. Regional aggregates are based on all countries and areas associated with the respective region, even if they are not included in the 202 reporting countries. Thus, the reported global population under 18 years of age, for example, is larger than the sum of the presented country values.

TABLE 2. CHILD MORTALITY

Each year, in *The State of the World's Children*, UNICEF presents a series of mortality estimates for children. These figures represent the best estimates available at the time of printing and are based on the work of the United Nations Inter-Agency Group for Child Mortality Estimation (UN IGME), which includes UNICEF, the World Health Organization (WHO), the World Bank Group and the UN Population Division. UN IGME mortality estimates are updated annually through a detailed review of all newly available data, which can result in changes to previously reported estimates. As a result, consecutive editions of *The State of the World's Children* should not be used for analysing mortality trends over time. Country-specific mortality indicators, based on the most recent UN IGME estimates, are presented in Table 2 and are available at <data.unicef.org/child-mortality/under-five> and <www.childmortality.org>, along with methodological notes.

TABLE 3. MATERNAL AND NEWBORN HEALTH

The maternal and newborn health table includes a combination of demographic and coverage indicators. The demographic indicators consist of life expectancy for females and maternal mortality estimates, including the number of maternal deaths, maternal mortality ratio and lifetime risk of maternal death.

The life expectancy indicator comes from the UN Population Division. The maternal mortality data are estimates generated by the United Nations Maternal Mortality Estimation Inter-agency Group (MMEIG), which includes WHO, UNICEF, the United Nations Population Fund (UNFPA), the World Bank Group, and the UN Population Division. MMEIG mortality estimates are updated regularly through a detailed review of all newly available data points. This process often results in adjustments to previously reported estimates. As a result, consecutive editions of *The State of the World's Children* should not be used for analysing maternal mortality trends over time.

Coverage encompasses indicators for family planning, antenatal care, delivery care and postnatal care for mother and baby. The data for these indicators come from national household survey programmes such as DHS and MICS and other reproductive health surveys. Regional and global estimates are calculated using a weighted-average method. The variables used for weighting are indicator-specific and applied to each country. They accord with the appropriate target population for each indicator (the denominator) and are derived from the latest edition of *World Population Prospects*. Only the most recent data points from 2016–2021 for each country were used to calculate regional and global aggregates.

The service coverage sub-index on reproductive, maternal, newborn and child health, which is a component of the Universal Health Coverage (UHC) index, has now been added to this table. It is defined as the average coverage of essential services based on eight tracer indicators related to interventions across reproductive, maternal, newborn and child health areas. The index is calculated as a weighted average of the included indicators and is reported on a scale from 0 to 100.

TABLE 4. CHILD HEALTH

The child health table includes a set of indicators that capture information on the coverage of effective interventions delivered to children under the age of 5 years and at the household level. These include a range of immunization indicators (described below) and indicators on interventions for the prevention or treatment of pneumonia, diarrhoea and malaria (the three leading killers of young children). The main data sources for the indicators on prevention and treatment of childhood illnesses are nationally representative household surveys such as the DHS, MICS and the Malaria Indicator Surveys (MIS). Regional and global estimates are calculated using a weighted-average method. Variables used for weighting are indicator-specific and applied to each country. They accord with the appropriate target population for each indicator (the denominator) and are derived from the latest edition of the *World Population Prospects*. Only the most recent data points from 2016–2021 for each country were used to calculate regional and global estimates. For indicators that capture information about households, the total population was used.

Immunization

The child health table presents WHO and UNICEF estimates of national immunization coverage. Since 2000, these estimates have been updated annually in July, following a consultation process during which countries are provided with draft reports for review and comment. As new empirical data are incorporated into the process for generating the estimates, the revised estimates supersede prior data releases. Coverage levels from earlier revisions are not comparable. A more detailed explanation of the process can be found at <data.unicef.org/child-health/immunization>. Regional averages for the reported antigens are computed as follows: For BCG, regional averages include only those countries where BCG is included in the national routine immunization schedule. For DTP, polio, measles, HepB, Hib, PCV and rotavirus vaccines, regional averages include all countries since these vaccines are universally recommended by WHO. For protection at birth (PAB) from tetanus, regional averages include only the countries where maternal and neonatal tetanus is endemic.

TABLE 5. ADOLESCENT HEALTH

This table contains a set of key indicators related to adolescent mortality, adolescent health and well-being. Mortality indicators include the adolescent mortality rate for ages 10–19 years, the number of adolescent deaths as well as the annual rate of reduction in the adolescent mortality rate for the period 2000–2020. Reproductive health indicators presented in this table include adolescent birth rate (for age groups 10–14 years and 15–19 years), early childbearing (which refers to women aged 20–24 years who gave birth before age 18), and demand for family planning satisfied with modern methods among adolescents aged 15–19 years. The following maternal health indicators are presented for adolescents aged 15–19 years: antenatal care with at least four visits and delivery-care indicators including skilled birth attendant, institutional deliveries and births by C-section. The following risk factors for non-communicable diseases (NCDs) are presented: alcohol use among adolescents aged 15–19 years, tobacco use among adolescents aged 13–15 years, and insufficient physical activity among school-going adolescents aged 11–17 years. Though vaccination against the human papillomavirus (HPV) can benefit boys and girls, HPV vaccination is presented for girls who received the last dose of the HPV vaccine per the national schedule. WHO/UNICEF produce two main coverage indicators for HPV vaccination. One is the HPV vaccination programme performance coverage that describes vaccination coverage according to a national schedule and the programme's eligibility criteria for each calendar year (the programme's target population up to 14 years of age). The second describes HPV vaccination coverage by 15 years of age, representing the proportion of the population turning 15 in the reporting year who have been vaccinated against HPV at any time between the ages of 9 and 14 years, at any time up to the calendar year in question. Data are always reported at the national level and may not necessarily show differences at the subnational level. Both indicators are calculated for the first dose (HPV1) and the full recommended schedule (HPVc), and by sex. For the vaccines currently on the market, the schedule depends on age. The general recommendation is a two-dose schedule, with the doses spaced a minimum of six months apart for individuals under 15 years of age at the time of the first dose. Meanwhile, a three-dose schedule (at 0, 1–2 and 6 months) is recommended for individuals 15 years of age or older, or who are immunocompromised or have an HIV infection. To establish denominators, the methodology uses as a default the UN Population Division country estimates. To deal with the different ways countries set and change eligibility criteria over time, a normalization process is used to translate eligibility into denominators. This includes translating school-grade eligibility in population cohorts and dealing with multiple cohort eligibility (changes) over time. For more details, see Laia Bruni et al. in *Preventive Medicine*, <doi.org/10.1016/j.ypmed.2020.106399>.

Two new indicators were added to the current edition of this table: adolescent birth rate for girls aged 10–14 years, sourced from the UN Population Division, and the percentage of adolescents and young women (aged 15–19 years) who make their own informed decisions regarding sexual relations, contraceptive use and reproductive health care, sourced from household surveys. The latter indicator is defined as the percentage of adolescents and young women aged 15–19 years (married or in union) who make their own decisions in all three selected areas. That is, they (1) decide on health care for themselves, either alone or jointly with their husbands or partners, (2) decide on use or non-use of contraception, either alone or jointly with their husbands or partners, and (3) can say no to sex with their husband/partner. When all three criteria are met, an adolescent girl or young woman is considered to have autonomy in reproductive health decision-making and to be empowered to exercise her reproductive rights.

TABLES 6 AND 7: HIV/AIDS

In 2022, the Joint United Nations Programme on HIV/AIDS (UNAIDS) released new global, regional and country-level HIV and AIDS estimates for 2021 that reflect the most up-to-date epidemiological estimates. The estimates also reflect coverage data for antiretroviral therapy (ART), prevention of mother-to-child transmission (PMTCT), and early infant diagnosis for HIV. The estimates are based on the most current available science and WHO programme guidelines. These guidelines have resulted in improvements in assumptions of the probability of HIV transmission from mother-to-child, fertility among women by age and HIV serostatus, net survival rates for children living with HIV, and more. Based on this refined methodology, UNAIDS has retrospectively generated new estimates of HIV prevalence, the number of people living with HIV and those needing treatment, AIDS-related deaths, new HIV infections, and other important trends in the HIV epidemic.

Key indicators on the HIV response for children are divided into two tables: Table 6. HIV/AIDS: Epidemiology and Table 7. HIV/AIDS: Intervention coverage.

Epidemiology

Table 6 includes key indicators used to measure trends in the HIV epidemic. Data are disaggregated by 10-year age groups (since children living with HIV under 10 years of age are all assumed to be infected through mother-to-child transmission). In addition, children aged 10–19 years living with HIV include new HIV infections that occur through sexual transmission and injection drug use, depending on the country context. Due to significant gender disparity among adolescents evident in HIV epidemic trends and programmatic response, disaggregates by sex are now included for all HIV/AIDS epidemiology indicators. For better comparison between countries and regions, the indicator on the number of new HIV infections has been replaced with HIV incidence per 1,000 uninfected population. Similarly, the number of AIDS-related deaths has been replaced with AIDS-related mortality per 100,000 population. These two indicators provide relative measures of new HIV infections and AIDS-related deaths and more accurately demonstrate the impact of the HIV response.

Interventions

Table 7 includes indicators on essential interventions in the HIV response for children. These coverage indicators have been revised from previous editions of *The State of the World's Children* to better reflect progress in current HIV/AIDS programmes and policy. For example, the indicator for early infant HIV diagnosis captures information on what percentage of HIV-exposed infants received an HIV test within two months of birth. All coverage indicators are calculated from the most recent and reliable data available from population-based surveys and programme service statistics.

Each coverage indicator is aggregated regionally or globally using a population-weighted average. Due to sometimes sparse data, indicators from population-based surveys are only aggregated if the data in that area represent at least 50 per cent of the adolescent population.

TABLES 8 AND 9: NUTRITION

Table 8 includes estimates of malnutrition at birth among pre-school-aged children, malnutrition among school-aged children and women of reproductive age as well as coverage of birth weighing and key micronutrient programmes. Table 9 includes feeding practices for infants and young children.

Estimates for low birthweight, stunting and overweight among pre-school-aged children, thinness and overweight among school-aged children, and maternal underweight and anaemia are from country models. For this reason, these may be different from survey-reported or aggregated administrative data estimates. For all other indicators, when raw data were available, the country-level estimates were re-analysed to conform to standard definitions and analysis methods and may therefore differ from survey-reported values.

Low birthweight

Estimates are based on methods updated as of 2019. Therefore, country, regional and global estimates may not be comparable with those published in editions of *The State of the World's Children* prior to 2019.

Unweighted at birth

This indicator represents the percentage of births without a birthweight in the data source. More information can be found at: <https://data.unicef.org/topic/nutrition/low-birthweight/> .

Stunting and overweight

UNICEF, WHO and the World Bank have continued to harmonize the country dataset of stunting and overweight estimates from household surveys. As of 2021, these have been used to generate country-modelled estimates. UNICEF, WHO and the World Bank transitioned from the use of survey estimates to represent country prevalence to the use of country-level modelled estimates for stunting and overweight. The methodology is based on the updated approach described in a UNICEF-WHO-World Bank publication called *Levels and Trends in Child*

Malnutrition: Key findings of the 2021 edition of the joint child malnutrition estimates. Technical notes from the background document for country consultations can be found at: <https://data.unicef.org/resources/jme-2021-country-consultations/>. The regional and global figures for stunting and overweight are population-weighted averages of the country-modelled estimates.

Wasting and severe wasting

Household survey-based estimates are used to report on country prevalence. UNICEF, WHO and the World Bank have continued to harmonize the country dataset of wasting and severe wasting estimates from household surveys, which are used to generate regional and global averages, using a model described by M. de Onis et al. in 'Methodology for Estimating Regional and Global Trends of Child Malnutrition', *International Journal of Epidemiology*, 33, 2004, pp. 1260–1270. For stunting, overweight, wasting and severe wasting, new time-series estimates are released every other year, which supersede all previous estimates and should not be compared.

Vitamin A supplementation

Emphasizing the importance of children receiving two high-dose vitamin A supplements annually (spaced 4–6 months apart), this report presents only a full coverage estimate for vitamin A supplementation. In the absence of a direct method to measure this indicator, full coverage is reported as the lower coverage estimate from semester 1 (January–June) and semester 2 (July–December) in a given year. Estimates for each semester can be found at: <https://data.unicef.org/topic/nutrition/vitamin-a-deficiency/>. The regional and global aggregates are comprised of the 64 countries indicated as priority countries for national-level programmes. Hence, the regional aggregates are published in cases where at least 50 per cent of the population coverage for the priority countries in each region has been met and when there are at least five priority countries in the region. In other words, estimates are not shown for Latin America and the Caribbean or Eastern Europe and Central Asia because each of these regions has only two priority countries.

Malnutrition among school-aged children

Indicators under this title reflect the importance of ending malnutrition among children of all ages. Country estimates for malnutrition among school-aged children are based on the NCD Risk Factor Collaboration (NCD-RisC), 'Worldwide Trends in Body-Mass Index, Underweight, Overweight, and Obesity from 1975 to 2016: A pooled analysis of 2,416 population-based measurement studies in 128.9 million children, adolescents, and adults', *The Lancet*, vol. 390, no. 10113, 2017, pp. 2627–2642.

Underweight women 18+ years

This indicator reflects the importance of maternal malnutrition if malnutrition among children is to be eliminated. Country estimates for underweight women are based on the NCD Risk Factor Collaboration (NCD-RisC), 'Worldwide Trends in Body-Mass Index, Underweight, Overweight, and Obesity from 1975 to 2016: A pooled analysis of 2,416 population-based measurement studies in 128.9 million children, adolescents, and adults', *The Lancet*, vol. 390, no. 10113, 2017, pp. 2627–2642.

Anaemia in women 15–49 years

This indicator also reflects the importance of maternal malnutrition if malnutrition among children is to be eliminated. Country estimates for anaemia are based on: World Health Organization, 'WHO Global Anaemia Estimates: Prevalence of anaemia in women of reproductive age (%)', Global Health Observatory (GHO) data, WHO, Geneva, 2021, <www.who.int/data/gho>.

Iodized salt

The definition of the indicator presented in this report changed in 2016. The indicator previously covered households consuming adequately iodized salt. Since 2016, the indicator measures the consumption of salt with any iodine. Therefore, country, regional and global prevalence estimates are not comparable to those published in previous editions of *The State of the World's Children*.

Infant and young child feeding

A total of 10 indicators are presented, including the following with recent definitional changes or that are new as described in the updated indicator guidance available at: <https://data.unicef.org/resources/indicators-for-assessing-infant-and-young-child-feeding-practices/>:

- Continued breastfeeding (12–23 months) replaces two previous indicators of continued breastfeeding at 1 year (12–15 months) and 2 years (20–23 months).

- Minimum dietary diversity (MDD) (6–23 months) is now defined as the percentage of children aged 6–23 months who received foods from at least five out of eight defined food groups during the previous day. The older version of this indicator reflected consumption of at least four out of seven defined food groups during the previous day.

- Minimum meal frequency (MMF) (6–23 months) has a revised indicator definition for non-breastfed children.

- Minimum acceptable diet (MAD) (6–23 months) is revised to align with the change to the MDD and MMF definitions.

- Zero vegetable or fruit consumption (6–23 months) is a new indicator.

Additionally, this table reflects two new indicators defined by UNICEF to assess child food poverty.

More information can be found at: <https://data.unicef.org/resources/child-food-poverty/>.

TABLE 10. EARLY CHILDHOOD DEVELOPMENT

Early childhood, which spans the period up to 8 years of age, is critical for cognitive, social, emotional and physical development. Optimal brain development requires a stimulating environment, adequate nutrients and social interaction with attentive caregivers. The early childhood development table presents data on some specific indicators with comparable and nationally representative data on children's development status, the quality of care and availability of learning materials at home, and access to early childhood care and education. The information in this table is best interpreted alongside data on other areas vital to early childhood development, such as nutrition and protection.

Early stimulation and responsive care by adults

Data on this indicator from the DHS were recalculated according to the MICS methodology for comparability. Therefore, the recalculated data presented here will differ from estimates in DHS national reports.

Learning materials at home: Playthings

Changes in the definition of this indicator were made between the third and fourth round of MICS (MICS3 and MICS4). To allow for comparability with MICS4 and subsequent rounds of MICS, data from MICS3 were recalculated according to the MICS4 indicator definition. Therefore, the recalculated data presented here will differ from estimates reported in MICS3 national reports.

TABLE 11: EDUCATION

This table contains a set of indicators on children's education: equitable access, school completion and learning outcomes.

This table first provides information about equitable access, as measured by the out-of-school children rate (SDG4.1.4). Estimates shown in this table were sourced from the database of the United Nations Educational, Scientific and Cultural Organization (UNESCO) Institute for Statistics (UIS). The out-of-school children rate identifies the segment of the population in the official age range for a given level of education who are not attending school. It can be used to formulate targeted policies to ensure equitable access to education.

In September 2019, UIS changed the methodology for capturing data on out-of-school children at the primary level. Primary school-aged children attending pre-primary education are now considered as in-school children.

Completion rate (SDG 4.1.2) measures the percentage of a cohort of children or young people aged 3–5 years older than the intended age for the last grade of each level of education who have completed that grade. Estimates were sourced from the UNICEF global database, calculated using MICS, DHS and other household surveys. By choosing an age group that is slightly older than the theoretical age group for completing each level of education, the indicator provides more robust measures on the share of children and adolescents completing each cycle of education.

This table also includes a set of indicators to monitor equitable learning outcomes, including the proportion of children and young people achieving at least a minimum proficiency in reading and mathematics (SDG 4.1.1) as well as the youth literacy rate (SDG 4.6.2). The minimum proficiency level is the benchmark of basic knowledge in a domain (i.e., mathematics and reading) measured through learning assessments. Estimates were based on the United Nations Statistics Division's database, an official SDG data source. The literacy rate shown in the table was sourced from the UIS database. It measures the basic literacy skills that the population should be equipped with through primary education. It is used to provide insight into the proportion of youth aged 15–24 years with a minimum level of proficiency in reading and writing; it also measures the effectiveness of primary education in each country.

Detailed information on the indicators included in this table can be found in the July 2017 UNESCO UIS publication, *Metadata for the Global and Thematic Indicators for the Follow-Up and Review of SDG4 and Education 2030*, July 2017.

TABLE 12. CHILD PROTECTION

Child protection refers to the prevention of and response to violence, exploitation and abuse of children in all contexts. There are many violations that children can be subjected to, but the lack of comparable data limits reporting on the full spectrum. In view of this, the child protection table presents data on a few issues for which comparable and nationally representative data are available.

Birth registration

Changes in the definition of birth registration were made from the second and third rounds of MICS (MICS2 and MICS3) to the fourth round (MICS4). To allow for comparability with later rounds, data from MICS2 and MICS3 on birth registration were recalculated according to the MICS4 indicator definition. Therefore, the recalculated data presented here may differ from estimates included in MICS2 and MICS3 national reports.

Child labour

This indicator has been replaced by the one used for SDG reporting on indicator 8.7.1. It reflects the proportion of children engaged in economic activities and/or household chores at/or above age-specific hourly thresholds (general production boundary basis). For the 5–11 year age group, the threshold refers to children who work at least one hour per week in economic activity and/or are involved in unpaid household services for more than 21 hours per week. For the 12–14 year age group, the threshold reflects children who work at least 14 hours per week in economic activity and/or are involved in unpaid household services for more than 21 hours per week. For the 15–17 year age group, it refers to children who work more than 43 hours per week in economic activity (no hourly threshold is set for unpaid household services for this age group). Country estimates compiled and presented in the global SDG database and reproduced in *The State of the World's Children* have been re-analysed by UNICEF and the International Labour Organization (ILO) in accordance with the definitions and criteria detailed above. This means that country data values will differ from those published in national survey reports.

Child marriage

This statistical table presents the share of individuals who were first married or in union before 18 years of age. While the practice is more widespread among girls, marriage in childhood is a rights violation for both sexes. Therefore, the prevalence of child marriage is shown for both males and females. A secondary indicator on child marriage, shown in the share of women married before 15 years of age, was featured in previous editions of *The State of the World's Children*. Starting with this edition, the indicator has been removed to allow space for data on other topics. The indicator continues to be monitored by UNICEF, and relevant data can be found at <data.unicef.org>.

Female genital mutilation (FGM)

Data on the prevalence of FGM among girls aged 0–14 years were recalculated for technical reasons and may differ from those presented in original DHS and MICS country reports. Beginning with the 2019 edition of *The State of the World's Children*, attitudes towards the practice are shown as the share of the population opposing (rather than supporting) FGM. This measure was shown for both males and females in previous editions of the report, but data for males have been removed, starting with this edition, to make room for data on other topics. The indicator continues to be monitored by UNICEF, and relevant data can be found at <data.unicef.org>.

Regional estimates on the prevalence of FGM and attitudes towards the practice are based on available data only from practising countries with nationally representative data. Since each region includes some countries that do not practise FGM, the data reflect the situation among those living in specific countries where the practice is ongoing.

Violent discipline

The reference age group for this indicator was revised, beginning with MICS5, to children aged 1–14 years. Therefore, estimates from MICS3 and MICS4 are not directly comparable since they refer to children aged 2–14 years.

Children in residential care and children in detention

Figures for these indicators are based on underlying data that rely on the strength of a country's data system and on the degree of coordination between the bodies and institutions that collect these data. Overall, there are several limitations in the availability, consistency and coverage of underlying country data based on administrative records. Therefore, data on these indicators are best interpreted as providing an indication, albeit approximate, of whether, and how well, a country's data system is able to generate and make available a count of these child populations. Accordingly, higher reported figures may actually reflect a more comprehensive system of identifying and monitoring such children and a greater capacity for the systematic collection of such data, rather than an indication of a larger population. Regional estimates should be interpreted with consideration of the wide variation in the number of children and the capacity of record-keeping and reporting systems among countries in the same region.

TABLE 13. SOCIAL PROTECTION AND EQUITY

This table provides information about social protection coverage and the magnitude of income inequality, both of which impact the context in which children live. Social protection indicators include mothers with newborns receiving cash benefits, the proportion of children covered by social protection, and the distribution of social protection benefits (among the 1st quintile, 5th quintile and bottom 40 per cent of households in terms of income). While the first two indicators capture the coverage of social protection, the third indicator reflects both incidence and distribution across quintiles. The table gives an overview of the social safety net that households – children in particular – have access to within each country.

Inequality indicators include the share of household income (1st quintile, 5th quintile, bottom 40 per cent), Gini index, Palma index, the vast majority income ratio, and gross domestic product (GDP) per capita. The first indicator captures the share of national income each quintile earns within a country. It illustrates the structure of income distribution per country, while the Gini coefficient expresses the extent of inequality and how it deviates from a perfectly equal income distribution. In contrast, the Palma index concentrates on the income difference between the richest 10 per cent and the poorest 40 per cent of a population. This indicator is more sensitive to the tails of distribution and extreme inequalities. Because changes in income inequality are mainly driven by changes in the income of the richest 10 per cent and the poorest 40 per cent, the Palma index offers insights on distributional changes of income inequality. The vast majority income ratio measures the income ratio of the first 80 per cent (vast majority) in the income ranking. GDP per capita complements those indicators as it measures the average standard of living in each country.

Data on social protection and equity indicators do not have an annual frequency and are extracted from the World Bank's *World Development Indicators, The Atlas of Social Protection Indicators of Resilience and Equity (ASPIRE),* and the ILO's *World Social Protection Report.*

TABLE 14. WASH

This table contains a set of indicators on access to basic water, sanitation and hygiene (WASH) services in households, schools and health-care facilities. The WASH estimates in this report come from the WHO/ UNICEF Joint Monitoring Programme for Water Supply, Sanitation and Hygiene (JMP). Full details of the JMP indicator definitions, data sources and methods used to produce national, regional and global estimates can be found at <www.washdata.org>. New estimates for each setting are released every two years. These supersede all previous estimates and should not be compared.

TABLE 15. ADOLESCENTS

The table on adolescents presents a selection of indicators on the well-being of adolescents across various domains of their lives: protection, education and learning as well as the transition to work. While adolescent well-being is broad and cannot be exhaustively captured in a small selection of indicators, the measures in Table 15 are meant to serve as an illustrative sample, and to complement adolescent-relevant indicators that appear throughout the other statistical tables in this publication. Adolescent health indicators are now presented in Table 5.

NEET and unemployment

Data on the degree to which adolescents are able to effectively transition to work, illustrated through the measures of those not in employment, education or training (NEET) and the unemployment rate among adolescents aged 15–19 years, are drawn from the ILO. Metadata and further notes on interpretation of these indicators are available through the 'Metadata' section of <ilo.org/ilostat>.

Some caution is warranted in interpreting these data since the standards for measuring labour statistics are in the midst of a revision that affects the comparability of the current dataset with previous versions. Data shown in this publication are drawn from the data series based on the 13th International Conference of Labour Statisticians. For more details, see the technical note on this topic prepared by the ILO, which maintains these datasets: *Quick guide to understanding the impact of the new statistical standards on ILOSTAT databases.*

TABLE 16. CHILDREN WITH DISABILITIES

This table presents a selection of indicators on child well-being across various domains: child protection, early childhood development, education, nutrition, social protection and equity as well as WASH. For each indicator, data are presented for children with and without disabilities. While measuring well-being is broad and cannot be exhaustively captured in a small selection of indicators, the data in Table 16 are meant to be illustrative of whether disparities exist between these two population groups. Some of the data in this table must be interpreted with caution due to caveats in the tools used to gather the information, as explained below.

Stunting and overweight

Collecting data on the growth of children with disabilities presents challenges. Anthropometric measurements in surveys are typically carried out by trained measurers and under uniform conditions, which include the use of standardized digital scales and measurement boards. Children with certain types of impairments may not grow in the same way as children who develop more typically. This may mean that their health and development cannot be properly measured by standard tools used in the context of household surveys. Moreover, measuring and weighing children with specific types of impairments may lead to larger measurement errors. Finally, it should be noted that the WHO Child Growth Standards were calculated based on children without physical impairments. Therefore, even when a child's height and weight can be collected, standard nutrition indicators (used to measure stunting and overweight) may be inappropriate to assess growth for children with certain disabilities, making findings more difficult to interpret.

Early childhood education and never attended school

A relevant consideration is the limitation of the data in providing a comprehensive account of all factors affecting a child's learning experience. While the indicators used here measure education uptake, they fall short in fully capturing the experiences of children with disabilities in obtaining an education and the barriers they face.

Another data limitation is the inability to distinguish between children who are in mainstream education and those who are in disability-specific educational settings. This is significant since many countries have highly segregated school systems for children with disabilities. For example, what is considered progression in a special education school may be significantly different from that in a mainstream school, fundamentally altering responses to what is considered 'at level' for the child. If this distinction could be captured, then the reported inequities between children with and without disabilities would likely be even greater.

Foundational learning skills
Data on foundational reading and numeracy skills are only generated for children who can complete three reading tasks and four numeracy tasks. Non-completion observations include children who started but were unable to finish the assessment tasks, who refused to take the assessment (or whose mothers did not permit them to take the assessment), or who could not participate in the assessment due to illness or an impairment. Inaccessibility could thus be a barrier to participation for some children (for example, if a child is blind or requires assistive technology or reasonable accommodations to participate and these could not be provided). Therefore, the results that show differences in foundational learning skills for children with and without disabilities should be interpreted with the understanding that children with certain difficulties are less likely to have been part of such an assessment.

Basic sanitation services on premises
The indicator provides information on the percentage of children aged 2–17 years living in a household with improved sanitation services not shared with other households and located in their own dwelling or in their own yard/plot. The definitions used for service levels and type of facilities are established by the JMP.

In assessing and measuring sanitation services, it is important to consider not only the types of facilities available to households but also whether they are easily accessible and/or shared with other households. The distinction between availability and access is particularly significant for children with disabilities since they often face unique and disproportionate barriers to access even when services are available. However, for indicators on the services, the key metric assessed is the type of facility used and whether it is in the household, shared with other households, or a distance away from the household. Therefore, while the data can demonstrate the availability of WASH services for households with children with disabilities, it is not possible from the current data to assess whether that translates into a usable facility and full accessibility for the children themselves. Further work is required to develop an international standard for measuring the accessibility of WASH facilities for children with disabilities.

Moreover, the data do not offer insights into non-household settings in which children with disabilities may find themselves (such as schools, residential care or health-care facilities and other public buildings).

Social transfers
While social protection encompasses a host of interventions beyond social transfers, there is a dearth of internationally comparable data about many, if not most, non-cash interventions. Also, for most countries, it is not possible to know whether the social transfer was in any way related to disability or was provided to the household based on other factors.

TABLE 17. WOMEN'S ECONOMIC EMPOWERMENT
This table was added in 2019 given the beneficial effects of women's economic empowerment on the well-being of children. It also reflects the intrinsic importance of women's economic empowerment as articulated in SDG 5: Achieve gender equality and empower all women and girls.

Social institutions and gender index (SIGI)
Discriminatory laws, attitudes and practices affect the life course of women and girls, restricting their ability to accumulate human, social and productive assets and to exercise agency and voice over choices that affect their well-being. The SIGI, a composite measure of gender discrimination in social institutions, produced by the Organisation for Economic Co-operation and Development, combines qualitative and quantitative data on discriminatory social institutions in four areas: discrimination in the family, restricted physical integrity, restricted access to productive and financial resources, and restricted civil liberties.

Legal frameworks that promote, enforce, and monitor gender equality in employment and economic benefits
Equality and non-discrimination on the basis of sex are core principles enshrined in international legal and policy frameworks, including the Convention on the Elimination of All Forms of Discrimination against Women (CEDAW) and the Beijing Declaration and Platform for Action. Removing discriminatory laws and putting in place legal frameworks that advance gender equality in employment are prerequisites for increasing women's paid and decent work and, in turn, their economic empowerment. The term 'legal frameworks' is defined broadly to encompass laws, mechanisms and policies/plans to promote, enforce and monitor gender equality. Data derived for this indicator, SDG 5.1.1, come from an assessment of a country's legal frameworks completed by national statistical offices and/or national women's machinery, and legal practitioners/researchers on gender equality.

Maternity/paternity leave benefits

Parental leave benefits are critical for supporting the health and well-being of children and women's economic empowerment, including infants' survival and healthy development as well as increased labour force participation and earnings for women. ILO Convention No. 183 provides for 14 weeks of paid maternity benefits to those women for whom the instrument applies. While no ILO standard exists specifically on paternity leave, paternity benefits permit working fathers to be more involved in the care of their children and the sharing of household responsibilities. It is important to note, however, that even in countries with legal rights to parental leave, not all workers will have access, such as those employed part-time or working in the informal economy.

Educational attainment

While primary education provides children with the foundation for a lifetime of learning, secondary education equips them with the knowledge and skills needed to become economically empowered adults. Compared to girls with only a primary education, girls with secondary education are less likely to marry as children and become pregnant as adolescents. And, while women with a primary education earn only marginally more than women with no education, women with secondary education earn twice as much, on average, than women who have not gone to school (see Wodon et al., 'Missed Opportunities: The high cost of not educating girls', *The Cost of Not Educating Girls Notes Series,* The World Bank, Washington D.C., 2018).

Labour force participation and unemployment rates

Equal access to the labour market is critical for women's economic empowerment. The labour force participation rate is calculated by expressing the number of persons in the labour force during a given reference period as a percentage of the working-age population (usually aged 15 years and older) in the same reference period. The unemployment rate conveys the percentage of persons (usually aged 15 years and older) in the labour force who are unemployed. This reflects the inability of an economy to generate employment for those who want to work but are not doing so, even though they are available for employment and actively seeking work. Information on unemployment by sex highlights the greater difficulty, in many cases, that women have in entering the labour market, which can be directly or indirectly linked to a country's gender norms.

Mobile phone ownership

Mobile phone ownership provides individuals with access to information, financial services, employment opportunities and social networks, and is an important asset for fostering women's economic empowerment as recognized in SDG5. In SDG5.b.1, an individual is considered to own a mobile phone if she/he has a mobile cellular phone device with at least one active SIM card for personal use. Mobile cellular phones supplied by employers that can be used for personal reasons (to make personal calls, access the Internet, etc.) are included. Individuals who have only an active SIM card(s) and not a mobile phone are excluded. Individuals who have a mobile phone for personal use that is not registered under his/her name are also included. An active SIM card is a SIM card that has been used in the last three months.

Financial inclusion

Measuring women's access to financial services, such as savings, insurance, payments, credit and remittances, is essential to understanding their economic empowerment. Access to financial services can also increase women's bargaining power in the household, with potential benefits for the well-being of children. As measured by SDG 8.10.2, having an account at a financial institution includes respondents who report having an account at a bank; who have an account at another type of financial institution, such as a credit union, microfinance institution, cooperative or the post office (if applicable); or who have a debit card in their own name. It also includes respondents who report receiving wages, government transfers or payments for agricultural products into an account at a financial institution in the past 12 months. In addition, it includes respondents who report having paid utility bills or school fees from an account at a financial institution in the past 12 months, or received wages or government transfers into a card in the past 12 months. Users of mobile money accounts include respondents who report personally using GSM Association (GSMA) Mobile Money for the Unbanked (MMU) services in the past 12 months to pay bills or to send or receive money. In addition, it includes respondents who report receiving wages, government transfers or payments for agricultural products through a mobile phone in the past 12 months.

Time use

A new indicator, the proportion of time spent on unpaid domestic and care work, has been added to this table to highlight discrepancies in how much time women and men spend on unpaid work, which has implications for their labour force participation and overall well-being. Data presented for this indicator are expressed as a proportion of time in a day, with the proportion of time spent on unpaid domestic and care work calculated by dividing the daily average number of hours spent on unpaid domestic and care work by 24 hours for the total relevant population. While own-use production work can be differentiated based on whether goods or services are produced, the indicator only considers the own-use production work of services or, in other words, the activities related to unpaid domestic services and unpaid caregiving services undertaken by households for their own use. Examples include food preparation, dishwashing, cleaning and upkeep of the dwelling, laundry, shopping, childcare, and care of the sick, elderly or disabled household and family members, among others. Comparisons across countries should be made with caution given that international comparability of time-use statistics is limited by a number of methodological considerations, including different target age populations.

TABLE 18. MIGRATION

This table was added in 2021 due to the significance of migration and displacement for children's well-being and the attention they have received recently. This attention culminated in the Global Compact for Migration and the Global Compact on Refugees, both endorsed by the United Nations General Assembly in 2018.

The data on international migration are based on the *International Migrant Stock,* published by the UN Population Division. The data provide the number of persons residing outside of their country of birth (for some countries, citizenship was used instead of country of birth, depending on data availability) at mid-year of the reference year. Refugees and asylum seekers are included in this population. The number of children under 18 years of age is estimated based on the five-age year groups of migrant stock published by the UN Population Division. For more details on the definition and methods for estimating the international migrant stock, see the UN Population Division's publication, *International Migrant Stock 2020.*

The data on refugees (including both refugees and persons living in refugee-like situations) and asylum seekers are based on the Refugee Population Statistics Database of the United Nations High Commissioner for Refugees (UNHCR) (see: <www. unhcr.org/refugee-statistics/>). The term 'refugee' is defined in the 1951 Convention amended by the 1967 Protocol. These numbers are stock numbers

and refer to the end of the reference year. Data for refugee children are estimated jointly with UNCHR and account for the lack of complete age coverage in many countries. Values for countries with high uncertainties around the point estimate are not shown, but are included in the regional age-related aggregates.

Data on internally displaced persons are based on the Global Internal Displacement Database (GIDD) maintained by the Internal Displacement Monitoring Center (IDMC). They refer to the number of internally displaced persons (IDPs) at the end of the reference year and the number of new internal displacements during the reference year (see: <https://www.internal-displacement.org/database>). The IDP numbers are stock data counting the number of persons living in internal displacement. The number of new displacements refers to the aggregate number of independent displacement events during the year; it can also include subsequent displacements of the same persons (during distinct events). For this reason, the number of 'new' displacements cannot be equated with the number of persons displaced. Due to the lack of age-disaggregated data, the number of IDP children and of new displacements of children are estimated using the age structure of the national population. This makes the implicit assumption that internal displacement happens randomly in terms of age and sex. Contrary to this, case studies have shown that women and children tend to be over-represented in the displaced population. As a consequence, the presented child-related data on internal displacement are likely to be an underestimation. Considering these issues, the age-disaggregated data on internal displacement are rounded to the second significant figure. Unrounded numbers are used to calculate regional aggregates.

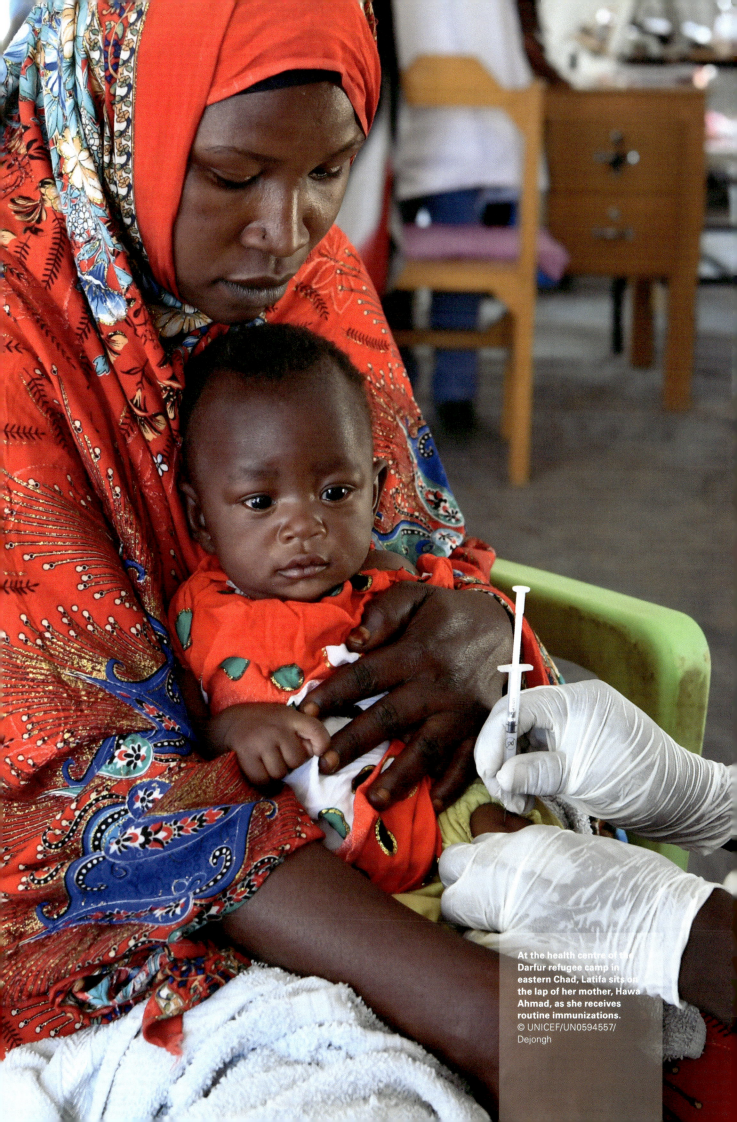

At the health centre of the Darfur refugee camp in eastern Chad, Latifa sits on the lap of her mother, Hawa Ahmad, as she receives routine immunizations.
© UNICEF/UN0594557/Dejongh

Number of under-five deaths and under-five mortality rate by country in 2021

Table ordered by the unrounded number of under-five deaths in 2021. Lower and upper bound refer to the lower and upper bound of 90 per cent uncertainty intervals.

HIGHEST BURDEN OF DEATH AMONG CHILDREN UNDER AGE 5

Countries and areas	Annual number of under-five deaths (thousands) 2021	Under-five mortality rate (deaths per 1,000 live births) in 2021		
		Median	Lower bound	Upper bound
Nigeria	852	111	82	152
India	709	31	28	34
Pakistan	399	63	51	79
Democratic Republic of the Congo	308	79	47	132
Ethiopia	178	47	36	60
Niger	124	115	93	144
United Republic of Tanzania	106	47	32	70
Indonesia	100	22	17	28
Angola	90	69	29	137
China	88	7	6	8
Mali	85	97	78	121
Sudan	83	55	37	81
Bangladesh	82	27	25	30
Somalia	80	112	51	248
Mozambique	79	70	45	110
Afghanistan	78	56	41	74
Chad	76	107	75	151
Uganda	69	42	29	60
Côte d'Ivoire	68	75	56	100
Cameroon	65	70	54	89
Burkina Faso	63	83	56	122
Philippines	63	26	18	36
Yemen	62	62	28	132
Madagascar	58	66	56	80
Kenya	54	37	30	46
Egypt	47	19	12	29
Guinea	45	99	80	123
Brazil	40	14	12	17
Ghana	39	44	33	59
South Africa	39	33	30	36
Benin	39	84	68	103
Myanmar	39	42	27	63
Zambia	38	58	41	80
South Sudan	31	99	35	229
Viet Nam	30	21	18	23
Iraq	29	25	18	33
Sierra Leone	27	105	85	128
Malawi	27	42	26	66
Mexico	26	13	11	16
Zimbabwe	24	50	34	72
United States	23	6	6	7
Burundi	23	53	32	85
Central African Republic	22	100	79	126
Algeria	22	22	20	25
Senegal	21	39	29	51
Togo	17	63	47	83
Nepal	16	27	21	36
Iran (Islamic Republic of)	16	13	7	22
Haiti	16	59	41	85
Rwanda	16	39	24	66
Liberia	12	76	56	104
Morocco	12	18	12	25
Uzbekistan	11	14	13	16
Türkiye	11	9	8	11
Venezuela (Bolivarian Republic of)	11	24	18	33
Papua New Guinea	11	43	29	63

Countries and areas	Annual number of under-five deaths (thousands) 2021	Under-five mortality rate (deaths per 1,000 live births) in 2021		
		Median	Lower bound	Upper bound
Colombia	9	13	8	20
Syrian Arab Republic	9	22	12	31
Guatemala	9	23	16	32
Peru	8	14	11	18
Tajikistan	8	31	18	54
Cambodia	8	25	12	51
Congo	8	43	24	77
Russian Federation	7	5	5	5
Lao People's Democratic Republic	7	43	29	61
Dominican Republic	7	33	24	44
Bolivia (Plurinational State of)	6	25	17	35
Mauritania	6	40	31	53
Turkmenistan	6	41	27	63
Thailand	5	8	7	11
Democratic People's Republic of Korea	5	15	12	20
Guinea-Bissau	5	74	43	122
Argentina	4	7	7	7
Saudi Arabia	4	7	5	9
Lesotho	4	73	51	108
Kazakhstan	4	10	10	11
Gambia	4	48	37	62
Eritrea	4	38	21	69
Malaysia	4	8	7	8
Equatorial Guinea	4	77	42	137
Ecuador	4	12	11	14
Honduras	4	17	13	22
Jordan	4	15	10	21
Tunisia	3	16	14	19
France	3	4	4	5
United Kingdom	3	4	4	4
Ukraine	3	8	8	9
Kyrgyzstan	3	17	17	18
Germany	3	4	3	4
Namibia	3	39	21	76
Gabon	3	40	24	67
Paraguay	3	18	9	38
Azerbaijan	2	19	11	32
State of Palestine	2	15	11	21
Botswana	2	35	10	116
Sri Lanka	2	7	5	9
Japan	2	2	2	2
Canada	2	5	5	5
Nicaragua	2	13	11	15
Timor-Leste	2	51	33	76
Poland	2	4	4	5
Eswatini	2	53	32	86
Chile	1	7	5	8
Djibouti	1	54	30	96
Libya	1	11	6	19
Romania	1	6	6	7
El Salvador	1	12	7	21
Comoros	1	50	37	67
Australia	1	4	4	4
Spain	1	3	3	3
Italy	1	3	2	3

LOWEST BURDEN OF DEATH AMONG CHILDREN UNDER AGE 5

Countries and areas	Annual number of under-five deaths (thousands) 2021	Under-five mortality rate (deaths per 1,000 live births) in 2021		
		Median	Lower bound	Upper bound
Mongolia	1	15	14	16
Panama	1	14	7	28
Oman	1	10	9	11
Republic of Korea	1	3	3	3
Lebanon	1	8	7	10
Netherlands (Kingdom of the)	1	4	4	4
United Arab Emirates	1	6	5	7
Israel	1	3	3	4
Republic of Moldova	1	14	10	20
Cuba	1	5	4	6
Fiji	1	28	25	31
Costa Rica	0	8	7	8
Belgium	0	4	4	5
Georgia	0	9	8	11
Guyana	0	28	16	48
Kuwait	0	9	8	10
Jamaica	0	12	6	24
Solomon Islands	0	19	12	30
Bulgaria	0	6	6	7
Serbia	0	5	5	6
Armenia	0	11	8	13
Hungary	0	4	4	5
Switzerland	0	4	4	4
Slovakia	0	6	5	6
Austria	0	4	3	4
Greece	0	4	3	4
New Zealand	0	5	4	5
Trinidad and Tobago	0	16	7	42
Czechia	0	3	3	3
Albania	0	9	9	10
Sweden	0	2	2	3
Bhutan	0	27	16	44
Portugal	0	3	3	3
Belarus	0	3	2	3
Mauritius	0	17	14	20
Denmark	0	4	3	4
Vanuatu	0	23	13	42
Uruguay	0	6	5	6
Suriname	0	17	11	28
Ireland	0	3	3	4
Kiribati	0	48	26	90
Croatia	0	5	4	5
Bosnia and Herzegovina	0	6	4	7
Qatar	0	5	5	6

Countries and areas	Annual number of under-five deaths (thousands) 2021	Under-five mortality rate (deaths per 1,000 live births) in 2021		
		Median	Lower bound	Upper bound
Cabo Verde	0	14	10	18
Bahrain	0	7	6	8
Norway	0	2	2	2
North Macedonia	0	5	4	7
Finland	0	2	2	2
Samoa	0	17	12	24
Sao Tome and Principe	0	15	9	27
Lithuania	0	3	3	4
Singapore	0	2	2	3
Belize	0	11	9	14
Brunei Darussalam	0	11	10	14
Latvia	0	4	3	4
Bahamas	0	13	11	15
Micronesia (Federated States of)	0	25	11	54
Saint Lucia	0	25	21	29
Maldives	0	6	5	7
Slovenia	0	2	2	3
Barbados	0	12	8	18
Cyprus	0	3	2	4
Dominica	0	36	31	42
Grenada	0	16	13	20
Estonia	0	2	2	2
Malta	0	6	5	7
Tonga	0	11	6	19
Marshall Islands	0	30	18	51
Seychelles	0	14	11	18
Saint Vincent and the Grenadines	0	14	10	19
Luxembourg	0	3	2	4
Montenegro	0	2	2	3
Iceland	0	3	2	3
Nauru	0	28	14	53
Saint Kitts and Nevis	0	15	10	22
Antigua and Barbuda	0	6	4	10
Tuvalu	0	21	12	37
Palau	0	16	8	34
Andorra	0	3	1	10
Cook Islands	0	7	4	13
Turks and Caicos Islands	0	4	3	8
British Virgin Islands	0	10	5	23
Anguilla	0	4	2	9
Monaco	0	3	2	5
Niue	0	24	10	57
Montserrat	0	5	2	14
San Marino	0	2	1	4

Cyprus: Some UN IGME indicators are calculated using population and live birth numbers from the 2022 Revision of World Population Prospects. The numbers for Cyprus refer to the whole country. However, the underlying data sent by the Health Monitoring Unit of the Cyprus Ministry of Health capture only the government-controlled area, whereas according to Eurostat, the population on 1 January 2022 was 904,705 (https://ec.europa.eu/eurostat/databrowser/view/tps00001).
Kosovo: All references to Kosovo in the UN IGME estimates should be understood to be in the context of United Nations Security Council resolution 1244 (1999).
Mozambique: UNAIDS estimates for Mozambique were not available at the time of publication.

Nicaragua: The UN IGME estimates are not the official statistics of Nicaragua. The most recent national official estimate of the under-five mortality rate available to the UN IGME comes from the vital registration system for 2020, with a rate of 12.6 deaths per 1,000 live births. Following a request from the Government of Nicaragua and per the objectives of the UN IGME, the UN IGME will continue to assess all data sources in the country relevant to child mortality estimation.
Uzbekistan: The most recent official national estimate of the under-five mortality rate in Uzbekistan is from the vital registration system, with a rate of 12.3 deaths per 1,000 live births for both sexes, in 2021.

FOR EVERY CHILD, VACCINATION

TABLE 1. DEMOGRAPHICS

Countries and areas	Population (thousands) 2021			Annual population growth rate (%)		Annual number of births (thousands) 2021	Total fertility (live births per woman) 2021	Life expectancy at birth (years)			Dependency ratio (%) 2021			Share of urban population (%) 2021	Annual growth rate of urban population (%)		Net migration rate (per 1,000 population) 2021
	Total	Under 18	Under 5	2000–2020	2020–2030 ᴬ			1970	2000	2021	Total dependency ratio	Child dependency ratio	Old age dependency ratio		2000–2020	2020–2030 ᴬ	
Afghanistan	40,099	20,298	6,491	3,3	2,3	1,441	4.6	37	55	62	85	80	4	26	4.1	3.5	-4.6
Albania	2,855	574	141	-0,5	-0,2	29	1.4	65	75	76	48	24	24	63	1.4	0.8	-3.7
Algeria	44,178	15,526	4,871	1,6	1,2	951	2.9	43	70	76	58	49	10	74	2.6	1.8	-0.4
Andorra	79	13	3	0,8	0,4	1	1.1	74	81	80	38	18	20	88	0.5	0.4	17.6
Angola	34,504	17,833	5,983	3,4	2,7	1,339	5.3	40	46	62	91	87	5	67	4.8	3.4	0.8
Anguilla	16	3	1	1,6	0,3	0	1.3	65	76	77	39	24	14	100	1.6	0.3	7.1
Antigua and Barbuda	93	21	5	1,0	0,5	1	1.6	70	75	78	41	27	14	24	-0.3	0.6	0.0
Argentina	45,277	12,669	3,333	0,9	0,5	629	1.9	66	74	75	54	36	18	92	1.1	0.6	0.1
Armenia	2,791	669	183	-0,6	-0,2	34	1.6	64	71	72	50	31	19	63	-0.7	0.2	-4.6
Australia	25,921	5,667	1,537	1,4	0,9	298	1.6	71	80	85	54	28	25	86	1.5	1.0	4.6
Austria	8,922	1,542	431	0,5	0,1	85	1.5	70	78	82	51	22	29	59	0.4	0.6	2.3
Azerbaijan	10,313	2,896	705	1,1	0,4	127	1.7	59	65	69	44	34	10	57	1.5	1.0	0.1
Bahamas	408	100	23	1,1	0,5	5	1.4	66	72	72	39	27	12	83	1.1	0.7	1.2
Bahrain	1,463	348	98	3,5	0,6	18	1.8	64	75	79	31	27	5	90	3.5	0.7	-6.2
Bangladesh	169,356	54,801	14,663	1,2	0,9	3,020	2.0	43	66	72	48	39	9	39	3.5	2.5	-1.0
Barbados	281	59	15	0,3	0,1	3	1.6	68	74	78	49	26	23	31	-0.1	0.5	-0.1
Belarus	9,578	1,901	474	-0,3	-0,4	89	1.5	71	69	72	51	25	25	80	0.3	0.0	1.4
Belgium	11,611	2,329	599	0,6	0,2	116	1.6	71	78	82	57	26	30	98	0.6	0.3	4.5
Belize	400	136	37	2,4	1,2	7	2.0	63	69	70	50	42	7	46	2.4	1.7	1.4
Benin	12,997	6,376	2,137	2,8	2,4	476	5.0	42	57	60	84	78	6	49	3.9	3.4	0.1
Bhutan	777	220	51	1,3	0,6	10	1.4	40	62	72	41	32	9	43	3.7	1.8	0.4
Bolivia (Plurinational State of)	12,079	4,470	1,272	1,6	1,2	264	2.6	47	62	64	56	49	8	70	2.2	1.7	-0.4
Bosnia and Herzegovina	3,271	588	154	-1,1	-0,6	28	1.3	67	74	75	49	22	27	49	-0.4	0.2	-7.9
Botswana	2,588	1,000	297	1,8	1,4	61	2.8	55	51	61	57	52	6	72	3.2	2.1	0.7
Brazil	214,326	53,465	14,241	0,9	0,4	2,761	1.6	57	70	73	43	29	14	87	1.2	0.7	0.1
British Virgin Islands	31	6	1	2,0	0,6	0	1.0	67	74	74	33	20	13	49	2.8	1.4	4.1
Brunei Darussalam	445	119	32	1,3	0,6	6	1.8	64	74	75	39	31	8	79	1.8	1.0	-0.4
Bulgaria	6,886	1,156	306	-0,7	-0,9	58	1.6	71	72	72	57	22	35	76	-0.3	-0.6	-1.3
Burkina Faso	22,101	11,244	3,568	2,8	2,2	786	4.8	39	51	59	87	83	5	31	5.4	4.0	-0.6
Burundi	12,551	6,655	2,054	3,1	2,3	438	5.1	43	48	62	95	90	5	14	5.6	4.6	-1.1
Cabo Verde	588	188	50	1,1	0,8	10	1.9	54	69	74	47	39	8	67	2.2	1.4	-2.2
Cambodia	16,589	5,756	1,613	1,4	0,9	321	2.3	39	59	70	53	45	8	25	2.7	2.5	-1.5
Cameroon	27,199	13,339	4,346	2,7	2,3	951	4.5	48	53	60	82	77	5	58	3.8	3.1	-0.4
Canada	38,155	7,215	1,901	1,0	0,7	374	1.5	73	79	83	52	24	28	82	1.1	0.9	5.1
Central African Republic	5,457	3,045	985	1,7	2,6	235	6.0	45	45	54	103	98	5	43	2.2	3.7	-15.6
Chad	17,180	9,343	3,218	3,3	2,7	745	6.3	41	47	53	99	95	4	24	3.7	4.0	0.5
Chile	19,493	4,313	1,151	1,1	0,3	229	1.5	62	77	79	45	27	18	88	1.2	0.4	5.9
China	1,425,893	300,092	74,790	0,6	-0,1	10,882	1.2	57	72	78	45	26	19	63	3.1	1.2	-0.1
Colombia	51,517	13,536	3,670	1,2	0,6	730	1.7	62	71	73	44	31	13	82	1.7	0.9	4.1
Comoros	822	363	114	1,9	1,6	24	4.0	45	59	63	74	67	7	30	2.2	2.5	-2.2
Congo	5,836	2,786	847	2,9	2,0	179	4.2	54	54	64	79	74	5	68	3.5	2.6	-0.8
Cook Islands	17	5	1	0,3	0,1	0	2.2	64	70	75	54	36	17	76	1.0	0.4	-9.4
Costa Rica	5,154	1,278	329	1,2	0,5	61	1.5	65	78	77	45	30	15	81	2.7	1.1	0.4
Côte d'Ivoire	27,478	13,379	4,202	2,2	2,2	933	4.4	44	51	59	79	75	4	52	3.1	3.1	-0.8
Croatia	4,060	691	180	-0,5	-0,6	35	1.5	69	75	78	57	22	34	58	-0.1	0.0	-2.6
Cuba	11,256	2,142	553	0,1	-0,2	100	1.4	68	76	74	46	23	23	77	0.2	-0.1	-0.6
Cyprus	1,244	236	67	1,3	0,5	13	1.3	69	77	81	44	23	21	67	1.1	0.7	1.6
Czechia	10,511	1,983	551	0,1	0,0	104	1.7	69	75	78	57	25	32	74	0.1	0.2	0.3
Democratic People's Republic of Korea	25,972	5,940	1,700	0,5	0,2	344	1.8	61	61	73	43	27	16	63	0.7	0.7	-0.1
Democratic Republic of the Congo	95,894	50,791	17,698	3,1	2,9	4,035	6.2	43	52	59	98	92	6	46	4.3	4.0	-0.7
Denmark	5,854	1,152	310	0,4	0,4	63	1.7	73	77	81	57	25	32	88	0.6	0.6	3.9
Djibouti	1,106	409	116	1,8	1,2	25	2.8	48	57	62	54	48	7	78	1.9	1.4	0.7
Dominica	72	18	5	0,2	0,4	1	1.6	65	73	73	41	28	13	71	0.7	0.8	0.8
Dominican Republic	11,118	3,626	1,015	1,2	0,8	205	2.3	56	69	73	53	42	11	83	2.6	1.3	-1.3
Ecuador	17,798	5,584	1,492	1,6	0,9	299	2.0	57	73	74	51	39	12	64	1.9	1.3	2.0
Egypt	109,262	41,988	12,368	1,9	1,4	2,465	2.9	50	68	70	61	53	8	43	1.9	1.8	-0.3
El Salvador	6,314	1,967	508	0,3	0,4	101	1.8	51	70	71	51	39	12	74	1.3	1.1	-4.3
Equatorial Guinea	1,634	722	230	4,0	2,0	50	4.3	30	53	61	72	67	5	74	5.9	2.5	4.0
Eritrea	3,620	1,712	486	1,9	1,7	104	3.9	41	56	67	78	71	7	42	4.0	3.0	-4.1
Estonia	1,329	260	71	-0,2	-0,3	14	1.7	70	71	77	58	26	32	69	-0.2	0.0	2.3
Eswatini	1,192	493	140	0,6	0,9	29	2.8	51	47	57	64	57	7	24	0.9	1.8	-4.1
Ethiopia	120,283	56,315	17,798	2,7	2,2	3,896	4.2	43	51	65	76	70	6	22	4.5	4.1	0.0

132   THE STATE OF THE WORLD'S CHILDREN 2023

TABLE 1. DEMOGRAPHICS

Countries and areas	Population (thousands) 2021			Annual population growth rate (%)		Annual number of births (thousands) 2021	Total fertility (live births per woman) 2021	Life expectancy at birth (years)			Dependency ratio (%) 2021			Share of urban population (%) 2021	Annual growth rate of urban population (%)		Net migration rate (per 1,000 population) 2021
	Total	Under 18	Under 5	2000–2020	2020–2030 ᴬ			1970	2000	2021	Total dependency ratio	Child dependency ratio	Old age dependency ratio		2000–2020	2020–2030 ᴬ	
Fiji	925	316	90	0,5	0,6	18	2.5	62	66	67	53	44	9	58	1.3	1.3	-6.5
Finland	5,536	1,036	244	0,3	0,1	47	1.4	70	78	82	62	25	37	86	0.5	0.2	2.7
France	64,531	13,568	3,408	0,5	0,1	677	1.8	72	79	82	63	28	35	81	0.8	0.4	0.3
Gabon	2,341	985	307	2,8	1,7	64	3.5	53	61	66	68	61	7	90	3.4	2.0	0.6
Gambia	2,640	1,331	412	2,8	2,2	88	4.7	40	57	62	85	80	5	63	4.1	3.0	-0.7
Georgia	3,758	920	261	-0,6	-0,3	50	2.1	64	70	72	55	33	23	60	0.0	0.4	-0.7
Germany	83,409	13,836	3,971	0,1	-0,1	763	1.5	71	78	81	56	22	35	78	0.3	0.1	3.8
Ghana	32,833	14,291	4,306	2,3	1,7	905	3.6	48	58	64	69	63	6	58	3.6	2.6	-0.3
Greece	10,445	1,794	433	-0,2	-0,4	79	1.4	73	78	80	58	22	35	80	0.2	-0.1	-1.4
Grenada	125	35	10	0,7	0,5	2	2.0	66	73	75	51	36	15	37	0.8	1.0	-0.7
Guatemala	17,608	6,930	1,927	1,9	1,3	372	2.4	49	67	69	61	53	8	52	2.5	2.1	-1.7
Guinea	13,532	6,562	2,097	2,2	2,1	466	4.4	39	52	59	82	76	6	37	3.0	3.1	-0.3
Guinea-Bissau	2,061	975	295	2,3	1,9	64	4.0	38	50	60	77	72	5	45	3.3	2.7	-0.7
Guyana	805	275	79	0,2	0,6	16	2.4	60	64	66	54	44	9	27	-0.1	1.1	-5.4
Haiti	11,448	4,397	1,277	1,4	1,1	269	2.8	47	58	63	58	51	7	58	3.7	2.2	-2.9
Holy See	1	-	-	-1,1	0,7	0	1.0	71	79	82	-	-	-	-	-	-	0.0
Honduras	10,278	3,784	1,056	2,0	1,3	217	2.4	54	69	70	53	47	6	59	3.2	2.2	-0.6
Hungary	9,710	1,707	468	-0,2	-0,1	92	1.6	69	72	75	54	22	31	72	0.3	0.3	2.0
Iceland	370	83	22	1,3	0,6	5	1.7	74	80	83	50	28	22	94	1.3	0.6	1.7
India	1,407,564	438,164	115,307	1,3	0,7	23,114	2.0	48	63	67	48	38	10	35	2.4	2.0	-0.2
Indonesia	273,753	83,188	22,414	1,1	0,7	4,496	2.2	53	66	68	48	38	10	57	2.6	1.6	-0.1
Iran (Islamic Republic of)	87,923	24,425	6,896	1,4	0,6	1,204	1.7	50	70	74	45	35	11	76	2.2	1.1	0.3
Iraq	43,534	19,352	5,691	2,6	2,0	1,192	3.5	60	67	70	71	65	6	71	2.8	2.3	-1.4
Ireland	4,987	1,189	305	1,3	0,6	59	1.8	71	77	82	53	31	23	64	1.6	1.0	3.1
Israel	8,900	2,930	890	1,7	1,3	174	3.0	71	79	82	67	47	20	93	1.8	1.4	1.9
Italy	59,240	9,203	2,161	0,2	-0,3	410	1.3	72	80	83	57	20	37	71	0.5	0.1	0.5
Jamaica	2,828	712	169	0,4	-0,1	33	1.4	67	71	71	38	28	10	57	0.8	0.6	-2.0
Japan	124,613	17,962	4,286	-0,1	-0,5	819	1.3	72	81	85	71	20	51	92	0.7	-0.4	0.7
Jordan	11,148	4,289	1,195	3,7	0,8	245	2.8	60	72	74	57	51	6	92	4.4	1.0	1.3
Kazakhstan	19,196	6,498	2,009	1,0	1,0	413	3.1	61	64	69	60	47	13	58	1.2	1.3	-1.0
Kenya	53,006	24,050	6,913	2,5	1,8	1,468	3.3	54	54	61	70	65	5	28	4.1	3.4	-1.0
Kiribati	129	53	17	1,7	1,5	4	3.3	55	64	67	66	60	6	56	2.9	2.5	-2.3
Kuwait	4,250	1,043	259	3,9	0,4	44	2.1	67	77	79	34	28	6	100	3.9	0.4	-8.6
Kyrgyzstan	6,528	2,574	805	1,3	1,3	158	3.0	58	65	70	64	56	7	37	1.5	2.3	-2.5
Lao People's Democratic Republic	7,425	2,739	790	1,4	1,2	163	2.5	44	58	68	55	48	7	37	3.8	2.7	-1.4
Latvia	1,874	348	93	-1,1	-1,0	17	1.6	70	70	74	59	25	34	68	-1.1	-0.8	-3.6
Lebanon	5,593	1,847	445	1,3	-1,7	84	2.1	67	74	75	59	44	15	89	1.4	-1.5	-20.4
Lesotho	2,281	916	275	0,6	0,9	60	3.0	51	48	53	62	55	7	29	2.5	2.4	-0.7
Liberia	5,193	2,492	745	2,7	1,9	163	4.1	41	51	61	80	74	6	53	3.5	2.8	-2.3
Libya	6,735	2,332	614	1,2	1,0	120	2.5	55	71	72	51	44	7	81	1.5	1.3	-0.1
Liechtenstein	39	7	2	0,8	0,5	0	1.5	65	77	83	50	22	28	14	0.5	1.2	5.9
Lithuania	2,787	499	140	-1,2	-0,9	27	1.6	71	72	74	56	24	32	68	-1.1	-0.5	-4.2
Luxembourg	639	122	33	1,8	0,9	7	1.4	70	78	83	44	23	21	92	2.2	1.1	10.9
Madagascar	28,916	13,292	4,151	2,6	2,1	895	3.9	48	58	64	75	69	6	39	4.3	3.6	0.0
Malawi	19,890	10,052	3,034	2,6	2,3	654	3.9	37	45	63	85	80	5	18	3.4	3.9	-0.1
Malaysia	33,574	9,311	2,572	1,8	0,9	511	1.8	63	73	75	43	33	10	78	2.8	1.4	1.4
Maldives	521	132	38	2,9	0,0	7	1.7	45	71	80	36	29	6	41	4.7	0.9	2.3
Mali	21,905	11,904	4,004	3,0	2,7	913	6.0	33	51	59	99	94	5	45	5.1	4.1	-1.0
Malta	527	82	24	1,2	0,5	5	1.2	69	78	84	47	19	28	95	1.3	0.5	20.0
Marshall Islands	42	16	4	-1,1	0,3	1	2.7	59	63	65	60	53	7	78	-0.5	0.6	-44.2
Mauritania	4,615	2,252	695	2,4	2,4	153	4.4	51	61	64	83	77	6	56	4.2	3.5	-0.3
Mauritius	1,299	272	66	0,3	0,1	13	1.4	61	72	74	41	23	17	41	0.1	0.3	-0.4
Mexico	126,705	38,144	9,893	1,2	0,6	1,882	1.8	61	74	70	49	37	12	81	1.6	0.9	-0.4
Micronesia (Federated States of)	113	42	11	0,0	0,8	2	2.7	61	70	71	58	48	9	23	0.1	1.6	-5.6
Monaco	37	6	2	0,6	-0,3	0	2.1	73	82	86	95	25	70	100	0.6	-0.3	5.6
Mongolia	3,348	1,220	380	1,4	1,1	72	2.8	53	63	71	58	51	7	69	2.3	1.4	0.0
Montenegro	628	136	37	0,0	-0,1	7	1.7	69	74	76	53	28	25	68	0.6	0.3	-0.2
Montserrat	4	1	0	-0,6	-0,4	0	1.6	64	75	76	44	19	25	9	6.4	0.3	-9.0
Morocco	37,077	11,779	3,285	1,2	0,8	651	2.3	49	67	74	52	41	11	64	2.0	1.5	-1.2
Mozambique	32,077	16,168	5,260	2,7	2,5	1,174	4.6	42	49	59	86	81	5	38	3.8	3.8	-0.3
Myanmar	53,798	16,125	4,491	0,8	0,6	920	2.2	51	60	66	46	36	10	31	1.4	1.6	-0.7
Namibia	2,530	1,060	333	1,5	1,4	69	3.3	54	52	59	67	61	7	53	3.8	2.8	-1.7
Nauru	13	6	2	0,8	0,7	0	3.5	60	59	64	70	66	4	100	0.8	0.7	-5.3

FOR EVERY CHILD, VACCINATION

TABLE 1. DEMOGRAPHICS

Countries and areas	Population (thousands) 2021			Annual population growth rate (%)		Annual number of births (thou-sands) 2021	Total fertility (live births per woman) 2021	Life expectancy at birth (years)			Dependency ratio (%) 2021			Share of urban population (%) 2021	Annual growth rate of urban population (%)		Net migration rate (per 1,000 population) 2021
	Total	Under 18	Under 5	2000–2020	2020–2030 ^			1970	2000	2021	Total depen-dency ratio	Child depen-dency ratio	Old age depen-dency ratio		2000–2020	2020–2030 ^	
Nepal	30,035	10,742	2,952	0,8	1,1	610	2.0	43	63	68	55	46	9	21	2.9	3.0	9.9
Netherlands (Kingdom of the)	17,502	3,309	866	0,4	0,3	180	1.6	74	78	82	55	24	31	93	1.3	0.5	3.3
New Zealand	5,130	1,159	310	1,3	0,7	64	1.8	71	79	82	53	29	24	87	1.3	0.9	7.5
Nicaragua	6,851	2,451	698	1,3	1,2	141	2.3	55	67	74	54	46	8	59	1.6	1.7	-1.5
Niger	25,253	14,056	4,972	3,5	3,4	1,144	6.8	36	49	62	105	100	5	17	3.6	4.4	-0.2
Nigeria	213,401	106,611	34,831	2,5	2,1	7,923	5.2	40	47	53	86	81	6	53	4.4	3.3	-0.4
Niue	2	1	0	-0,3	0,0	0	2.4	64	67	71	70	45	25	47	1.3	1.2	-2.0
North Macedonia	2,103	408	105	0,2	-0,2	20	1.4	64	73	74	45	23	21	59	0.2	0.5	-0.2
Norway	5,403	1,108	280	0,9	0,6	54	1.5	74	79	83	54	26	28	83	1.3	0.9	2.0
Oman	4,520	1,369	443	3,2	1,0	83	2.6	48	73	73	42	38	4	87	4.0	1.6	-4.6
Pakistan	231,402	100,538	29,604	1,8	1,7	6,375	3.5	55	62	66	70	63	7	37	2.4	2.5	-2.0
Palau	18	5	1	-0,4	0,0	0	2.4	56	66	66	44	30	14	81	0.2	0.4	0.2
Panama	4,351	1,366	385	1,7	1,1	77	2.3	65	74	76	54	41	13	69	2.2	1.6	1.3
Papua New Guinea	9,949	4,057	1,207	2,7	1,6	254	3.2	52	62	65	60	55	5	13	2.8	2.8	1.1
Paraguay	6,704	2,305	682	1,2	1,0	138	2.5	63	70	70	54	45	10	62	1.8	1.5	-1.2
Peru	33,715	10,639	2,917	1,1	0,9	594	2.2	47	70	72	53	40	13	79	1.4	1.1	2.0
Philippines	113,880	41,441	11,923	1,7	1,3	2,485	2.7	62	69	69	56	48	8	48	1.9	2.0	-0.7
Poland	38,308	6,982	1,908	0,0	0,1	363	1.5	70	74	76	52	23	29	60	-0.1	0.3	-0.1
Portugal	10,290	1,690	433	0,0	-0,2	80	1.4	67	77	81	56	21	35	67	0.9	0.5	2.7
Qatar	2,688	475	145	6,9	0,3	27	1.8	67	75	79	21	19	2	99	7.1	0.3	-11.4
Republic of Korea	51,830	7,517	1,651	0,5	-0,1	289	0.9	62	76	84	40	17	23	81	0.6	0.0	0.8
Republic of Moldova	3,062	709	202	-1,5	0,3	38	1.8	64	66	69	50	30	20	43	-1.7	0.8	-4.7
Romania	19,329	3,722	1,029	-0,6	-0,2	195	1.7	68	71	74	54	25	29	54	-0.5	0.2	-0.7
Russian Federation	145,103	30,178	7,890	0,0	-0,3	1,397	1.5	68	65	69	50	27	23	75	0.1	0.0	2.2
Rwanda	13,462	6,162	1,889	2,3	2,0	404	3.8	47	47	66	73	67	5	18	3.0	3.1	-0.5
Saint Kitts and Nevis	48	11	3	0,2	0,1	1	1.5	61	70	72	42	28	14	31	-0.1	0.6	-1.9
Saint Lucia	180	40	10	0,6	0,2	2	1.4	64	71	71	38	25	13	19	-1.3	0.9	0.0
Saint Vincent and the Grenadines	104	27	7	-0,4	0,0	1	1.8	69	71	70	49	33	16	53	0.4	0.7	-3.6
Samoa	219	96	29	0,7	1,3	6	3.9	60	71	73	75	66	9	18	-0.2	1.0	-4.0
San Marino	34	5	1	1,1	-0,1	0	1.1	74	80	81	50	20	30	98	1.3	-0.1	1.2
Sao Tome and Principe	223	105	30	2,0	1,7	6	3.8	57	62	68	78	71	7	75	3.6	2.4	-3.5
Saudi Arabia	35,950	11,026	3,187	2,4	1,1	629	2.4	53	72	77	40	37	4	85	2.7	1.3	-4.3
Senegal	16,877	8,168	2,571	2,5	2,3	550	4.4	41	57	67	82	76	6	49	3.4	3.2	-0.6
Serbia	7,297	1,253	345	-0,4	-0,7	68	1.5	66	71	74	54	22	32	57	0.0	-0.2	0.0
Seychelles	106	29	9	1,3	0,5	2	2.3	58	70	71	45	34	11	58	1.9	1.1	1.4
Sierra Leone	8,421	3,880	1,188	2,8	1,9	264	4.0	39	45	60	74	69	5	43	3.7	2.8	-0.2
Singapore	5,941	860	246	1,8	0,5	42	1.0	69	79	83	35	16	19	100	1.8	0.5	3.3
Slovakia	5,448	1,026	289	0,1	0,2	54	1.6	70	73	75	49	24	26	54	-0.1	0.5	0.3
Slovenia	2,119	380	101	0,3	-0,1	19	1.6	68	76	81	55	24	32	55	0.7	0.5	2.2
Solomon Islands	708	323	101	2,3	1,9	21	4.0	56	67	70	75	69	6	25	4.4	3.5	-1.1
Somalia	17,066	9,212	3,200	3,0	2,7	744	6.3	46	51	55	99	94	5	47	4.6	3.8	-1.0
South Africa	59,392	19,961	5,813	1,1	0,9	1,177	2.4	56	58	62	53	44	9	68	1.9	1.5	0.2
South Sudan	10,748	5,621	1,486	2,6	1,5	313	4.5	26	46	55	91	85	5	21	3.6	3.2	-3.0
Spain	47,487	8,198	1,897	0,7	-0,1	358	1.3	72	79	83	52	21	30	81	1.0	0.2	5.8
Sri Lanka	21,773	6,120	1,562	0,7	0,2	306	2.0	65	70	76	52	35	17	19	0.8	1.3	-4.2
State of Palestine	5,133	2,339	712	2,2	2,0	145	3.5	55	70	73	74	68	6	77	2.5	2.4	-2.4
Sudan	45,657	21,570	7,084	2,5	2,3	1,534	4.5	46	58	65	80	74	6	36	2.9	3.3	-0.3
Suriname	613	195	54	1,1	0,8	11	2.3	60	66	70	51	40	11	66	1.1	1.0	-0.8
Sweden	10,467	2,215	595	0,7	0,5	113	1.7	75	80	83	61	28	32	88	1.0	0.8	7.7
Switzerland	8,691	1,560	436	0,9	0,5	87	1.5	73	80	84	52	23	29	74	0.9	0.7	2.8
Syrian Arab Republic	21,324	8,679	1,892	1,2	3,3	427	2.7	61	71	72	60	53	7	56	1.5	4.3	10.0
Tajikistan	9,750	4,093	1,269	2,0	1,6	261	3.2	57	63	72	66	60	6	28	2.2	2.7	-0.4
Thailand	71,601	13,764	3,379	0,6	0,1	644	1.3	58	72	79	43	23	21	52	2.9	1.2	0.0
Timor-Leste	1,321	562	157	1,9	1,3	33	3.1	37	59	68	68	59	9	32	3.1	2.3	-1.5
Togo	8,645	4,035	1,270	2,5	2,0	275	4.3	46	55	62	77	71	5	43	3.7	3.2	-0.1
Tokelau	2	1	0	0,4	1,0	0	2.7	62	72	75	60	47	13	0	-	-	0.0
Tonga	106	44	12	0,1	0,7	2	3.2	63	69	71	69	59	10	23	0.1	1.0	-8.9
Trinidad and Tobago	1,526	353	92	0,6	0,2	18	1.6	65	69	73	44	28	16	53	0.4	0.4	1.7
Tunisia	12,263	3,574	1,035	1,0	0,7	197	2.1	54	74	74	51	38	13	70	1.4	1.1	-0.7
Türkiye	84,775	23,673	6,610	1,3	0,5	1,245	1.9	57	72	76	47	34	12	77	2.1	1.0	-0.8
Turkmenistan	6,342	2,282	688	1,5	1,1	137	2.7	58	65	69	57	49	8	53	2.1	2.0	-0.7
Turks and Caicos Islands	45	9	3	4,1	0,8	1	1.7	56	74	75	37	23	14	94	4.6	1.0	15.2
Tuvalu	11	4	1	0,7	0,7	0	3.2	55	63	65	61	51	10	65	2.2	1.5	-1.3

134   THE STATE OF THE WORLD'S CHILDREN 2023

TABLE 1. DEMOGRAPHICS

Countries and areas	Population (thousands) 2021			Annual population growth rate (%)		Annual number of births (thousands) 2021	Total fertility (live births per woman) 2021	Life expectancy at birth (years)			Dependency ratio (%) 2021			Share of urban population (%) 2021	Annual growth rate of urban population (%)		Net migration rate (per 1,000 population) 2021
	Total	Under 18	Under 5	2000–2020	2020–2030 ^A			1970	2000	2021	Total dependency ratio	Child dependency ratio	Old age dependency ratio		2000–2020	2020–2030 ^A	
Uganda	45,854	24,092	7,690	2,9	2,5	1,687	4.6	50	48	63	88	85	3	26	5.4	4.5	0.9
Ukraine	43,531	7,898	1,798	-0,5	-1,2	336	1.3	69	68	72	48	23	26	70	-0.3	-1.0	0.0
United Arab Emirates	9,365	1,599	482	5,0	0,7	97	1.5	60	74	79	20	18	2	87	5.4	0.9	-0.3
United Kingdom	67,281	14,169	3,652	0,6	0,3	677	1.6	72	78	81	58	28	30	84	0.9	0.5	3.0
United Republic of Tanzania	63,588	32,079	10,537	2,8	2,6	2,303	4.7	46	52	66	88	82	6	36	4.9	4.3	-0.1
United States	336,998	74,735	19,164	0,8	0,4	3,723	1.7	71	77	77	54	28	26	83	1.0	0.7	1.7
Uruguay	3,426	811	195	0,2	0,0	36	1.5	69	75	75	54	30	24	96	0.4	0.1	-0.4
Uzbekistan	34,081	11,809	3,847	1,4	1,2	803	2.9	61	66	71	54	46	8	50	1.8	1.5	-1.2
Vanuatu	319	145	45	2,3	2,1	9	3.7	55	69	70	76	70	7	26	3.1	2.7	-0.6
Venezuela (Bolivarian Republic of)	28,200	9,560	2,396	0,7	1,1	452	2.2	64	72	71	58	44	13	88	0.8	1.1	-18.5
Viet Nam	97,468	26,183	7,368	1,0	0,6	1,463	1.9	56	72	74	46	33	13	38	3.0	2.1	0.0
Yemen	32,982	15,348	4,714	2,6	1,9	1,009	3.8	41	63	64	74	69	5	39	4.4	3.4	-3.1
Zambia	19,473	9,768	3,073	3,1	2,4	672	4.3	51	45	61	82	79	3	45	4.3	3.5	0.5
Zimbabwe	15,994	7,622	2,300	1,3	1,8	489	3.5	57	45	59	79	73	6	32	1.1	2.4	-1.6
SUMMARY																	
East Asia and Pacific	2,351,075	544,718	141,163	0,7	0,2	24,171	1.5	57	72	76	47	28	18	61	2.5	1.1	0.0
Europe and Central Asia	921,948	196,265	52,835	0,3	0,1	10,098	1.7	68	72	76	54	28	26	73	0.6	0.4	1.4
Eastern Europe and Central Asia	425,237	104,630	29,039	0,3	0,1	5,528	1.9	64	67	71	51	32	19	67	0.6	0.4	0.2
Western Europe	496,711	91,635	23,795	0,3	0,0	4,570	1.5	71	78	81	56	24	32	77	0.6	0.3	2.4
Latin America and Caribbean	651,297	185,463	49,512	1,1	0,6	9,662	1.9	58	71	72	48	35	13	81	1.4	0.9	-0.4
Middle East and North Africa	484,290	170,267	49,223	1,9	1,3	9,763	2.7	51	69	73	55	47	8	66	2.5	1.6	-0.8
North America	375,153	81,950	21,066	0,8	0,5	4,097	1.6	71	77	78	54	28	26	83	1.0	0.7	2.0
South Asia	1,901,529	631,014	170,669	1,4	0,9	34,882	2.2	48	63	67	51	42	10	35	2.5	2.2	-0.5
Sub-Saharan Africa	1,182,308	575,568	185,103	2,6	2,2	40,950	4.6	44	51	60	82	77	6	42	3.9	3.4	-0.4
Eastern and Southern Africa	608,005	286,706	90,099	2,5	2,1	19,573	4.1	47	51	63	78	72	6	36	3.6	3.3	-0.2
West and Central Africa	574,303	288,861	95,003	2,7	2,3	21,377	5.2	41	50	57	87	82	5	48	4.1	3.4	-0.6
Least developed countries	1,099,569	500,147	157,433	2,3	2,0	34,449	4.0	43	55	64	74	68	6	35	3.9	3.4	-0.5
World	**7,909,295**	**2,392,419**	**671,477**	**1,2**	**0,8**	**133,975**	**2.3**	**56**	**66**	**71**	**54**	**39**	**15**	**57**	**2.0**	**1.4**	**0.0**

For a complete list of countries and areas in the regions, subregions and country categories, see page on Regional Classifications or visit <data.unicef.org/regionalclassifications>.

It is not advisable to compare data from consecutive editions of *The State of the World's Children* report.

Sex disaggregated data available at United Nations, Department of Economic and Social Affairs, Population Division (2022). *2022 Revision of World Population Prospects.*

NOTES

- Data not available.

Regional and global values are based on more countries and areas than listed here. Therefore, country values don't add up to the corresponding regional values and global value.

^A Based on medium-fertility variant projections.

MAIN DATA SOURCES

All demographic data – United Nations, Department of Economic and Social Affairs, Population Division (2022). *2022 Revision of World Population Prospects.*

Urban data – United Nations Department of Economic and Social Affairs, Population Division, World Urbanization Prospects: The 2018 revision. Adjusted based on the *2022 Revision of World Population Prospects.*

Last update – December 2022.

DEFINITIONS OF THE INDICATORS

Population (thousands) – Total population

Annual population growth rate – Average exponential rate of growth of the population over one year. It is calculated as ln(Pt/P0)/T where P0 is the population at the beginning of the time period, Pt the population at the end of the time period, and T the length of the period. It is expressed as a percentage.

Annual number of births – Annual number of births for the reference year. Data are presented in thousands.

Total fertility – The average number of live births a hypothetical cohort of women would have at the end of their reproductive period if they were subject during their whole lives to the fertility rates of a given period and if they were not subject to mortality. It is expressed as live births per woman.

Dependency ratios – The total dependency ratio is the ratio of the sum of the population aged 0–14 and that aged 65+ to the population aged 15–64. The child dependency ratio is the ratio of the population aged 0–14 to the population aged 15–64. The old-age dependency ratio is the ratio of the population aged 65 years or over to the population aged 15–64. All ratios are presented as number of dependants per 100 persons of working age (15–64).

Life expectancy at birth – Number of years newborn children would live if subject to the mortality risks prevailing for the cross section of population at the time of their birth.

Share of urban population – Urban population as a percentage of the total population.

Annual growth rate of urban population – Average annual exponential rate of growth of the urban population over a given period, expressed as a percentage.

Net migration rate – The number of immigrants minus the number of emigrants over a period, divided by the person-years lived by the population of the receiving country over that period. It is expressed as net number of migrants per 1,000 population.

FOR EVERY CHILD, VACCINATION

135

TABLE 2. CHILD MORTALITY

Countries and areas	Under-five mortality rate			Annual rate of reduction in under-five mortality rate	Under-five mortality rate 2021		Infant mortality rate		Neonatal mortality rate			Mortality rate among children aged 5–14 years		Stillbirth rate		Annual rate of reduction in stillbirth rate	Under-five deaths	Neonatal deaths	Neonatal deaths as a percentage of under-five deaths	Deaths among children aged 5–14 years	Stillbirths
	1990	2000	2021	2000–2021	Male	Female	1990	2021	1990	2000	2021	1990	2021	2000	2021	2000–2021	2021	2021	2021	2021	2021
Afghanistan	178	129	56	4.0	59	52	121	43	74	61	34	19	4	35	26	1.5	77,811	49,061	63	4,396	37,980
Albania	41	27	9	5.0	10	9	35	8	13	12	7	6	2	7	4	2.3	279	209	75	59	128
Algeria	52	42	22	3.0	24	21	44	19	24	22	16	9	3	20	10	3.5	21,567	14,888	69	2,475	9,429
Andorra	13	8	3	4.8	3	2	9	3	7	4	1	3	1	4	2	2.3	2	1	50	0	1
Angola	224	205	69	5.2	75	63	132	47	54	50	27	55	16	28	19	1.8	89,896	35,644	40	15,451	26,351
Anguilla	17	10	4	4.1	4	4	14	4	9	5	2	3	1	-	-	-	1	0	0	0	-
Antigua and Barbuda	14	16	6	4.4	7	6	11	5	8	10	3	3	2	9	5	2.6	7	4	57	2	6
Argentina	29	20	7	5.0	8	6	25	6	15	11	5	3	1	8	4	2.8	4,410	3,232	73	1,064	2,719
Armenia	49	31	11	5.0	12	10	42	10	23	16	6	3	2	20	11	3.0	372	190	51	74	369
Australia	9	6	4	2.4	4	3	8	3	5	4	2	2	1	4	2	2.1	1,111	706	64	239	714
Austria	10	6	4	1.9	4	3	8	3	5	3	2	2	1	3	2	0.7	308	198	64	64	207
Azerbaijan	95	75	19	6.6	20	17	76	17	31	34	10	6	3	19	9	3.7	2,435	1,210	50	553	1,117
Bahamas	23	16	13	1.0	14	12	20	11	14	8	7	4	2	12	11	0.4	61	33	54	13	53
Bahrain	23	12	7	2.8	7	7	20	6	15	5	3	4	2	8	6	1.7	128	52	41	36	102
Bangladesh	146	86	27	5.5	29	25	101	23	66	44	16	24	5	41	21	3.3	82,081	48,319	59	13,637	63,199
Barbados	18	15	12	1.1	13	11	16	11	12	9	8	3	2	8	8	0.5	36	24	67	5	23
Belarus	15	13	3	7.4	3	2	12	2	10	5	1	4	1	5	2	4.1	251	78	31	122	195
Belgium	10	6	4	1.7	5	4	8	3	5	3	2	2	1	3	3	0.7	476	283	59	102	342
Belize	38	24	11	3.6	12	10	31	10	19	12	7	5	3	10	7	1.9	80	53	66	21	50
Benin	173	137	84	2.3	89	77	104	55	45	39	29	42	19	28	20	1.6	38,680	13,907	36	6,514	9,713
Bhutan	127	77	27	5.1	29	24	89	22	42	32	15	17	7	17	9	3.0	263	144	55	95	88
Bolivia (Plurinational State of)	121	76	25	5.3	27	22	84	20	41	29	13	12	4	16	9	2.7	6,484	3,477	54	988	2,333
Bosnia and Herzegovina	18	10	6	2.7	6	5	16	5	11	7	4	3	1	4	3	2.0	159	113	71	40	74
Botswana	45	74	35	3.6	38	31	34	28	18	8	18	19	7	11	15	-1.5	2,131	1,098	52	383	912
Brazil	63	35	14	4.2	16	13	53	13	26	19	8	4	2	10	7	1.8	40,107	23,391	58	6,566	19,411
British Virgin Islands	19	16	10	1.9	11	9	17	10	10	8	5	3	2	-	-	-	2	1	50	1	-
Brunei Darussalam	13	10	11	-0.5	12	10	10	10	6	5	6	4	2	5	5	0.2	72	38	53	13	30
Bulgaria	18	17	6	4.8	7	6	15	5	8	8	3	4	2	8	5	1.6	377	175	46	106	317
Burkina Faso	199	179	83	3.7	87	78	99	52	46	41	25	38	17	29	20	1.7	63,466	19,832	31	10,688	16,351
Burundi	170	155	53	5.1	57	48	103	38	39	37	20	59	19	29	18	2.2	22,715	8,943	39	7,263	8,130
Cabo Verde	60	38	14	4.9	15	12	47	12	20	19	8	6	2	15	9	2.2	136	84	62	20	92
Cambodia	116	106	25	6.9	28	22	85	21	40	35	13	32	4	25	11	3.7	8,013	4,119	51	1,431	3,705
Cameroon	136	144	70	3.5	75	64	85	47	40	35	26	32	21	24	19	1.1	64,977	24,360	37	15,529	18,288
Canada	8	6	5	1.0	5	5	7	4	4	4	3	2	1	3	3	0.7	1,873	1,274	68	368	1,041
Central African Republic	177	166	100	2.4	107	93	115	75	51	43	32	30	23	31	26	0.8	22,387	7,483	33	3,924	6,337
Chad	212	184	107	2.6	114	100	112	66	52	44	32	49	23	32	25	1.2	76,471	24,070	31	11,491	19,317
Chile	19	11	7	2.4	7	6	16	6	9	6	4	3	1	4	3	2.2	1,492	981	66	308	609
China	54	37	7	7.9	7	7	43	5	30	21	3	7	2	15	5	5.3	88,271	34,850	39	31,781	53,551
Colombia	36	25	13	3.2	14	11	29	11	18	14	7	5	2	9	7	1.2	9,382	5,106	54	1,748	5,255
Comoros	126	96	50	3.2	52	47	89	39	50	40	26	16	5	30	24	0.9	1,192	622	52	109	600
Congo	91	114	43	4.6	47	39	60	32	27	30	18	31	7	21	16	1.4	7,604	3,297	43	1,050	2,868
Cook Islands	24	18	7	4.4	7	7	20	6	13	10	4	5	2	10	5	3.4	2	1	50	0	1
Costa Rica	17	13	8	2.6	8	7	14	6	9	8	5	3	2	5	4	0.8	479	328	68	121	260
Côte d'Ivoire	153	143	75	3.1	83	67	104	56	49	46	32	28	24	30	22	1.4	68,056	30,095	44	17,524	21,042
Croatia	13	8	5	2.8	5	4	11	4	8	6	3	3	1	5	3	2.5	165	97	59	50	105
Cuba	14	9	5	2.7	5	4	11	4	7	4	2	4	2	11	7	2.2	526	239	45	222	703
Cyprus	11	7	3	4.1	3	3	10	2	6	4	2	2	1	4	3	2.5	36	21	58	15	33
Czechia	12	5	3	3.3	3	2	10	2	7	3	1	2	1	3	3	0.2	293	150	51	97	285
Democratic People's Republic of Korea	43	60	15	6.5	17	14	33	10	22	27	8	8	3	15	8	2.9	5,297	2,835	54	1,122	2,878
Democratic Republic of the Congo	186	160	79	3.4	85	72	120	62	42	39	26	37	20	32	28	0.6	307,593	106,733	35	54,698	114,852
Denmark	9	6	4	2.2	4	3	7	3	4	3	2	2	1	3	2	2.4	222	156	70	41	121
Djibouti	118	101	54	2.9	59	49	92	46	49	44	30	26	12	36	27	1.4	1,316	725	55	279	674
Dominica	16	17	36	-3.6	39	33	13	32	10	13	28	4	3	11	15	-1.5	34	27	79	3	15
Dominican Republic	60	40	33	0.9	36	30	46	27	24	23	23	7	3	15	13	0.8	6,799	4,705	69	641	2,640
Ecuador	54	30	12	4.1	14	11	42	11	22	14	7	7	2	16	9	2.7	3,722	1,989	53	755	2,670
Egypt	86	47	19	4.3	20	18	63	16	33	22	10	11	4	17	9	3.0	46,892	24,704	53	9,740	22,876
El Salvador	60	33	12	4.7	14	11	46	11	23	15	6	6	4	20	9	3.9	1,268	618	49	422	906
Equatorial Guinea	179	156	77	3.4	83	70	121	57	50	46	28	35	15	19	15	1.1	3,768	1,416	38	634	758
Eritrea	153	85	38	3.8	43	33	94	29	35	27	17	41	7	21	16	1.4	3,892	1,799	46	674	1,704
Estonia	18	11	2	8.1	2	2	14	2	10	5	1	5	1	5	2	4.1	28	12	43	15	26
Eswatini	68	112	53	3.6	57	48	52	41	23	29	23	11	11	16	14	0.6	1,526	670	44	314	416

136   THE STATE OF THE WORLD'S CHILDREN 2023

TABLE 2. CHILD MORTALITY

Countries and areas	Under-five mortality rate			Annual rate of reduction in under-five mortality rate	Under-five mortality rate 2021		Infant mortality rate		Neonatal mortality rate			Mortality rate among children aged 5–14 years		Stillbirth rate		Annual rate of reduction in stillbirth rate	Under-five deaths	Neonatal deaths	Neonatal deaths as a percentage of under-five deaths	Deaths among children aged 5–14 years	Stillbirths
	1990	2000	2021	2000–2021	Male	Female	1990	2021	1990	2000	2021	1990	2021	2000	2021	2000–2021	2021	2021	2021	2021	2021
Ethiopia	201	140	47	5.2	52	41	120	34	59	48	26	74	7	33	21	2.2	177,737	101,951	57	21,616	81,798
Fiji	29	23	28	-1.0	30	25	24	23	13	10	14	12	5	10	9	0.6	501	247	49	88	165
Finland	7	4	2	3.2	2	2	6	2	4	2	1	2	1	3	2	1.5	102	60	59	44	91
France	9	5	4	1.0	5	4	7	3	4	3	3	2	1	5	3	2.3	2,985	1,713	57	564	2,083
Gabon	92	84	40	3.6	44	36	60	29	31	28	19	18	12	18	14	1.1	2,512	1,203	48	629	908
Gambia	167	114	48	4.1	53	43	81	34	50	40	25	33	10	27	21	1.3	4,138	2,221	54	730	1,887
Georgia	48	37	9	6.5	11	8	41	8	25	23	5	4	2	16	6	4.9	474	272	57	96	288
Germany	9	5	4	1.9	4	3	7	3	3	3	2	2	1	3	3	0.3	2,723	1,673	61	569	2,115
Ghana	128	100	44	3.9	48	39	80	33	42	36	23	25	10	28	21	1.3	39,423	20,641	52	8,049	19,787
Greece	10	6	4	2.6	4	3	9	3	6	4	2	2	1	5	3	1.8	299	178	60	78	245
Grenada	22	15	16	-0.2	17	15	18	14	12	8	10	5	4	9	9	-0.2	32	20	63	8	18
Guatemala	80	52	23	3.9	25	21	60	20	28	21	11	13	3	20	13	1.9	8,704	4,021	46	1,311	5,030
Guinea	233	166	99	2.5	106	91	138	64	62	46	31	43	18	30	23	1.2	44,995	14,486	32	6,529	11,089
Guinea-Bissau	223	174	74	4.1	80	68	132	50	64	55	34	45	13	46	31	1.8	4,693	2,197	47	722	2,064
Guyana	61	47	28	2.5	31	24	47	23	31	27	17	5	5	19	13	1.7	450	276	61	71	217
Haiti	145	104	59	2.7	64	53	100	45	39	30	24	28	12	21	18	0.8	15,748	6,540	42	2,904	4,859
Holy See	-	-	-	-	-	-	-	-	-	-	-	-	-	-	-	-	-	-	-	-	-
Honduras	58	37	17	3.9	18	15	45	14	22	18	10	9	5	14	8	2.7	3,570	2,059	58	1,012	1,797
Hungary	17	10	4	4.4	4	4	15	3	11	6	2	3	1	4	4	0.8	369	191	52	88	330
Iceland	6	4	3	2.0	3	2	5	2	3	2	1	2	1	3	2	2.0	12	6	50	3	8
India	127	92	31	5.2	30	31	89	25	57	45	19	21	4	30	12	4.2	709,366	441,801	62	100,307	286,482
Indonesia	84	52	22	4.1	24	20	62	19	31	23	11	13	5	15	9	2.5	100,012	50,931	51	22,469	41,163
Iran (Islamic Republic of)	57	36	13	5.0	13	12	45	11	25	19	8	14	3	12	7	2.6	15,806	9,719	61	4,456	8,746
Iraq	54	44	25	2.8	27	22	42	21	26	24	14	11	5	17	12	1.9	28,890	16,772	58	5,673	14,091
Ireland	9	7	3	3.9	3	3	8	3	5	4	2	2	1	5	3	3.2	187	121	65	41	148
Israel	12	7	3	3.4	4	3	10	3	6	4	2	2	1	4	3	2.1	589	302	51	126	480
Italy	10	6	3	3.6	3	2	8	2	6	3	1	2	1	3	2	1.1	1,081	604	56	333	915
Jamaica	28	21	12	2.5	14	11	23	11	18	17	10	4	3	18	14	1.2	414	342	83	103	483
Japan	6	5	2	3.2	2	2	5	2	3	2	1	2	1	3	2	2.3	1,930	667	35	758	1,292
Jordan	36	27	15	2.9	16	13	30	13	20	16	9	5	2	12	9	1.5	3,545	2,087	59	580	2,221
Kazakhstan	52	43	10	6.8	12	9	44	9	23	24	5	6	3	11	8	1.5	4,295	2,081	48	938	3,384
Kenya	102	99	37	4.7	40	34	65	28	27	27	18	16	9	20	19	0.3	54,038	27,040	50	12,259	27,720
Kiribati	92	68	48	1.6	52	44	67	38	35	28	21	15	9	18	14	1.1	168	73	43	28	50
Kuwait	18	13	9	1.8	10	8	15	7	10	7	5	5	2	7	5	1.0	434	217	50	114	242
Kyrgyzstan	65	50	17	5.0	19	15	54	16	24	20	12	6	3	11	6	2.5	2,774	1,881	68	390	1,018
Lao People's Democratic Republic	154	107	43	4.4	47	38	106	34	47	38	21	42	7	23	16	1.7	6,939	3,434	49	1,031	2,666
Latvia	17	14	4	6.4	4	3	13	3	8	7	2	5	1	6	3	2.7	65	35	54	19	58
Lebanon	32	20	8	4.2	9	8	27	7	20	12	5	6	2	11	6	2.9	724	404	56	216	505
Lesotho	84	107	73	1.8	79	66	68	57	39	36	35	16	8	37	27	1.5	4,312	2,100	49	423	1,632
Liberia	264	189	76	4.3	82	70	176	57	60	48	30	32	17	30	23	1.3	12,187	4,866	40	2,377	3,806
Libya	42	28	11	4.6	12	10	36	9	21	15	6	8	3	12	7	2.5	1,306	692	53	357	827
Liechtenstein	-	-	-	-	-	-	-	-	-	-	-	-	-	-	-	-	-	-	-	-	-
Lithuania	15	11	3	5.6	4	3	12	3	8	5	2	4	1	5	3	3.0	91	51	56	37	69
Luxembourg	9	5	3	2.4	3	2	7	2	4	2	2	2	0	4	4	-0.1	18	11	61	2	24
Madagascar	156	105	66	2.2	71	61	95	45	39	31	24	36	21	20	18	0.5	57,839	21,571	37	15,623	16,743
Malawi	245	174	42	6.8	46	37	142	31	51	39	19	38	12	22	16	1.5	26,800	12,608	47	6,771	10,668
Malaysia	17	10	8	1.4	8	7	14	6	8	5	4	5	2	5	5	-0.3	3,866	2,153	56	908	2,590
Maldives	86	39	6	9.0	6	5	63	5	39	22	4	9	1	15	5	5.4	44	30	68	11	36
Mali	231	188	97	3.1	102	92	120	62	67	51	33	40	21	32	23	1.5	85,222	30,484	36	13,891	21,858
Malta	11	8	6	1.3	6	5	10	5	8	5	4	1	1	4	3	1.3	27	18	67	4	14
Marshall Islands	47	42	30	1.7	33	26	38	25	18	19	14	9	6	14	11	0.9	26	11	42	6	9
Mauritania	117	99	40	4.2	45	36	71	32	45	39	23	20	8	25	17	1.9	6,070	3,463	57	1,014	2,604
Mauritius	23	19	17	0.6	18	15	20	15	15	12	11	3	2	13	10	0.9	223	142	64	26	140
Mexico	45	28	13	3.6	14	12	36	11	22	14	8	5	2	10	7	1.8	25,592	15,274	60	5,372	12,531
Micronesia (Federated States of)	49	38	25	2.1	28	22	39	21	24	20	13	9	5	14	11	1.2	58	31	53	12	27
Monaco	8	5	3	2.7	3	3	4	1	4	3	2	2	1	3	2	2.8	1	0	0	0	1
Mongolia	107	64	15	7.0	16	13	77	13	30	23	8	11	3	12	4	4.8	1,074	541	50	222	316
Montenegro	16	14	2	8.7	2	2	15	2	11	8	1	2	1	5	3	2.0	16	7	44	7	24
Montserrat	17	11	5	3.5	5	5	15	5	9	6	3	3	1	-	-	-	0	0	0	0	-
Morocco	81	52	18	5.1	20	16	64	15	37	28	11	9	2	21	13	2.1	11,788	7,239	61	1,626	8,722
Mozambique	246	171	70	4.3	74	65	163	51	62	47	28	61	13	25	17	1.8	79,353	32,279	41	11,828	20,723
Myanmar	115	89	42	3.6	46	38	82	34	48	37	22	29	4	20	15	1.6	38,581	19,939	52	3,763	13,579

FOR EVERY CHILD, VACCINATION

TABLE 2. CHILD MORTALITY

Countries and areas	Under-five mortality rate			Annual rate of reduction in under-five mortality rate	Under-five mortality rate 2021		Infant mortality rate		Neonatal mortality rate			Mortality rate among children aged 5–14 years		Stillbirth rate		Annual rate of reduction in stillbirth rate	Under-five deaths	Neonatal deaths	Neonatal deaths as a percentage of under-five deaths	Deaths among children aged 5–14 years	Stillbirths
	1990	2000	2021	2000–2021	Male	Female	1990	2021	1990	2000	2021	1990	2021	2000	2021	2000–2021	2021	2021	2021	2021	2021
Namibia	73	77	39	3.2	43	35	49	29	28	24	19	14	13	18	17	0.2	2,703	1,352	50	756	1,222
Nauru	67	43	28	2.1	30	25	51	23	32	26	18	12	6	14	12	0.9	10	6	60	2	4
Nepal	139	79	27	5.1	29	25	96	23	58	39	16	26	5	30	16	3.1	16,392	9,853	60	2,775	9,739
Netherlands (Kingdom of the)	8	6	4	2.0	4	4	7	4	5	4	3	2	1	5	2	4.0	713	482	68	133	402
New Zealand	11	7	5	2.1	5	4	9	4	4	4	3	3	1	4	3	1.6	297	162	55	67	167
Nicaragua	67	39	13	5.1	15	12	51	11	23	17	7	7	3	15	10	2.1	1,868	1,036	55	447	1,396
Niger	332	229	115	3.3	119	111	134	60	55	44	34	64	33	26	21	0.9	124,291	38,501	31	25,100	25,078
Nigeria	209	182	111	2.4	117	104	124	71	50	46	35	38	20	29	22	1.2	852,298	276,463	32	116,311	182,307
Niue	25	32	24	1.4	27	22	21	20	13	17	13	5	5	13	10	1.2	1	0	0	0	0
North Macedonia	37	16	5	5.2	6	5	33	5	17	9	3	3	2	11	4	5.0	108	69	64	35	77
Norway	9	5	2	3.8	2	2	7	2	4	3	1	2	1	4	2	2.7	117	69	59	41	113
Oman	39	16	10	2.3	11	9	32	9	17	7	5	8	2	8	6	1.4	870	380	44	180	474
Pakistan	140	108	63	2.5	68	59	107	53	64	57	39	14	8	38	31	1.0	399,429	251,307	63	42,924	203,374
Palau	35	28	16	2.7	18	14	30	15	19	15	9	7	4	10	7	1.6	4	2	50	0	2
Panama	31	26	14	3.0	15	12	26	12	18	15	8	5	3	12	8	2.1	1,067	596	56	232	582
Papua New Guinea	85	71	43	2.4	46	39	62	34	32	30	21	14	8	18	15	0.9	10,765	5,382	50	1,839	3,811
Paraguay	46	34	18	3.0	20	16	36	16	22	18	10	7	3	17	10	2.4	2,512	1,335	53	332	1,400
Peru	80	38	14	4.7	15	13	57	11	28	16	7	10	2	14	7	3.5	8,333	4,235	51	1,475	3,962
Philippines	57	38	26	1.8	28	23	40	20	19	17	12	8	5	14	10	1.5	63,392	30,500	48	10,575	25,531
Poland	17	9	4	3.6	5	4	15	4	11	6	3	3	1	4	3	2.4	1,614	1,005	62	376	941
Portugal	15	7	3	4.0	3	3	12	3	7	3	2	4	1	4	2	2.8	255	137	54	78	180
Qatar	21	12	5	4.1	6	5	18	5	11	7	3	4	1	7	3	4.1	152	88	58	37	73
Republic of Korea	16	8	3	4.6	3	3	13	2	7	3	1	4	1	3	2	2.8	860	400	47	341	505
Republic of Moldova	33	31	14	3.8	16	13	28	12	19	21	11	5	2	12	7	2.6	552	402	73	98	268
Romania	31	21	6	5.7	7	6	24	5	16	10	3	5	2	6	3	2.7	1,281	632	49	341	665
Russian Federation	22	19	5	6.4	6	5	17	4	11	9	2	5	2	7	3	3.4	7,347	2,857	39	3,103	4,616
Rwanda	150	185	39	7.4	43	36	92	30	41	44	18	62	15	28	17	2.5	15,638	7,070	45	5,184	6,876
Saint Kitts and Nevis	30	24	15	2.3	16	13	25	12	19	17	10	5	3	11	8	1.7	9	6	67	2	5
Saint Lucia	22	18	25	-1.4	27	22	18	22	12	12	13	5	3	14	11	0.9	52	27	52	7	23
Saint Vincent and the Grenadines	24	22	14	2.3	15	12	20	13	13	13	8	4	5	10	12	-0.7	19	11	58	7	16
Samoa	30	21	17	1.1	18	15	25	14	13	9	7	5	2	9	8	1.0	99	39	39	13	46
San Marino	14	6	2	5.6	2	2	12	2	7	3	1	3	1	3	2	2.8	0	0	0	0	0
Sao Tome and Principe	109	82	15	8.0	17	14	69	12	26	22	8	22	3	16	9	2.8	97	48	49	19	56
Saudi Arabia	44	22	7	5.7	7	7	35	6	22	12	3	8	2	9	4	3.3	4,350	2,060	47	1,018	2,680
Senegal	139	130	39	5.8	42	35	71	29	40	38	21	34	8	26	19	1.4	20,831	11,590	56	3,608	10,713
Serbia	28	13	5	4.0	6	5	24	5	17	8	4	3	1	5	5	0.4	374	240	64	80	327
Seychelles	16	14	14	0.0	15	13	14	12	11	9	9	4	2	9	9	-0.3	23	14	61	4	15
Sierra Leone	261	226	105	3.7	111	98	155	78	52	48	31	42	25	33	23	1.7	27,155	8,166	30	5,444	6,254
Singapore	8	4	2	2.9	2	2	6	2	4	2	1	2	1	3	2	2.2	87	32	37	29	79
Slovakia	15	10	6	2.6	6	5	13	5	9	5	3	3	1	4	3	1.2	312	152	49	69	168
Slovenia	10	5	2	4.4	2	2	9	2	6	3	1	2	1	4	3	1.6	42	24	57	15	49
Solomon Islands	38	31	19	2.3	20	17	31	16	15	13	8	7	4	12	9	1.4	393	160	41	73	196
Somalia	180	173	112	2.1	117	105	109	71	45	45	36	39	25	33	28	0.7	79,723	26,719	34	12,490	21,450
South Africa	62	71	33	3.7	35	30	48	26	22	17	11	7	6	21	16	1.2	38,868	12,979	33	6,240	19,337
South Sudan	251	182	99	2.9	104	94	149	64	64	56	40	54	22	31	26	0.9	31,312	12,408	40	7,502	8,312
Spain	9	5	3	2.7	3	3	7	3	5	3	2	2	1	3	2	2.0	1,089	637	58	322	776
Sri Lanka	23	17	7	4.3	7	6	19	6	14	10	4	6	2	11	6	2.7	2,088	1,179	56	527	1,849
State of Palestine	45	30	15	3.4	16	13	36	13	23	17	9	5	3	14	9	1.8	2,147	1,350	63	449	1,377
Sudan	132	104	55	3.1	60	50	82	39	43	37	27	26	8	28	22	1.1	82,570	40,883	50	9,027	34,499
Suriname	45	31	17	2.9	19	15	39	15	21	17	11	5	4	14	11	1.2	190	119	63	42	123
Sweden	7	4	2	2.4	3	2	6	2	4	2	1	1	1	4	2	2.0	279	153	55	85	278
Switzerland	8	6	4	1.8	4	4	7	3	4	3	3	2	1	3	2	0.6	332	235	71	60	211
Syrian Arab Republic	37	23	22	0.2	24	20	30	18	17	12	11	10	5	12	11	0.4	9,057	4,621	51	2,432	4,615
Tajikistan	103	84	31	4.7	35	27	81	28	31	28	14	8	2	14	9	2.0	8,189	3,540	43	469	2,403
Thailand	37	22	8	4.6	9	7	30	7	21	12	5	6	4	10	5	2.7	5,429	3,035	56	3,357	3,531
Timor-Leste	176	111	51	3.8	55	46	132	43	57	39	22	26	9	22	14	2.0	1,653	733	44	290	481
Togo	148	120	63	3.1	68	57	91	43	44	37	24	33	12	27	21	1.3	16,919	6,618	39	2,600	5,872
Tokelau	-	-	-	-	-	-	-	-	-	-	-	-	-	-	-	-	-	-	-	-	-
Tonga	22	17	11	2.0	12	10	19	10	10	7	5	3	2	8	6	1.3	27	12	44	5	16
Trinidad and Tobago	30	28	16	2.6	18	15	27	15	20	18	10	4	2	12	9	1.5	294	184	63	44	157
Tunisia	55	30	16	2.9	18	15	43	14	28	18	12	7	3	15	11	1.7	3,281	2,278	69	636	2,097
Türkiye	74	38	9	6.9	10	8	56	8	32	19	5	9	2	11	4	4.7	11,390	5,883	52	2,341	5,280

TABLE 2. CHILD MORTALITY

Countries and areas	Under-five mortality rate			Annual rate of reduction in under-five mortality rate	Under-five mortality rate 2021		Infant mortality rate		Neonatal mortality rate			Mortality rate among children aged 5–14 years		Stillbirth rate		Annual rate of reduction in stillbirth rate	Under-five deaths	Neonatal deaths	Neonatal deaths as a percent-age of under-five deaths	Deaths among children aged 5–14 years	Stillbirths
	1990	2000	2021	2000–2021	Male	Female	1990	2021	1990	2000	2021	1990	2021	2000	2021	2000–2021	2021	2021	2021	2021	2021
Turkmenistan	79	70	41	2.5	47	35	65	36	27	30	23	7	4	11	9	0.8	5,728	3,217	56	473	1,309
Turks and Caicos Islands	14	9	4	3.1	5	4	11	4	8	5	2	3	1	-	-	-	2	1	50	0	-
Tuvalu	53	42	21	3.3	23	19	41	18	28	24	10	10	5	15	9	2.4	6	3	50	1	2
Uganda	183	146	42	5.9	47	37	107	31	40	33	19	29	13	23	15	2.0	69,025	32,037	46	17,089	25,855
Ukraine	19	18	8	3.8	9	7	16	7	12	11	5	4	2	7	5	1.7	2,834	1,622	57	802	1,669
United Arab Emirates	17	11	6	2.7	7	6	14	5	8	6	3	4	2	8	5	2.8	618	337	55	148	454
United Kingdom	9	7	4	2.1	5	4	8	4	4	4	3	2	1	4	3	2.4	2,864	1,893	66	585	1,836
United Republic of Tanzania	167	130	47	4.8	51	43	100	34	40	34	20	27	13	26	18	1.7	105,694	46,050	44	22,341	42,873
United States	11	8	6	1.4	7	6	9	5	6	5	3	2	1	3	3	0.9	23,162	12,169	53	5,703	10,196
Uruguay	23	17	6	5.1	6	5	20	5	12	8	4	3	1	7	5	2.0	211	143	68	70	173
Uzbekistan	70	61	14	6.9	16	12	58	13	30	28	8	7	3	12	6	3.4	11,404	6,172	54	2,043	4,740
Vanuatu	36	29	23	1.0	25	21	30	20	17	12	10	7	5	12	11	0.5	216	93	43	40	101
Venezuela (Bolivarian Republic of)	30	22	24	-0.6	26	22	25	21	13	11	15	4	4	10	11	-0.5	11,322	6,779	60	2,006	4,882
Viet Nam	52	30	21	1.8	24	17	37	16	24	15	11	10	3	11	8	1.6	30,455	15,404	51	3,982	11,822
Yemen	126	95	62	2.0	66	58	89	47	44	37	28	18	7	24	23	0.1	61,914	28,554	46	5,902	24,195
Zambia	182	156	58	4.7	62	53	108	40	37	35	25	27	10	22	14	2.1	37,822	16,492	44	5,558	9,703
Zimbabwe	80	96	50	3.2	54	45	51	36	23	28	25	13	11	23	11	0.8	23,960	12,211	51	4,684	9,711

SUMMARY

	1990	2000	2021	2000–2021	Male	Female	1990	2021	1990	2000	2021	1990	2021	2000	2021	2000–2021	2021	2021	2021	2021	2021
East Asia and Pacific	57	39	15	4.7	16	13	44	12	28	20	7	9	3	14	7	3.3	369,615	176,539	48	84,485	169,030
Europe and Central Asia	31	21	8	4.9	8	7	25	7	14	10	4	4	1	7	4	2.6	77,934	41,355	53	16,158	40,443
Eastern Europe and Central Asia	47	35	11	5.7	12	10	37	9	20	17	6	6	2	10	5	3.1	60,992	31,086	51	12,277	28,373
Western Europe	10	6	4	2.5	4	3	9	3	6	3	2	2	1	4	3	1.8	16,942	10,269	61	3,880	12,070
Latin America and Caribbean	55	33	16	3.5	17	14	44	14	23	16	9	6	3	11	8	1.8	155,279	87,212	56	28,325	75,307
Middle East and North Africa	66	43	22	3.3	24	20	50	18	28	21	12	11	4	16	11	2.0	214,058	116,744	55	36,201	104,206
North America	11	8	6	1.4	7	6	9	5	6	5	3	2	1	3	3	0.9	25,035	13,443	54	6,071	11,237
South Asia	130	93	37	4.4	38	36	92	31	59	46	23	20	5	32	17	3.0	1,287,474	801,694	62	164,672	602,747
Sub-Saharan Africa	179	151	73	3.5	78	67	107	50	45	40	27	37	15	28	21	1.3	2,904,277	1,107,631	38	492,989	881,965
Eastern and Southern Africa	163	135	53	4.5	57	48	100	38	43	38	23	37	12	26	19	1.5	1,010,308	455,407	45	183,894	378,064
West and Central Africa	197	168	91	2.9	97	85	114	61	48	43	31	37	19	29	23	1.1	1,893,969	652,224	34	309,095	503,901
Least developed countries	176	136	61	3.8	66	56	109	44	52	42	25	37	13	30	21	1.7	2,051,993	865,498	42	344,903	737,181
World	**93**	**76**	**38**	**3.3**	**40**	**36**	**65**	**28**	**37**	**31**	**18**	**14**	**6**	**21**	**14**	**2.0**	**5,033,672**	**2,344,618**	**47**	**828,902**	**1,884,935**

For a complete list of countries and areas in the regions, subregions and country categories, see page on Regional Classifications or visit <data.unicef.org/regionalclassifications>.

It is not advisable to compare data from consecutive editions of *The State of the World's Children* report.

NOTES
- Data not available.

MAIN DATA SOURCES
United Nations Inter-agency Group for Child Mortality Estimation (UNICEF, World Health Organization, United Nations Population Division and the World Bank Group). Last update: Janurary 2023.

DEFINITIONS OF THE INDICATORS

Under-five mortality rate – Probability of dying between birth and exactly 5 years of age, expressed per 1,000 live births.

Annual rate of reduction in under-five mortality rate – The annual percentage reduction in the under-five mortality rate (U5MR) defined as ARR=100*(ln(U5MRt2/U5MRt1)/(t1-t2)), where t1=2000 and t2=2021.

Infant mortality rate – Probability of dying between birth and exactly 1 year of age, expressed per 1,000 live births.

Neonatal mortality rate – Probability of dying during the first 28 days of life, expressed per 1,000 live births.

Mortality rate (children aged 5 to 14 years) – Probability of dying at age 5–14 years expressed per 1,000 children aged 5.

Under-five deaths – Number of deaths among children under 5 years of age.

Neonatal deaths – Number of deaths occurring within the first 28 days of life.

Neonatal deaths as a percentage of under-five deaths – The percentage of under-five deaths occurring within the first 28 days of life.

Deaths among children aged 5–14 years – Number of deaths among children aged 5 -14.

Stillbirth rate – Stillbirth rate (SBR) is defined as the number of babies born with no sign of life at 28 weeks or more of gestation per 1,000 total births.

Annual rate of reduction in stillbirth rate – The annual percentage reduction in the stillbirth rate (SBR) defined as ARR=100*(ln(SBRt2/SBRt1)/(t1-t2)), where t1=2000 and t2=2021.

Stillbirths – Number of stillbirths.

FOR EVERY CHILD, VACCINATION

139

TABLE 3. MATERNAL AND NEWBORN HEALTH

Countries and areas	Life expectancy at birth (years): female 2021	Universal health coverage 2019 — Service Coverage sub-index on reproductive, maternal, newborn and child health	Demand for family planning satisfied with modern methods (%) 2016–2021 R	Antenatal care (%) 2016–2021 R — At least one visit	At least four visits	Delivery care (%) 2016–2021 R — Skilled birth attendant	Institutional delivery	C-section	Postnatal health check (%) 2016–2021 R — For newborns	For mothers	Maternal mortality 2020 C — Number of maternal deaths	Maternal mortality ratio	Lifetime risk of maternal death (1 in X)
Afghanistan	65	37	42	65	28	62	63	7	19	37	8,700	620	32
Albania	79	62	6	88	78	100	99	31	86	88	2	8	8,700
Algeria	78	75	77 x	95	70	99	99	25	92	88	760	78	410
Andorra	84	-	-	-	-	100	-	-	-	-	-	-	-
Angola	64	39	30	82	61	50	46	4	21	23	2,900	222	79
Anguilla	80	-	-	-	-	100	-	-	-	-	-	-	-
Antigua and Barbuda	81	72	-	100 x	100 x	99	-	-	-	-	0	21	2,700
Argentina	79	73	-	95	90	99	100	47	98	97	290	45	1,100
Armenia	77	69	40	100	96	100	99	18	98	97	10	27	2,100
Australia	86	87	-	98 x	92 x	99	99 x	31 x	-	-	9	3	19,000
Austria	84	82	-	-	-	98	99 x	24 x	-	-	4	5	14,000
Azerbaijan	73	65	22 x	92 x	96 x	100	96 x	26 x	-	83 x	54	41	1,400
Bahamas	75	70	-	98 x	85 x	99	-	-	-	-	4	77	940
Bahrain	80	71	-	100 x	100 x	100	98 x	-	-	-	3	16	3,000
Bangladesh	74	51	77	75	37	59	53	36	67	65	3,700	123	390
Barbados	79	74	70 x	93 x	88 x	98	100 x	21 x	98 x	97 x	1	39	1,900
Belarus	78	74	73 x	100	100	100	100	31	100	99	1	1	65,000
Belgium	84	85	-	-	-	-	-	18 x	-	-	5	5	12,000
Belize	74	67	65	97	93	95	96	34	96	96	9	130	380
Benin	61	38	28	83	52	78	84	5	64	66	2,500	523	36
Bhutan	74	62	85 x	98 x	85 x	96	94	12 x	30 x	41 x	6	60	970
Bolivia (Plurinational State of)	67	67	50	96	86	81	80	33	-	56	420	161	230
Bosnia and Herzegovina	78	65	22 x	87 x	84 x	100	100 x	14 x	-	-	2	6	13,000
Botswana	64	54	-	94 x	73 x	100	100 x	-	-	-	120	186	180
Brazil	76	75	89 x	97 x	93	99	99	56	-	-	2,000	72	800
British Virgin Islands	78	-	-	-	-	-	-	-	-	-	-	-	-
Brunei Darussalam	77	77	-	99 x	93 x	100	100 x	-	-	-	3	44	1,300
Bulgaria	76	70	-	-	-	100 x	100	47	-	-	4	7	10,000
Burkina Faso	61	43	53	93 x	47 x	80 x	82 x	4 x	33 x	74 x	2,000	264	77
Burundi	64	44	40	99	49	85	84	4 x	49	51	2,200	494	38
Cabo Verde	79	69	73 x	99	86	97	97	11 x	-	87	4	42	1,100
Cambodia	72	61	57 x	95 x	76 x	89 x	83 x	6 x	79 x	90 x	710	218	170
Cameroon	62	44	45	87	65	69	67	4	60	59	4,100	438	46
Canada	85	89	-	100 x	99 x	98	98 x	26 x	-	-	41	11	6,500
Central African Republic	56	32	28	52	41	40	58	2	59	57	1,900	835	19
Chad	54	28	18	55 x	31 x	39	27	1	27	26	7,800	1,063	15
Chile	81	80	-	-	-	100	100 x	50 x	-	-	34	15	3,800
China	81	82	97 x	100	93	100	100	41 x	-	-	2,800	23	3,100
Colombia	76	78	87	97	90	99	97	43	-	-	550	75	780
Comoros	66	44	29 x	92 x	49 x	82 x	76 x	10 x	14 x	49 x	52	217	110
Congo	65	40	43 x	94 x	79 x	91 x	92 x	5 x	86 x	80 x	500	282	82
Cook Islands	79	-	-	100 x	-	100 x	100 x	-	-	-	-	-	-
Costa Rica	80	78	81	98	94	99	98	28	97	92	14	22	2,600
Côte d'Ivoire	60	45	44	93	51	74	70	3	83	80	4,400	480	46
Croatia	81	73	-	-	98	100	-	24	-	-	2	5	15,000
Cuba	76	80	87	99	79	100	100	31	100	100	42	39	1,800
Cyprus	83	79	-	99 x	-	99	97 x	-	-	-	9	68	1,000
Czechia	81	78	86 x	-	-	100	100 x	20 x	-	-	4	3	17,000
Democratic People's Republic of Korea	76	68	90	100	94	100	92	13	99	98	370	107	550
Democratic Republic of the Congo	62	39	33	82	43	85	82	5	57	50	22,000	547	29
Denmark	83	85	-	-	-	95	-	21 x	-	-	3	5	12,000
Djibouti	65	48	-	88 x	23 x	87 x	87 x	11 x	-	-	56	234	160
Dominica	76	-	-	100 x	-	100	-	-	-	-	-	-	-
Dominican Republic	76	66	82 x	98	93	99	98	63	94	90	220	107	390
Ecuador	78	80	79 x	84 x	58 x	97	93 x	46 x	-	-	200	66	740
Egypt	73	70	80 x	90 x	83 x	92 x	87 x	52 x	14 x	82 x	420	17	1,900
El Salvador	75	76	80 x	96 x	90 x	100	98 x	32 x	97 x	94 x	44	43	1,100
Equatorial Guinea	63	43	21 x	91 x	67 x	68 x	67 x	7 x	-	-	110	212	100
Eritrea	69	50	21 x	89 x	57 x	34 x	34 x	3 x	-	5 x	330	322	77
Estonia	81	78	-	-	97 x	100	99	-	-	-	1	5	11,000
Eswatini	61	58	83 x	99 x	76 x	88 x	88 x	12 x	90 x	88 x	69	240	130
Ethiopia	68	38	64	74	43	50	48	2	35	34	10,000	267	86

140   THE STATE OF THE WORLD'S CHILDREN 2023

TABLE 3. MATERNAL AND NEWBORN HEALTH

Countries and areas	Life expectancy at birth (years): female 2021	Universal health coverage 2019 — Service Coverage sub-index on reproductive, maternal, newborn and child health	Demand for family planning satisfied with modern methods (%) 2016–2021 [R]	Antenatal care (%) 2016–2021 [R] — At least one visit	Antenatal care (%) 2016–2021 [R] — At least four visits	Delivery care (%) 2016–2021 [R] — Skilled birth attendant	Delivery care (%) 2016–2021 [R] — Institutional delivery	Delivery care (%) 2016–2021 [R] — C-section	Postnatal health check (%) 2016–2021 [R] — For newborns	Postnatal health check (%) 2016–2021 [R] — For mothers	Maternal mortality 2020 [C] — Number of maternal deaths	Maternal mortality 2020 [C] — Maternal mortality ratio	Maternal mortality 2020 [C] — Lifetime risk of maternal death (1 in X)
Fiji	69	61	-	98	89	100	100	20	98	94	7	38	960
Finland	85	83	-	100 x	-	100	100 x	16 x	-	-	4	8	8,600
France	86	84	96 x	100 x	99 x	98	98 x	21 x	-	-	54	8	7,300
Gabon	69	49	44 x	95 x	78 x	89 x	90 x	10 x	25 x	60 x	140	227	120
Gambia	64	48	40	98	79	84	84	4	83	88	400	458	47
Georgia	77	65	51	98 x	85	100	99	41	-	-	14	28	1,700
Germany	83	86	-	100 x	99 x	96	99 x	29 x	-	-	34	4	13,000
Ghana	66	45	40	97	85	79	78	13	91	85	2,400	263	100
Greece	83	78	-	-	-	100	-	-	-	-	6	8	9,400
Grenada	78	70	-	100 x	-	100	-	-	-	-	0	21	2,300
Guatemala	73	57	66 x	91 x	86 x	70	65 x	26 x	8 x	78 x	360	96	380
Guinea	60	37	38	81	35	55	53	3	43	49	2,600	553	37
Guinea-Bissau	62	37	60	97	81	54	50	3	57	53	460	725	32
Guyana	69	74	52 x	91 x	87 x	95	93 x	17 x	95 x	93 x	18	112	330
Haiti	66	47	45	91	67	42	39	5	38	31	950	350	94
Holy See	-	-	-	-	-	-	-	-	-	-	-	-	-
Honduras	73	63	76 x	96	88	94	92	25	94	92	160	72	510
Hungary	78	73	-	-	-	100	-	31 x	-	-	14	15	4,800
Iceland	84	87	-	-	-	97	-	17 x	-	-	0	3	18,000
India	69	61	73	85	59	89	89	22	82	61	24,000	103	470
Indonesia	70	59	77	98	77	95	79	17	76	87	7,800	173	280
Iran (Islamic Republic of)	77	77	69 x	97 x	94 x	99 x	95 x	55 x	-	-	270	22	2,600
Iraq	72	55	54	88	68	96	87	33	78	83	900	76	350
Ireland	84	83	-	100 x	-	100	100 x	25 x	-	-	3	5	12,000
Israel	84	84	-	-	-	-	-	-	-	-	5	3	11,000
Italy	85	83	-	99 x	68 x	100	100 x	40 x	-	-	19	5	21,000
Jamaica	73	70	83 x	98 x	86 x	100	99	21 x	-	-	33	99	730
Japan	88	85	-	-	-	100	100 x	-	-	-	36	4	22,000
Jordan	77	60	57	98	92	100	98	26	86	83	100	41	780
Kazakhstan	73	76	73	99 x	95 x	100	99 x	15 x	99 x	98 x	57	13	2,400
Kenya	64	56	74	93	59	70	61 x	9 x	36 x	53 x	7,700	530	52
Kiribati	69	51	53	89	67	92	86	9	91	86	3	76	390
Kuwait	82	70	-	100 x	-	100	99 x	-	-	-	4	7	8,000
Kyrgyzstan	74	70	65	100	94	100	100	8	98	96	81	50	580
Lao People's Democratic Republic	70	50	72	78	62	64	65	6	47	47	220	132	280
Latvia	78	72	-	92 x	-	100	98 x	-	-	-	3	18	3,900
Lebanon	77	72	-	96 x	-	98 x	100 x	-	-	-	18	21	2,300
Lesotho	56	48	83	91	77	87	89	10 x	82	84	330	566	55
Liberia	62	42	41	98	87	84	80	5	76	80	1,100	652	35
Libya	74	60	24 x	93 x	-	100 x	100 x	-	-	-	88	72	580
Liechtenstein	85	-	-	-	-	-	-	-	-	-	-	-	-
Lithuania	79	70	-	100 x	-	100	-	-	-	-	2	9	6,700
Luxembourg	85	86	-	-	97 x	100 x	100 x	29 x	-	-	0	6	11,000
Madagascar	67	35	66	85	51	46	39	2	78	72	3,500	392	59
Malawi	67	48	74	97	51	96	97	8	88	84	2,500	381	60
Malaysia	77	76	-	97 x	97	100	99 x	21	-	-	110	21	2,300
Maldives	81	69	29	99	82	100	95	40	82	80	4	57	840
Mali	60	42	41	80	43	67	67	3	54	56	3,900	440	37
Malta	86	81	-	100 x	-	100	100 x	31	-	-	0	3	25,000
Marshall Islands	67	-	81 x	81 x	77 x	92	85 x	9 x	-	-	-	-	-
Mauritania	66	40	30 x	87 x	63 x	69 x	69 x	5 x	58 x	57 x	700	464	45
Mauritius	77	65	41 x	-	-	100	98 x	-	-	-	11	84	860
Mexico	75	74	80 x	99 x	94 x	97	97 x	41 x	95 x	95 x	1,200	59	820
Micronesia (Federated States of)	75	48	-	80 x	-	100 x	87 x	11 x	-	-	1	74	490
Monaco	88	-	-	-	-	-	-	-	-	-	-	-	-
Mongolia	76	63	64	99	89	99	98	26	98	94	29	39	820
Montenegro	80	67	33	97	94	99	99	24	96	86	0	6	9,300
Montserrat	77	-	-	-	-	100	-	-	-	-	-	-	-
Morocco	76	73	72	89	54	87	86	21	-	-	470	71	580
Mozambique	62	47	56 x	94	51	73 x	55 x	4 x	28 x	-	1,500	127	160
Myanmar	69	61	75	81	59	60	37	17	36	71	1,700	179	270
Namibia	63	62	80 x	97 x	63 x	88 x	87 x	14 x	20 x	69 x	150	215	130
Nauru	67	-	43 x	95 x	40 x	97 x	99 x	8 x	-	-	-	-	-

FOR EVERY CHILD, VACCINATION

141

TABLE 3. MATERNAL AND NEWBORN HEALTH

Countries and areas	Life expectancy at birth (years): female 2021	Universal health coverage 2019 — Service Coverage sub-index on reproductive, maternal, newborn and child health	Demand for family planning satisfied with modern methods (%) 2016–2021 R	Antenatal care (%) 2016–2021 R — At least one visit	At least four visits	Delivery care (%) 2016–2021 R — Skilled birth attendant	Institutional delivery	C-section	Postnatal health check (%) 2016–2021 R — For newborns	For mothers	Maternal mortality 2020 C — Number of maternal deaths	Maternal mortality ratio	Lifetime risk of maternal death (1 in X)
Nepal	70	53	62	89	78	77	78	15	69	68	1,100	174	240
Netherlands (Kingdom of the)	83	86	-	-	-	-	-	14 x	-	-	7	4	13,000
New Zealand	84	86	-	-	-	96	97 x	23 x	-	-	4	7	8,200
Nicaragua	77	70	90 x	95 x	88 x	94	71 x	30 x	-	-	110	78	470
Niger	63	37	46	84	37	44	44	1 x	13 x	34	4,900	441	31
Nigeria	53	44	36	67	57	43	39	3	38	42	82,000	1,047	19
Niue	73	-	-	100 x	-	100 x	-	-	-	-	-	-	-
North Macedonia	76	68	30	97	96	100	99	38	99	94	1	3	24,000
Norway	85	86	-	-	-	99	99 x	16 x	-	-	1	2	43,000
Oman	75	69	40 x	99 x	74	100	99 x	19 x	98 x	95 x	15	17	1,900
Pakistan	69	45	49	91	52	68	70	23	64	69	9,800	154	170
Palau	71	-	-	90 x	81 x	97	100 x	-	-	-	-	-	-
Panama	80	77	65 x	99 x	88 x	95	96 x	32 x	93 x	92 x	38	50	840
Papua New Guinea	68	33	49	76	49	56	55	3	45	46	490	192	150
Paraguay	73	61	79	99	86	98	93	46	96	94	99	71	510
Peru	75	78	67	98	96	96	95	36	96 x	97	410	69	600
Philippines	72	55	56	94	87	84	78	13	86	86	1,900	78	410
Poland	80	74	-	-	-	100	100 x	21 x	-	-	7	2	37,000
Portugal	84	84	-	100 x	-	99	99 x	31 x	-	-	10	12	6,100
Qatar	81	74	69 x	91 x	85 x	100	99 x	20 x	-	-	2	8	6,300
Republic of Korea	87	87	-	-	97 x	100 x	100 x	32 x	-	-	24	8	18,000
Republic of Moldova	74	67	64	99 x	95 x	100	99 x	16 x	-	-	5	12	4,700
Romania	78	71	47 x	72	76 x	93	95 x	34 x	-	-	20	10	5,700
Russian Federation	75	75	72 x	-	-	100	99 x	13 x	-	-	200	14	5,300
Rwanda	68	54	63 x	98	47	94	93	13 x	19 x	70	1,000	259	95
Saint Kitts and Nevis	75	-	-	100 x	-	100	-	-	-	-	-	-	-
Saint Lucia	75	72	72 x	97 x	90 x	100	100 x	19 x	100 x	90 x	1	73	790
Saint Vincent and the Grenadines	72	73	-	100 x	100 x	99	-	-	-	-	1	62	940
Samoa	76	53	39 x	94	70	89	89	8	85	83	4	59	380
San Marino	84	-	-	-	-	-	-	-	-	-	-	-	-
Sao Tome and Principe	70	60	58	98	84 x	97	95	10	92	84	9	146	170
Saudi Arabia	79	73	-	97 x	-	99	-	-	-	-	110	16	2,500
Senegal	69	49	53	98	56	75	80	7	81	80	1,400	261	80
Serbia	77	71	38	99	97	100	100	32	-	-	7	10	7,100
Seychelles	76	70	-	-	-	100	-	-	-	-	0	3	15,000
Sierra Leone	61	39	53	98	79	87	83	4	83	86	1,200	443	52
Singapore	85	86	-	-	-	100	100	-	-	-	3	7	13,000
Slovakia	78	77	-	97 x	-	98	-	24 x	-	-	3	5	15,000
Slovenia	84	80	-	100 x	-	100 x	100 x	-	-	-	1	5	16,000
Solomon Islands	72	50	38 x	89 x	69 x	86 x	85 x	6 x	16 x	69 x	26	122	200
Somalia	57	27	-	26 x	6 x	9 x	9 x	-	-	-	4,500	621	25
South Africa	65	67	80	94	76	97	96	26	86	84	1,500	127	300
South Sudan	57	32	4 x	62 x	17 x	19 x	12 x	1 x	-	-	3,800	1,223	20
Spain	86	86	-	-	-	100	-	26 x	-	-	12	3	28,000
Sri Lanka	80	67	74	99	93 x	100	100	32 x	-	99	89	29	1,700
State of Palestine	76	-	61	99	95	100	99	26	92	89	30	20	1,200
Sudan	68	44	30 x	79 x	51 x	78 x	28 x	9 x	28 x	27 x	4,100	270	78
Suriname	74	67	58	85	68	98	93	16	94	91	11	96	430
Sweden	85	87	87	100 x	-	-	-	-	-	-	5	5	13,000
Switzerland	86	87	-	-	-	-	-	30 x	-	-	6	7	7,800
Syrian Arab Republic	75	56	53 x	88 x	64 x	96 x	78 x	26 x	-	-	120	30	1,200
Tajikistan	74	66	52	92	64	95	88	5	90	92	44	17	1,600
Thailand	83	83	88	99	90	99	99	35	-	-	190	29	2,500
Timor-Leste	70	53	46	84	77	57	49	4	31	35	67	204	140
Togo	62	44	40	78	55	69	80	9	80	81	1,100	399	59
Tokelau	76	-	-	-	-	-	-	-	-	-	-	-	-
Tonga	74	56	50	98	89	98	98	14	98	95	3	126	230
Trinidad and Tobago	76	73	58 x	95 x	100 x	100	98 x	22 x	96 x	92 x	5	27	2,200
Tunisia	77	70	63	95	84	100	100	43	97	89	74	37	1,300
Türkiye	79	79	60	96	90	97	99	52	68	79	220	17	2,800
Turkmenistan	73	73	80	100	98	100	100	8	100	100	7	5	6,300
Turks and Caicos Islands	78	-	-	97	93	100	97	55	99	95	-	-	-
Tuvalu	69	-	41 x	94	60	100	99	20	97	89	-	-	-

142

THE STATE OF THE WORLD'S CHILDREN 2023

TABLE 3. MATERNAL AND NEWBORN HEALTH

Countries and areas	Life expectancy at birth (years): female 2021	Universal health coverage 2019 — Service Coverage sub-index on reproductive, maternal, newborn and child health	Demand for family planning satisfied with modern methods (%) 2016–2021 [R]	Antenatal care (%) 2016–2021 [R] — At least one visit	Antenatal care (%) — At least four visits	Delivery care (%) 2016–2021 [R] — Skilled birth attendant	Delivery care (%) — Institutional delivery	Delivery care (%) — C-section	Postnatal health check (%) 2016–2021 [R] — For newborns	Postnatal health check (%) — For mothers	Maternal mortality 2020 [C] — Number of maternal deaths	Maternal mortality — Maternal mortality ratio	Maternal mortality — Lifetime risk of maternal death (1 in X)
Uganda	65	50	55	95	57	74	73	6	56	54	4,700	284	66
Ukraine	77	73	68 x	99 x	87 x	100 x	99 x	12 x	99 x	96 x	56	17	5,800
United Arab Emirates	81	78	-	100 x	-	99	100 x	-	-	-	9	9	6,100
United Kingdom	83	88	87 x	-	-	-	-	26 x	-	-	67	10	5,800
United Republic of Tanzania	68	46	55	98	62	64	63	6	43	34	5,400	238	83
United States	80	83	78	-	97 x	99	-	31 x	-	-	770	21	2,700
Uruguay	79	79	-	97 x	77 x	100	100 x	30 x	-	-	7	19	3,900
Uzbekistan	73	71	-	99 x	-	100	100	17	-	-	250	30	1,100
Vanuatu	73	52	51 x	76 x	52 x	89 x	89 x	12 x	-	-	8	94	260
Venezuela (Bolivarian Republic of)	75	70	-	98 x	84 x	99	99 x	52 x	-	-	1,200	259	160
Viet Nam	78	70	70 x	97	88	96	96	34	89	88	1,800	124	390
Yemen	67	44	41 x	60 x	25 x	45 x	30 x	5 x	11 x	20 x	1,900	183	130
Zambia	64	55	66	97	64	80	84	5	72	70	890	135	160
Zimbabwe	62	55	85 x	93	72	86	86	9	91	82	1,700	357	71

SUMMARY

East Asia and Pacific	80	77	88	97	87	95	89	-	-	-	18,000	74	840
Europe and Central Asia	80	73	74	-	-	98	-	-	-	-	1,300	13	4,500
Eastern Europe and Central Asia	76	74	67	-	-	99	98	32	-	-	1,000	19	2,900
Western Europe	84	84	82	-	-	98	-	-	-	-	290	6	11,000
Latin America and Caribbean	76	74	83	96	90 j	95	94	47	-	84 j	8,400	88	570
Middle East and North Africa	75	69	70	-	-	-	-	-	-	-	5,200	56	660
North America	81	84	83	-	-	99	-	-	-	-	810	20	2,900
South Asia	69	58	73	85	55	81	81	22	74	62	47,000	138	320
Sub-Saharan Africa	62	36	53	83	54	62	60	5	52	50	206,000	536	41
Eastern and Southern Africa	65	47	63	89	56	66	64	6	52	50	59,000	324	71
West and Central Africa	58	42	38	78	53	60	58	4	52	51	147,000	724	27
Least developed countries	66	45	59	84	49	66	62	9	51	50	-	-	-
World	**74**	**67**	**78**	**88**	**65**	**82**	**78**	**18**	**67**	**62**	**287,000**	**223**	**210**

For a complete list of countries and areas in the regions, subregions and country categories, see page on Regional Classifications or visit <data.unicef.org/regionalclassifications>.

It is not advisable to compare data from consecutive editions of *The State of the World's Children* report.

NOTES

- Data not available.

ʲ Excludes Brazil and Mexico.

[R] Data refer to the most recent year available during the period specified in the column heading.

ˣ Data refer to years or periods other than those specified in the column heading. Such data are not included in the calculation of regional and global averages. Estimates from data years prior to 2000 are not displayed.

[C] Maternal mortality estimates are from the 2023 United Nations inter-agency maternal mortality estimates. Periodically, the United Nations Maternal Mortality Estimation Inter-agency Group (WHO, UNICEF, UNFPA, the World Bank and the United Nations Population Division) produces internationally comparable sets of maternal mortality data that account for the well-documented problems of under-reporting and misclassification of maternal deaths, including also estimates for countries with no data. Please note that owing to an evolving methodology, these values are not comparable with previously reported maternal mortality ratio 'adjusted' values.

MAIN DATA SOURCES

Life expectancy – United Nations Population Division, *2022 Revision of World Population Prospects.*

Universal health coverage Service Coverage sub-index on reproductive, maternal, newborn and child health – WHO, based on DHS, MICS and other national household surveys. Last update: February 2022.

Demand for family planning satisfied with modern methods – United Nations, Department of Economic and Social Affairs, Population Division, United Nations Population Fund (UNFPA), based on Demographic and Health Surveys (DHS), Multiple Indicator Cluster Surveys (MICS), Reproductive Health Surveys, other national surveys, and National Health Information Systems (HIS). Last Update: August 2022.

Antenatal care (at least one visit) – DHS, MICS and other national household surveys. Last update: September 2022.

Antenatal care (at least four visits) – DHS, MICS and other national household surveys. Last update: September 2022.

Skilled birth attendant – Joint UNICEF/WHO SAB database, based on DHS, MICS and other national household surveys as well as national administrative data. Last update: September 2022.

Institutional delivery – DHS, MICS and other national household surveys. Last update: September 2022.

C-section – DHS, MICS and other national household surveys. Last update: September 2022.

Postnatal health check for newborn and mother – DHS, MICS and other national household surveys. Last update: September 2022.

Number of maternal deaths – United Nations Maternal Mortality Estimation Inter-agency Group (WHO, UNICEF, UNFPA, the World Bank and the United Nations Population Division). Last Update: February 2023.

Maternal mortality ratio – United Nations Maternal Mortality Estimation Inter-agency Group (WHO, UNICEF, UNFPA, the World Bank and the United Nations Population Division). Last Update: February 2023.

Lifetime risk of maternal death – United Nations Maternal Mortality Estimation Inter-agency Group (WHO, UNICEF, UNFPA, the World Bank and the United Nations Population Division). Last Update: February 2023.

DEFINITIONS OF THE INDICATORS

Life expectancy at birth – Number of years newborn female children would live if subject to the mortality risks prevailing for the cross section of population at the time of their birth.

Universal health coverage Service Coverage sub-index on reproductive, maternal, newborn and child health – Average coverage of essential services based on eight tracer indicators related to interventions across reproductive, maternal, newborn and child health areas. The index is calculated as a weighted average of the included indicators and is reported on a scale of 0 to 100.

Demand for family planning satisfied with modern methods – Percentage of adolescent girls and women (aged 15–49) who have their need for family planning satisfied with modern methods.

Antenatal care (at least one visit) – Percentage of adolescent girls and women (aged 15–49) attended at least once during pregnancy by skilled health personnel (typically a doctor, nurse or midwife).

Antenatal care (at least four visits) – Percentage of adolescent girls and women (aged 15–49) attended by any provider at least four times.

Skilled birth attendant – Percentage of births from adolescent girls and women (aged 15–49) attended by skilled health personnel (typically a doctor, nurse or midwife).

Institutional delivery – Percentage of adolescent girls and women (aged 15–49) who gave birth in a health facility.

C-section – Percentage of births delivered by Caesarean section. NB: C-section rates between 10 per cent and 15 per cent are expected with adequate levels of emergency obstetric care.

Postnatal health check for newborn – Percentage of last live births in the last two years who received a health check within two days after delivery. NB: For MICS, health check refers to a health check while in facility or at home following delivery or a postnatal visit.

Postnatal health check for mother – Percentage of adolescent girls and women (aged 15–49) who received a health check within 2 days after delivery of their most recent live birth in the last 2 years. NB: For MICS, health check refers to a health check while in facility or at home following delivery or a postnatal visit.

Number of maternal deaths – Number of deaths of women from pregnancy-related causes (modelled estimates).

Maternal mortality ratio – Number of deaths of women from pregnancy-related causes per 100,000 live births during the same time period (modelled estimates).

Lifetime risk of maternal death – Lifetime risk of maternal death takes into account both the probability of becoming pregnant and the probability of dying as a result of that pregnancy, accumulated across a woman's reproductive years (modelled estimates).

FOR EVERY CHILD, VACCINATION

143

TABLE 4. CHILD HEALTH

Countries and areas	Intervention coverage											2016–2021 [R]				
	Immunization for vaccine preventable diseases (%) 2021 [J]											Pneumonia	Diarrhoea	Malaria		
	BCG	DTP1	DTP3	Polio3	MCV1	MCV2 [F]	HepB3	Hib3	Rota	PCV3	Protection at birth (PAB) against tetanus [G]	Care seeking for children with symptoms of Acute Respiratory Infection (%)	Treatment with oral rehydration salts (%)	Care seeking for children with fever (%)	Children sleeping under ITNs (%)	Households with at least one ITN (%)
Afghanistan	84	74	66	71	63	44	66	66	59	65	65	68	40	62	5 x	26 x
Albania	99	98	98	98	87	92	98	98	98	89	96	82	35	60	-	-
Algeria	99	96	91	91	80	77	91	91	-	91	98	47	27	-	-	-
Andorra	-	99	99	98	99	97	98	98	-	95	-	-	-	-	-	-
Angola	56	57	45	43	36	32	41	41	36	34	68	49	43	51	22	31
Anguilla	-	-	-	-	-	-	-	-	-	-	-	-	-	-	-	-
Antigua and Barbuda	-	93	92	92	85	76	92	92	-	-	-	-	-	-	-	-
Argentina	81	82	76	74	81	79	76	76	74	74	-	94	15	71	-	-
Armenia	98	96	93	93	94	94	93	93	92	93	-	92	37	71	-	-
Australia	-	98	95	95	93	94	95	95	95	96	-	-	-	-	-	-
Austria	-	95	85	85	95	88	85	85	61	-	-	-	-	-	-	-
Azerbaijan	95	92	89	93	93	90	89	89	-	90	-	33 x	8 x	-	1 x	-
Bahamas	-	79	75	75	82	82	75	75	75	82	100	-	-	-	-	-
Bahrain	-	99	98	99	99	99	98	98	99	99	100	-	-	-	-	-
Bangladesh	99	99	98	98	97	93	98	98	-	99	98	46	72	56	-	-
Barbados	-	83	82	84	77	70	82	82	-	83	-	-	-	-	-	-
Belarus	98	98	98	97	98	98	98	98	-	-	-	93	53	84	-	-
Belgium	-	98	98	98	96	85	97	97	86	94	-	-	-	-	-	-
Belize	84	83	83	83	79	77	83	83	-	-	93	67	55	71	-	-
Benin	88	84	76	75	68	-	76	76	76	73	81	29	22	53	70	85
Bhutan	99	99	98	98	97	91	98	98	-	95	90	74 x	61 x	-	-	-
Bolivia (Plurinational State of)	78	75	70	70	75	56	70	70	71	70	89	81	40	-	-	-
Bosnia and Herzegovina	95	89	73	73	68	76	80	62	-	-	-	87 x	36 x	-	-	-
Botswana	98	98	95	96	97	70	95	95	85	90	91	14 x	43 x	75 x	31 x	53 x
Brazil	63	74	68	68	73	46	68	68	69	69	96	50 x	-	-	-	-
British Virgin Islands	-	-	-	-	-	-	-	-	-	-	-	-	-	-	-	-
Brunei Darussalam	99	99	99	99	99	99	99	99	-	-	97	-	-	-	-	-
Bulgaria	97	92	89	89	89	86	89	89	45	86	-	-	-	-	-	-
Burkina Faso	98	95	91	91	88	71	91	91	91	66	95	56 x	40 x	74	54	75
Burundi	95	96	94	94	90	85	94	94	94	94	87	59	36	70	40	46
Cabo Verde	98	93	93	94	95	86	94	94	-	-	95	-	-	-	-	-
Cambodia	95	94	92	93	84	71	92	92	-	90	93	69 x	35 x	61 x	4 x	5 x
Cameroon	77	76	69	70	62	35	69	69	65	67	83	30	18	61	60	73
Canada	-	94	92	92	90	83	84	92	84	84	-	-	-	-	-	-
Central African Republic	61	54	42	46	41	-	42	42	-	40	65	35	23	32	51	61
Chad	67	73	58	58	55	-	58	58	-	-	75	18	17	32	54	66
Chile	98	99	95	95	92	58	98	95	-	92	-	-	-	-	-	-
China	99	99	99	99	99	99	99	-	-	-	-	-	-	-	-	-
Colombia	87	90	86	86	86	86	86	86	86	84	97	64 x	54 x	54 x	-	3 x
Comoros	96	95	85	89	82	19	85	85	-	-	83	38 x	38 x	45 x	41 x	59 x
Congo	81	81	77	75	68	31	77	77	23	75	87	28 x	27 x	51 x	61 x	66 x
Cook Islands	99	99	98	98	99	98	98	98	-	-	-	-	-	-	-	-
Costa Rica	88	99	99	99	89	69	94	99	91	92	-	80	56	74	-	-
Côte d'Ivoire	93	85	76	73	68	1	76	76	58	57	86	44	17	45	60	76
Croatia	97	98	92	92	89	90	90	92	-	75	-	-	-	-	-	-
Cuba	99	99	99	98	99	99	99	99	-	-	-	90	35	85	-	-
Cyprus	-	98	96	96	86	88	94	92	-	81	-	-	-	-	-	-
Czechia	-	98	94	94	97	90	94	94	-	-	-	-	-	-	-	-
Democratic People's Republic of Korea	95	42	41	0	42	41	41	41	-	-	98	86	74	-	-	-
Democratic Republic of the Congo	67	81	65	65	55	-	65	65	52	63	80	34	24	46	51	63
Denmark	-	98	97	97	95	94	-	97	-	96	-	-	-	-	-	-
Djibouti	61	70	59	59	50	48	59	59	66	59	98	94 x	94 x	-	20 x	32 x
Dominica	89	96	92	92	92	88	92	92	-	-	-	-	-	-	-	-
Dominican Republic	99	99	84	83	88	60	83	83	80	71	99	85	53	79	-	-
Ecuador	75	78	72	62	65	58	68	68	60	62	90	-	46 x	-	-	-
Egypt	97	97	96	96	96	96	96	96	-	-	88	68 x	28 x	68 x	-	-
El Salvador	78	72	79	79	86	71	79	80	78	94	92	80	70	-	-	-
Equatorial Guinea	85	77	53	55	53	17	53	53	-	-	60	54 x	40 x	62 x	23 x	38 x
Eritrea	97	97	95	95	93	85	95	95	96	95	99	45 x	43 x	-	20 x	71 x
Estonia	90	91	90	89	89	84	84	89	80	-	-	-	-	-	-	-
Eswatini	97	86	77	61	80	69	77	77	85	63	90	60 x	84 x	63 x	2 x	10 x
Ethiopia	68	70	65	68	54	46	65	65	65	61	90	30	30	35	45 x	64 x
Fiji	99	99	99	99	96	94	99	99	99	99	96	-	54	68	-	-

144 THE STATE OF THE WORLD'S CHILDREN 2023

TABLE 4. CHILD HEALTH

Countries and areas	Intervention coverage																				
	Immunization for vaccine preventable diseases (%) 2021 [J]											2016–2021 [R]									
												Pneumonia		Diarrhoea		Malaria					
	BCG	DTP1	DTP3	Polio3	MCV1	MCV2 [F]	HepB3	Hib3	Rota	PCV3	Protec-tion at birth (PAB) against tetanus [G]	Care seeking for children with symptoms of Acute Respiratory Infection (%)		Treatment with oral rehydration salts (%)		Care seeking for children with fever (%)		Children sleeping under ITNs (%)		Households with at least one ITN (%)	
Finland	-	98	89	89	93	93	-	89	80	82	-	-		-		-		-		-	
France	-	99	96	96	92	86	91	95	-	92	-	-		-		-		-		-	
Gabon	86	76	75	69	64	-	75	75	-	-	83	68	x	26	x	67	x	39	x	36	x
Gambia	81	82	82	89	79	67	82	82	79	78	95	70		44		64		44		77	
Georgia	96	97	85	85	90	81	85	85	76	82	-	74	x	42		67		-		-	
Germany	-	98	91	91	97	93	87	90	68	82	-	-		-		-		-		-	
Ghana	99	99	98	98	94	83	98	98	96	98	90	56		48		69		54		74	
Greece	-	99	99	99	97	83	96	99	20	96	-	-		-		-		-		-	
Grenada	-	79	72	72	83	79	72	72	-	-	-	-		-		-		-		-	
Guatemala	84	89	79	67	81	72	79	79	64	72	91	52	x	49	x	50	x	-		-	
Guinea	72	62	47	48	47	-	47	47	-	-	83	69		55		61		38		63	
Guinea-Bissau	34	81	67	23	63	-	67	67	72	67	80	48		30		52		94		97	
Guyana	89	98	91	80	94	83	91	91	93	99	99	84	x	43	x	71	x	7	x	5	x
Haiti	73	75	51	51	65	41	51	51	48	51	80	37		39		40		18		31	
Holy See	-	-	-	-	-	-	-	-	-	-	-	-		-		-		-		-	
Honduras	82	82	77	77	81	75	77	77	80	77	99	70		53		61		-		-	
Hungary	99	99	99	99	99	99	-	99	-	99	-	-		-		-		-		-	
Iceland	-	97	92	92	92	10	-	92	-	92	-	-		-		-		-		-	
India	84	88	85	85	89	82	85	85	83	25	90	56		61		80		4		8	
Indonesia	81	74	67	68	72	50	67	67	-	1	83	75		36		90		3	x	3	x
Iran (Islamic Republic of)	99	98	98	98	99	98	98	98	-	-	97	76	x	61	x	-		-		-	
Iraq	94	89	78	78	75	84	78	78	41	0	73	44		25		75		-		-	
Ireland	0	98	94	94	90	-	93	93	91	85	-	-		-		-		-		-	
Israel	-	99	98	98	99	93	96	98	80	95	-	-		-		-		-		-	
Italy	-	94	94	94	92	86	94	94	63	91	-	-		-		-		-		-	
Jamaica	97	93	90	90	88	85	89	89	-	-	91	82	x	64	x	-		-		-	
Japan	95	98	96	96	98	95	92	95	-	95	-	-		-		-		-		-	
Jordan	76	78	77	76	76	90	77	77	75	-	92	61		44		68		-		-	
Kazakhstan	94	98	95	95	97	96	95	95	-	93	-	81	x	62	x	-		-		-	
Kenya	97	99	91	91	89	57	91	91	91	92	85	66	x	54	x	64		42		49	
Kiribati	96	99	92	91	80	58	94	95	80	99	93	87		61		27	x	69		86	
Kuwait	99	99	94	94	94	94	94	94	75	96	99	-		-		-		-		-	
Kyrgyzstan	97	89	89	90	93	97	89	88	90	90	-	60	x	36		48		-		-	
Lao People's Democratic Republic	80	85	75	74	73	50	75	75	-	74	93	40		56		58		50		61	
Latvia	96	96	94	94	97	85	94	93	84	92	-	-		-		-		-		-	
Lebanon	-	88	67	64	67	59	67	67	-	70	-	74	x	44	x	-		-		-	
Lesotho	96	92	87	87	90	82	87	87	74	87	85	58		40		61	x	-		-	
Liberia	81	81	66	64	58	35	66	66	68	65	90	78		54		81		44		55	
Libya	74	74	73	73	73	72	73	73	73	73	-	-		-		-		-		-	
Liechtenstein	-	-	-	-	-	-	-	-	-	-	-	-		-		-		-		-	
Lithuania	93	93	90	90	88	88	90	90	48	82	-	-		-		-		-		-	
Luxembourg	-	99	99	99	99	90	96	99	89	96	-	-		-		-		-		-	
Madagascar	52	65	55	52	39	24	55	55	48	54	75	40		19		48		62		78	
Malawi	89	95	93	89	90	74	93	93	92	93	90	71		51		64		68		74	
Malaysia	99	98	95	95	96	84	94	94	-	95	-	92		45		-		-		-	
Maldives	99	97	96	97	99	96	96	96	-	-	99	74	x	75		86		-		-	
Mali	83	82	77	72	70	33	77	77	70	77	87	35		21		53		79		85	
Malta	-	99	99	99	90	93	99	99	-	99	-	-		-		-		-		-	
Marshall Islands	83	97	86	85	85	58	89	72	53	61	-	-		38	x	63	x	-		-	
Mauritania	79	75	68	66	63	-	68	68	53	65	83	34	x	25	x	35	x	32	x	49	x
Mauritius	95	93	92	93	77	64	92	92	86	94	97	-		-		-		-		-	
Mexico	99	83	78	78	99	97	80	78	77	83	98	73	x	61	x	-		-		-	
Micronesia (Federated States of)	59	95	72	72	64	38	79	56	42	70	-	-		-		-		-		-	
Monaco	-	99	99	99	88	80	99	99	-	-	-	-		-		-		-		-	
Mongolia	99	97	95	97	95	94	95	95	-	95	-	76		58		-		-		-	
Montenegro	76	94	83	83	18	79	51	83	-	-	-	89	x	16	x	74	x	-		-	
Montserrat	-	-	-	-	-	-	-	-	-	-	-	-		-		-		-		-	
Morocco	99	99	99	99	99	99	99	99	98	98	90	70		22	x	-		-		-	
Mozambique	79	67	61	67	84	70	61	61	73	70	84	57	x	46	x	69		73		82	
Myanmar	48	45	37	43	44	42	37	37	33	40	88	58		62		65		19		27	
Namibia	99	97	93	92	90	63	93	93	90	78	90	68	x	72	x	63	x	6	x	24	x
Nauru	99	99	98	98	98	97	98	98	60	59	-	69	x	23	x	51	x	-		-	
Nepal	95	92	91	91	90	87	91	91	76	84	91	82		60		73		-		-	
Netherlands (Kingdom of the)	-	98	95	95	93	90	93	94	-	93	-	-		-		-		-		-	

FOR EVERY CHILD, VACCINATION

145

TABLE 4. CHILD HEALTH

Countries and areas	Immunization for vaccine preventable diseases (%) 2021 [J]										Protection at birth (PAB) against tetanus [G]	Pneumonia — Care seeking for children with symptoms of Acute Respiratory Infection (%)		Diarrhoea — Treatment with oral rehydration salts (%)		Malaria — Care seeking for children with fever (%)		Malaria — Children sleeping under ITNs (%)		Malaria — Households with at least one ITN (%)	
	BCG	DTP1	DTP3	Polio3	MCV1	MCV2 [F]	HepB3	Hib3	Rota	PCV3											
New Zealand	-	93	90	90	91	82	90	90	90	95	-	-		-		-		-		-	
Nicaragua	86	88	87	88	83	83	87	87	87	87	92	67	x	95	x	-		-		-	
Niger	95	94	82	82	80	66	82	82	85	82	83	59	x	41	x	75	x	96	x	87	x
Nigeria	75	70	56	53	59	36	56	56	-	52	65	40		40		73		52		61	
Niue	88	99	99	99	99	99	99	99	99	99	-	-		-		-		-		-	
North Macedonia	93	89	81	81	70	80	79	81	65	53	-	93	x	62	x	-		-		-	
Norway	-	98	97	97	97	95	96	97	96	96	-	-		-		-		-		-	
Oman	99	99	99	99	99	99	99	99	-	99	99	56	x	59	x	-		-		-	
Pakistan	93	90	83	83	81	79	83	83	87	83	86	71		37		81		0		4	
Palau	-	99	95	95	93	84	96	89	82	77	-	-		-		-		-		-	
Panama	99	93	74	74	80	97	74	74	86	74	-	82	x	52	x	-		-		-	
Papua New Guinea	42	39	31	32	38	20	31	31	-	32	67	63		30		50		52		69	
Paraguay	79	79	70	66	68	67	70	70	68	62	96	89		28		86		-		-	
Peru	87	90	82	79	78	60	82	82	82	75	95	50		22		46		-		-	
Philippines	47	57	57	56	57	55	57	57	-	51	91	66		45		55		-		-	
Poland	91	99	90	91	80	95	90	90	-	62	-	-		-		-		-		-	
Portugal	-	99	99	99	98	95	99	99	-	98	-	-		-		-		-		-	
Qatar	99	99	98	98	99	99	98	98	98	98	-	-		-		-		-		-	
Republic of Korea	98	98	98	98	98	96	98	98	-	98	-	-		-		-		-		-	
Republic of Moldova	98	87	87	88	83	92	87	87	60	78	-	79	x	42	x	-		-		-	
Romania	97	95	86	86	86	75	86	86	-	85	-	-		-		-		-		-	
Russian Federation	95	97	97	97	97	96	97	-	-	89	-	-		-		-		-		-	
Rwanda	89	90	88	88	87	85	88	88	89	88	97	54	x	34		62		56		66	
Saint Kitts and Nevis	96	97	96	96	96	94	96	96			-	-		-		-		-		-	
Saint Lucia	81	89	80	75	77	66	80	80			-	-		-		-		-		-	
Saint Vincent and the Grenadines	99	99	97	99	99	99	97	97			-	-		-		-		-		-	
Samoa	92	96	85	80	62	50	85	85	30	3	-	72		59		63		-		-	
San Marino	-	91	90	90	89	81	90	90	-	82	-	-		-		-		-		-	
Sao Tome and Principe	93	97	97	93	77	69	97	97	78	97	99	82		42		62		63		78	
Saudi Arabia	94	97	97	97	98	97	97	97	97	97	-	-		-		-		-		-	
Senegal	87	87	85	78	87	75	86	86	84	86	96	48		26		63		46		75	
Serbia	98	97	92	92	78	84	87	92	-	87	-	90	x	36	x	-		-		-	
Seychelles	99	99	94	94	94	86	94	94	98	95	100	-		-		-		-		-	
Sierra Leone	74	94	92	90	87	67	92	92	75	90	93	76		85		75		59		68	
Singapore	98	98	96	96	95	84	96	96	-	82	-	-		-		-		-		-	
Slovakia	-	97	97	97	95	96	97	97	-	97	-	-		-		-		-		-	
Slovenia	-	92	86	86	95	91	86	86	-	58	-	-		-		-		-		-	
Solomon Islands	83	95	87	84	67	40	87	87	75	86	90	79	x	37	x	62	x	70	x	86	x
Somalia	37	52	42	47	46	4	42	42	-	-	60	13	x	13	x	-		11	x	19	x
South Africa	86	91	86	86	87	82	86	86	85	87	88	66		51		68		-		-	
South Sudan	52	51	49	50	49	-	49	49	-	-	65	48	x	39	x	57	x	42		63	
Spain	-	96	92	92	95	91	92	91	58	92	-	-		-		-		-		-	
Sri Lanka	99	96	96	96	97	97	96	96	-	-	99	52		54		92		4		6	
State of Palestine	99	99	95	95	98	99	95	95	87	95	-	77		35		-		-		-	
Sudan	80	94	84	85	81	63	84	84	84	85	81	48	x	20	x	-		30	x	25	x
Suriname	-	81	72	72	58	43	72	72	-	-	95	89		46		52		43	x	61	x
Sweden	24	98	98	98	97	91	98	98	84	97	-	-		-		-		-		-	
Switzerland	-	97	96	96	95	94	73	95	-	88	-	-		-		-		-		-	
Syrian Arab Republic	76	65	48	52	59	53	48	48	-	-	90	77	x	50	x	-		-		-	
Tajikistan	98	97	97	97	97	96	97	97	97	-	-	69		62		44		1	x	2	x
Thailand	99	99	97	97	96	87	97	76	71	-	99	80		73		76		-		-	
Timor-Leste	88	87	86	86	79	78	86	86	80	-	85	70		70		58		55		64	
Togo	98	88	83	81	70	50	83	83	80	83	85	39		14		54		61		71	
Tokelau	-	-	-	-	-	-	-	-	-	-	-	-		-		-		-		-	
Tonga	99	99	99	99	99	99	99	99	-	67	-	-		-		82		-		-	
Trinidad and Tobago	-	95	94	94	93	88	94	94	-	95	-	74	x	45	x	-		-		-	
Tunisia	85	99	97	97	95	98	95	97	-	96	97	98		40		74		-		-	
Türkiye	95	95	95	95	96	93	96	95	-	96	97	45	x	-		-		-		-	
Turkmenistan	98	99	97	97	97	98	97	97	97	97	-	51	x	47		59		-		-	
Turks and Caicos Islands	-	-	-	-	-	-	-	-	-	-	-	-		-		75		-		-	
Tuvalu	99	99	94	87	93	84	94	94	59	-	-	-		46		76		-		-	
Uganda	83	97	91	91	90	-	91	91	87	91	83	71		47		87		60		83	
Ukraine	86	91	78	78	88	86	77	87	-	-	-	92	x	59	x	-		-		-	
United Arab Emirates	99	96	96	96	99	96	95	96	91	95	-	-		-		-		-		-	

146

THE STATE OF THE WORLD'S CHILDREN 2023

TABLE 4. CHILD HEALTH

Countries and areas	Intervention coverage																				
	Immunization for vaccine preventable diseases (%) 2021 [J]											2016–2021 [R]									
												Pneumonia		Diarrhoea		Malaria					
	BCG	DTP1	DTP3	Polio3	MCV1	MCV2 [F]	HepB3	Hib3	Rota	PCV3	Protection at birth (PAB) against tetanus [G]	Care seeking for children with symptoms of Acute Respiratory Infection (%)		Treatment with oral rehydration salts (%)		Care seeking for children with fever (%)		Children sleeping under ITNs (%)		Households with at least one ITN (%)	
United Kingdom	-	97	93	93	91	87	93	93	91	91	-	-		-		-		-		-	
United Republic of Tanzania	75	82	81	70	76	62	81	81	77	80	90	55		45		75		55		78	
United States	-	97	93	92	91	95	91	90	75	82	-	-		-		-		-		-	
Uruguay	99	95	89	89	96	84	89	89	-	94	-	91	x	-		-		-		-	
Uzbekistan	99	99	98	99	99	99	98	98	80	98	-	68	x	28	x	-		-		-	
Vanuatu	76	71	62	62	50	-	62	62	9	2	78	72	x	48	x	57	x	51	x	83	x
Venezuela (Bolivarian Republic of)	68	73	56	50	68	37	56	56	0	0	67	72	x	38	x	-		-		-	
Viet Nam	88	87	83	81	89	85	83	83	-	-	96	73		58		-		9	x	10	x
Yemen	70	82	72	66	71	52	72	72	73	72	73	34	x	25	x	33	x	-		-	
Zambia	92	94	91	87	90	81	91	91	87	89	83	75		67		77		52		78	
Zimbabwe	88	93	86	86	85	74	86	86	88	86	87	48		33		50	x	15		37	
SUMMARY																					
East Asia and Pacific	86	86	83	83	85	82	83	38	5	15	88 h	-		-		-		-		-	
Europe and Central Asia	92	97	94	94	94	91	91	80	33	82		-		-		-		-		-	
Eastern Europe and Central Asia	95	96	94	94	95	94	94	70	24	80		-		-		-		-		-	
Western Europe	68	97	94	94	93	89	87	93	45	84		-		-		-		-		-	
Latin America and Caribbean	81	82	75	73	81	68	75	75	67	70	94	73	j	31	j	-		-		-	
Middle East and North Africa	92	93	88	88	88	87	88	88	32	38	87	-		-		-		-		-	
North America	-	97	93	92	91	94	90	90	76	82	-	-		-		-		-		-	
South Asia	87	89	85	85	87	81	85	85	75	44	89	59		57		77		4		7	
Sub-Saharan Africa	77	79	71	69	68	40	71	71	54	65	80	45		36		61		53		66	
Eastern and Southern Africa	76	81	75	74	71	51	74	74	71	71	84	51		40		60		51		66	
West and Central Africa	78	78	67	65	64	31	67	67	38	60	76	40		33		61		54		67	
Least developed countries	77	81	73	73	69	45	73	73	57	68	84	48		41		57		52		65	
World	**84**	**86**	**81**	**80**	**81**	**71**	**80**	**71**	**49**	**51**	**86 h**	**56**		**46**		**70**		**-**		**-**	

For a complete list of countries and areas in the regions, subregions and country categories, see page on Regional Classifications or visit <data.unicef.org/regionalclassifications>. Sex disaggregated data for specific child health indicators are available at https://data.unicef.org/topic/child-health/immunization/.

It is not advisable to compare data from consecutive editions of *The State of the World's Children* report.

NOTES

- Data not available.

[J] Excludes Brazil and Mexico.

[h] Excludes China.

[R] Data refer to the most recent year available during the period specified in the column heading.

[x] Data refer to years or periods other than those specified in the column heading. Such data are not included in the calculation of regional and global averages. Estimates from data years prior to 2000 are not displayed.

[F] Generally, the second dose of measles–containing vaccine (MCV2) is recommended for administration during the second year of life; however, in many countries, MCV2 is scheduled after the second year. *2022 Revision of World Population Prospects.* estimates of the second year of life target population were used to calculate regional and global aggregates.

[G] WHO and UNICEF use a complex process employing administrative data, surveys (routine and supplemental), serosurveys, and information on other vaccines to calculate the percentage of births that can be considered as protected against tetanus because pregnant women were given two doses or more of tetanus toxoid (TT) vaccine.

[J] For the calculation of regional and global vaccination coverage, the national coverage is considered to be 0 per cent for the countries that did not introduce the vaccine in their national schedule or did not report coverage, with the exception of BCG, which is only recommended in countries or settings with a high incidence of tuberculosis or high leprosy burden. *2022 Revision of World Population Prospects.* estimates of target populations were used in the calculation of global and regional aggregates.

MAIN DATA SOURCES

Immunization – WHO and UNICEF estimates of national immunization coverage, 2021 revision. Last update: July 2022.

Care seeking for children with symptoms of Acute Respiratory Infection (ARI) – DHS, MICS and other national household surveys. Last update: September 2022.

Diarrhoea treatment with oral rehydration salts (ORS) – DHS, MICS and other national household surveys. Last update: September 2022.

Care seeking for children with fever – DHS, MICS, MIS and other national household surveys. Last update: September 2022.

Children sleeping under ITNs – DHS, MICS, MIS and other national household surveys. Last update: September 2022.

Households with at least one ITN – DHS, MICS, MIS and other national household surveys. Last update: September 2022.

DEFINITIONS OF THE INDICATORS

BCG – Percentage of live births who received bacilli Calmette–Guérin (vaccine against tuberculosis).

DTP1 – Percentage of surviving infants who received the first dose of diphtheria, pertussis and tetanus vaccine.

DTP3 – Percentage of surviving infants who received three doses of diphtheria, pertussis and tetanus vaccine.

Polio3 – Percentage of surviving infants who received three doses of the polio vaccine.

MCV1 – Percentage of surviving infants who received the first dose of the measles–containing vaccine.

MCV2 – Percentage of children who received the second dose of measles–containing vaccine as per national schedule.

HepB3 – Percentage of surviving infants who received three doses of hepatitis B vaccine.

Hib3 – Percentage of surviving infants who received three doses of Haemophilus influenzae type b vaccine.

Rota – Percentage of surviving infants who received the last dose of rotavirus vaccine as recommended.

PCV3 – Percentage of surviving infants who received three doses of pneumococcal conjugate vaccine.

Protection at birth (PAB) – Percentage of newborns protected at birth against tetanus with tetanus toxoid.

Care seeking for children with symptoms of Acute Respiratory Infection – Percentage of children under age 5 with symptoms of pneumonia (cough and fast or difficult breathing due to a problem in the chest) in the two weeks preceding the survey for whom advice or treatment was sought from a health facility or provider.

Diarrhoea treatment with oral rehydration salts – Percentage of children under age 5 who had diarrhoea in the two weeks preceding the survey and who received oral rehydration salts (ORS packets or pre–packaged ORS fluids).

Care seeking for children with fever – Percentage of children under age 5 with fever for whom advice or treatment was sought from a health facility or provider. Excludes drug vendor, stores, shops and traditional healer. In some countries, particularly non–malaria endemic countries, pharmacies have also been excluded from the calculation.

Children sleeping under ITNs – Percentage of children under age 5 who slept under an insecticide–treated mosquito net the night prior to the survey.

Households with at least one ITN – Percentage of households with at least one insecticide–treated mosquito net.

FOR EVERY CHILD, VACCINATION

TABLE 5. ADOLESCENT HEALTH

Countries and areas	Adolescent mortality rate 2021 (Aged 10–19) Total	Adolescent deaths 2021 (Aged 10–19) Total	Annual rate of reduction in the adolescent mortality rate 2000–2021 (Aged 10–19) Total	Adolescent birth rate 2016–2021 (Aged 10–14) Female	Adolescent birth rate 2016–2021 (Aged 15–19) Female	Births by age 18 (%) 2016–2021 (Women aged 20–24 who gave birth before age 18) Female	Demand for family planning satisfied with modern methods (%) 2016–2021 (Aged 15–19) Female	Informed decisions regarding sexual relations, contraceptive use and reproductive health care (%) 2016–2021 (Aged 15–19) Female	Antenatal care (%) (At least 4 visits) 2016–2021 (Aged 15–19) Female	Skilled birth attendant (%) 2016–2021 (Aged 15–19) Female	Girls vaccinated against HPV (%) 2021 Female	Alcohol use 2016 Male	Alcohol use 2016 Female	Tobacco use 2015–2020 Male	Tobacco use 2015–2020 Female	Insufficient physical activity among school going adolescents (aged 11–17) 2016 Male	Insufficient physical activity among school going adolescents (aged 11–17) 2016 Female
Afghanistan	14	13,833	-0.4	0 x	62	20 x	21	-	19	58	-	1	0	10 x	6 x	88	88
Albania	3	91	3.3	0	14	3	6	47	72	100	-	51	24	-	-	68	81
Algeria	4	2,651	2.6	0	12	1	57	-	69	97	-	2	1	17 x	3 x	76	91
Andorra	2	1	3.4	0	3	-	-	-	-	-	83	77	51	-	-	-	-
Angola	18	14,283	3.7	11 x	163 x	38	15	29	56	50	-	46	21	-	-	-	-
Anguilla	3	0	2.2	3 x	40 x	-	-	-	-	-	-	-	-	-	-	-	-
Antigua and Barbuda	3	4	2.6	0	30	-	-	-	-	-	2	48	22	8	7	74	85
Argentina	3	2,421	2.2	1	41	14	76	-	85	97	53	68	40	19	21	80	90
Armenia	3	103	-0.2	0	19	1	7 x	56	93	100	8	24	9	-	-	73	83
Australia	2	622	2.3	0	9	-	-	-	-	-	66	81	57	-	-	87	91
Austria	2	147	3.3	0	5	-	-	-	-	-	-	80	56	-	-	71	85
Azerbaijan	5	798	0.1	0	42	4 x	13 x	-	40 x	99 x	-	18	7	-	-	-	-
Bahamas	4	29	2.0	0 x	29 x	-	-	-	-	-	-	41	18	16 x	8 x	81	88
Bahrain	3	45	2.2	0	13	-	-	-	-	-	-	5	2	27	10	75	87
Bangladesh	5	14,869	3.2	1	74	24	71	47	35	62	-	2	1	13 x	2 x	63	69
Barbados	3	12	1.8	1 x	50 x	7 x	56 x	-	-	-	28	50	24	17 x	11 x	77	87
Belarus	2	209	4.7	0	12	3 x	66 x	-	99	100	-	66	49	10	10	-	-
Belgium	1	184	4.0	0	5	-	-	-	-	-	70	79	53	-	-	79	88
Belize	5	43	2.0	1	55	17	47	-	92	97	4	38	16	17 x	8 x	76	84
Benin	18	5,110	0.7	2	108	19	13	12	47	78	-	22	8	7	2	71	81
Bhutan	10	137	1.5	0	8	15 x	52 x	-	66 x	40 x	88	24	9	31	14	83	85
Bolivia (Plurinational State of)	6	1,508	3.0	3 x	71 x	20 x	34 x	-	81	90	36	43	19	14	8	82	89
Bosnia and Herzegovina	2	78	1.1	0	10	-	-	-	-	100 x	-	47	22	23	17	-	-
Botswana	7	374	3.0	0	53	-	-	-	-	-	22	28	11	27 x	21 x	86	89
Brazil	6	19,031	0.9	3	49	-	-	-	89	-	67	37	16	7	7	78	89
British Virgin Islands	4	2	1.1	-	14 x	-	-	-	-	-	-	-	-	-	-	-	-
Brunei Darussalam	2	13	4.0	-	10	-	-	-	-	-	89	30	19	14	4	81	94
Bulgaria	3	209	1.6	2	39	5 x	-	-	-	-	3	68	40	-	-	67	80
Burkina Faso	13	6,611	2.8	3	124	28 x	42	-	52 x	83 x	-	35	13	-	-	-	-
Burundi	16	4,980	5.1	1 x	58 x	13	55	34	52	91	-	28	11	21 x	17 x	-	-
Cabo Verde	3	30	3.8	1	57	22 x	68 x	-	-	87 x	-	30	12	-	-	-	-
Cambodia	5	1,533	4.7	0 x	30 x	7 x	46 x	-	71 x	91 x	-	28	11	3	2	90	93
Cameroon	20	12,254	0.8	3	122	28	24	19	58	67	5	38	15	14 x	6 x	-	-
Canada	2	930	1.7	0	7	-	-	-	-	-	87	65	37	-	-	70	82
Central African Republic	22	3,284	1.3	8	184	43	14	-	45	43	-	35	14	-	-	-	-
Chad	25	10,289	1.3	4	139	44	11	-	34 x	42	-	19	7	21 x	14 x	-	-
Chile	3	725	1.1	1	23	-	-	-	-	-	57	68	40	-	-	84	91
China	2	36,785	3.8	-	6	-	-	-	-	-	-	53	28	-	-	80	89
Colombia	5	4,304	3.2	2	53	20	72	-	86	99	11	35	15	21	20	81	87
Comoros	5	90	3.8	2 x	38	17 x	20 x	-	38 x	82 x	-	3	1	16	8	-	-
Congo	8	1,023	4.6	3 x	111 x	26 x	28 x	-	77 x	92 x	-	50	24	28 x	20 x	-	-
Cook Islands	6	1	2.5	0	42	-	-	-	-	-	-	49	23	30	14	78	88
Costa Rica	3	249	1.3	1	33	13	78	-	92	98	59	33	14	10 x	8 x	76	88
Côte d'Ivoire	20	13,547	0.5	5 x	119	25	18	-	47	76	41	36	14	-	-	-	-
Croatia	3	102	1.4	0	9	-	-	-	-	-	-	61	33	-	-	70	84
Cuba	3	374	1.8	1	51	10	76	-	76	100	-	44	20	13	10	-	-
Cyprus	2	21	4.4	0	7	-	-	-	-	-	-	69	41	-	-	-	-
Czechia	2	182	3.0	0	10	-	-	-	-	-	-	77	51	-	-	73	82
Democratic People's Republic of Korea	5	1,817	3.9	0 x	1	-	-	-	-	-	-	38	17	-	-	-	-
Democratic Republic of the Congo	26	56,702	0.4	3	109	25	19	-	46	87	-	34	14	-	-	-	-

TABLE 5. ADOLESCENT HEALTH

Countries and areas	Adolescent mortality rate 2021 — Aged 10–19 Total	Adolescent deaths 2021 — Aged 10–19 Total	Annual rate of reduction in the adolescent mortality rate 2000–2021 — Aged 10–19 Total	Adolescent birth rate 2016–2021 R — Aged 10–14 Female	Adolescent birth rate 2016–2021 R — Aged 15–19 Female	Births by age 18 (%) 2016–2021 R — Women aged 20–24 years who gave birth before age 18 Female	Demand for family planning satisfied with modern methods (%) 2016–2021 R — Aged 15–19 Female	Informed decisions regarding sexual relations, contraceptive use and reproductive health care (%) 2016–2021 R — Aged 15–19 Female	Antenatal care (%) (At least 4 visits) 2016–2021 R — Aged 15–19 Female	Skilled birth attendant (%) 2016–2021 R — Aged 15–19 Female	Girls vaccinated against HPV (%) 2021 Female	Alcohol use 2016 Male	Alcohol use 2016 Female	Tobacco use 2015–2020 R Male	Tobacco use 2015–2020 R Female	Insufficient physical activity among school going adolescents (aged 11–17) 2016 Male	Insufficient physical activity — Female
Denmark	1	87	3.7	0	2	-	-	-	-	-	80	77	51	-	-	82	87
Djibouti	15	349	2.1	0 x	21 x	-	-	-	19 x	83 x	-	16	6	18 x	11 x	81	89
Dominica	3	4	1.9	1 x	47 x	-	-	-	-	-	68	43	19	30 x	20 x	82	86
Dominican Republic	6	1,101	2.6	1	51	20	71	-	90	98	8	40	18	8	6	-	-
Ecuador	4	1,392	2.9	2	58	-	81	-	-	-	3	44	20	15	11	83	90
Egypt	6	11,468	0.9	1 x	47	7 x	64 x	-	87 x	93 x	-	2	1	18 x	8 x	82	93
El Salvador	7	779	1.4	2	52	18 x	70 x	-	90 x	99 x	24	27	11	15	11	83	90
Equatorial Guinea	17	552	2.3	-	176 x	42 x	20 x	-	-	70 x	-	73	46	25 x	17 x	-	-
Eritrea	12	1,040	2.9	1 x	76 x	19 x	6 x	-	40 x	30 x	-	17	6	8 x	5 x	-	-
Estonia	2	30	4.5	0	9	-	-	-	-	-	57	75	49	-	-	81	88
Eswatini	11	280	1.0	1 x	87 x	17 x	34 x	-	68 x	89 x	-	25	10	16 x	9 x	-	-
Ethiopia	11	29,171	5.6	1	74	21	75	36	36	55	75	20	7	-	-	-	-
Fiji	7	113	1.7	0	23	4	-	44	-	-	-	14	5	12	7	81	86
Finland	2	134	1.7	0	4	-	-	-	-	-	-	75	48	-	-	69	82
France	1	1,081	3.7	0	8	-	-	-	-	-	37	78	52	-	-	82	92
Gabon	13	617	1.8	7 x	91 x	28 x	24 x	-	76 x	91 x	-	66	38	9 x	9 x	-	-
Gambia	12	777	2.9	1	65	14	13	13	76	86	30	23	9	18	5	-	-
Georgia	4	177	-0.2	0	27	6	27	66	-	100 x	12	33	13	-	-	-	-
Germany	1	1,141	3.2	0	7	-	-	-	-	-	47	82	58	-	-	80	88
Ghana	11	8,053	1.8	1	78	18	29	-	78	75	-	22	8	9	8	87	88
Greece	1	157	3.8	0	9	-	-	-	-	-	-	67	39	-	-	80	89
Grenada	4	8	0.7	1 x	36 x	-	-	-	-	-	-	47	22	13	7	82	87
Guatemala	8	3,048	1.0	2	63	20 x	50 x	-	85 x	70 x	15	24	9	20	14	84	89
Guinea	19	5,808	2.0	4	120	39	33	16	36	59	-	18	7	31 x	20 x	-	-
Guinea-Bissau	16	769	2.2	2	84	27	24	-	81	62	-	25	10	-	-	-	-
Guyana	8	122	-0.2	0 x	74 x	16 x	17 x	-	86 x	94 x	2	37	15	19	10	82	86
Haiti	11	2,689	2.5	1 x	55 x	14	31	47	55	37	-	32	13	20 x	19 x	-	-
Holy See	-	-	-	-	-	-	-	-	-	-	-	-	-	-	-	-	-
Honduras	7	1,500	1.1	3	97	22 x	74	-	85	94	53	26	10	10	6	80	88
Hungary	2	178	2.6	0	21	-	-	-	-	-	82	68	40	16	15	73	86
Iceland	2	8	3.1	0	4	-	-	-	-	-	90	73	45	-	-	75	85
India	6	149,611	4.2	0 x	12	8	27	-	59	90	-	35	14	-	-	72	76
Indonesia	7	29,806	1.7	0	36	7	82	-	65	87	-	19	7	-	-	85	87
Iran (Islamic Republic of)	6	7,300	1.0	1	28	5 x	-	-	-	-	-	3	1	13	8	-	-
Iraq	7	6,234	1.1	2	70	14	44	-	76	97	-	2	1	20	11	80	90
Ireland	1	78	5.3	0	6	-	-	-	-	-	71	83	60	-	-	64	81
Israel	2	217	2.9	0	8	-	-	-	-	-	55	55	27	-	-	80	90
Italy	1	661	4.3	0	4	-	-	-	-	-	-	65	36	-	-	86	91
Jamaica	5	220	1.3	0	52	15 x	-	-	85 x	97 x	2	32	13	16	15	-	-
Japan	1	1,661	1.9	0	3	-	-	-	-	-	-	59	31	-	-	-	-
Jordan	4	910	1.5	0	27	5	31	43	93	100	-	2	1	34 x	14 x	81	88
Kazakhstan	4	1,240	3.0	0	25	2 x	64 x	-	98 x	99 x	-	37	16	-	-	-	-
Kenya	10	12,823	2.3	1	81	23 x	75	-	58	65 x	44	20	7	13 x	7 x	85	89
Kiribati	11	27	1.0	2	51	8	30	-	66	96	-	10	3	53	43	79	86
Kuwait	3	148	1.9	0	6	-	-	-	-	-	-	0	0	24	10	79	90
Kyrgyzstan	5	554	0.9	0	34	3	29	-	82	100	-	22	8	10	2	-	-
Lao People's Democratic Republic	9	1,289	4.6	3	83	18	60	-	52	56	42	37	16	16	6	78	91
Latvia	3	49	4.0	0	11	-	-	-	-	-	42	78	52	25	21	76	84
Lebanon	3	349	2.5	0 x	12	-	-	-	-	-	-	5	2	35	28	76	88
Lesotho	14	636	1.9	0	91	14 x	60	-	71	90	-	15	5	26 x	22 x	-	-
Liberia	20	2,508	1.1	4	128	34	16	45	86	84	30	27	10	9	11	-	-

FOR EVERY CHILD, VACCINATION

TABLE 5. ADOLESCENT HEALTH

Countries and areas	Adolescent mortality rate 2021 — Total (Aged 10–19)	Adolescent deaths 2021 — Total (Aged 10–19)	Annual rate of reduction in the adolescent mortality rate 2000–2021 — Total (Aged 10–19)	Adolescent birth rate 2016–2021 [R] — Female (Aged 10–14)	Adolescent birth rate 2016–2021 [R] — Female (Aged 15–19)	Births by age 18 (%) 2016–2021 [R] — Women aged 20–24 years who gave birth before age 18	Demand for family planning satisfied with modern methods (%) 2016–2021 [R] — Female (Aged 15–19)	Informed decisions regarding sexual relations, contraceptive use and reproductive health care (%) 2016–2021 [R] — Female (Aged 15–19)	Antenatal care (%) (At least 4 visits) 2016–2021 [R] — Female (Aged 15–19)	Skilled birth attendant (%) 2016–2021 [R] — Female (Aged 15–19)	Girls vaccinated against HPV (%) 2021 — Female	Risk factors (%) — Alcohol use 2016 — Male	Risk factors (%) — Alcohol use 2016 — Female	Risk factors (%) — Tobacco use 2015–2020 — Male	Risk factors (%) — Tobacco use 2015–2020 — Female	Risk factors (%) — Insufficient physical activity among school going adolescents (aged 11–17) 2016 — Male	Risk factors (%) — Insufficient physical activity among school going adolescents (aged 11–17) 2016 — Female
Libya	4	548	1.8	0 x	11 x	-	-	-	-	-	-	0	0	11 x	5 x	78	89
Liechtenstein	-	-	-	1	1	-	-	-	-	-	-	-	-	-	-	-	-
Lithuania	3	72	3.5	0	10	-	-	-	-	-	66	82	59	-	-	76	85
Luxembourg	1	9	2.5	0	4	-	-	-	-	-	-	93	80	-	-	73	85
Madagascar	18	12,027	0.9	7	151	36	68	65	45	42	-	18	6	17	7	-	-
Malawi	12	5,970	4.2	3 x	102	29	69	36	50	97	12	21	8	17 x	11 x	-	-
Malaysia	3	1,684	2.9	0	9	-	-	-	94	98	14	26	10	32	10	81	91
Maldives	3	19	2.2	0	6	1	10	45	87	99	41	6	2	16 x	7 x	78	86
Mali	18	9,639	1.5	7	164	37	31	3	42	71	-	19	7	23 x	9 x	-	-
Malta	2	6	2.6	0	12	-	-	-	-	-	99	64	36	-	-	77	86
Marshall Islands	8	7	1.0	0 x	85 x	21 x	40 x	-	-	94 x	27	-	-	37	21	-	-
Mauritania	10	1,094	0.9	8 x	84 x	22 x	20	20	56 x	67 x	-	1	0	20	19	83	91
Mauritius	4	74	0.4	1	24	-	-	-	-	-	55	28	11	23	14	76	88
Mexico	6	12,749	-0.3	1	71	21 x	63	-	94 x	99 x	1	40	17	22 x	18 x	79	88
Micronesia (Federated States of)	7	17	1.3	1 x	44 x	-	-	-	-	-	32	13	4	34	25	-	-
Monaco	2	0	1.9	-	-	-	-	-	-	-	-	-	-	-	-	-	-
Mongolia	5	254	2.2	0	27	4	53	-	90	100	-	29	12	21	7	74	83
Montenegro	2	16	2.2	0	10	3	-	-	-	-	-	54	27	-	-	-	-
Montserrat	3	0	2.4	0	81 x	-	-	-	-	-	-	-	-	-	-	-	-
Morocco	3	1,866	3.2	0	23	8 x	75	-	45	92	-	2	1	7	4	85	90
Mozambique	15	11,103	3.4	6	180	40 x	34 x	-	55 x	75 x	-	18	7	5	6	83	91
Myanmar	6	5,232	5.2	0	21	5	73	53	47	61	-	24	9	26	4	84	90
Namibia	13	688	1.2	4 x	64	15 x	47 x	-	58 x	88 x	-	27	10	14 x	9 x	86	88
Nauru	8	2	1.3	0 x	94 x	22 x	-	-	-	91 x	-	19	7	26 x	27 x	84	90
Nepal	6	3,964	2.7	0	63	14	30	24	80	81	-	25	9	10	5	82	85
Netherlands (Kingdom of the)	1	273	2.9	0	3	-	-	-	-	-	66	74	47	-	-	77	84
New Zealand	3	165	2.7	0	13	-	-	-	-	-	48	76	51	-	-	85	93
Nicaragua	6	740	2.3	5 x	103	28 x	87 x	-	84 x	88 x	-	29	11	16	12	-	-
Niger	22	13,663	1.9	4	154	48 x	22	-	35	43	-	17	6	12 x	6 x	-	-
Nigeria	15	73,790	2.1	2	106	28	15	9	47	31	-	52	22	-	-	-	-
Niue	7	0	0.8	-	20 x	-	-	-	-	-	76	30	12	23	19	86	88
North Macedonia	2	54	2.1	0	16	4	-	-	-	100 x	21	53	26	-	-	74	84
Norway	2	105	3.2	0	2	-	-	-	-	-	93	81	57	-	-	79	89
Oman	4	215	1.4	0	8	2 x	17 x	-	-	99 x	-	5	2	9	4	78	90
Pakistan	9	45,440	1.2	0	54	7	23	11	44	76	-	1	0	13 x	7 x	85	89
Palau	9	2	0.5	0	34	-	-	-	-	-	21	-	-	48	37	76	82
Panama	5	380	0.7	3	68	-	72 x	-	84 x	99 x	-	45	21	8	7	-	-
Papua New Guinea	10	2,079	1.5	1	68	14 x	33	37	54	61	-	11	4	40	28	-	-
Paraguay	6	737	1.6	1	72 x	-	83	-	92	97	17	33	13	9	7	79	88
Peru	3	2,033	3.8	1	50	11	63	-	93	94	53	51	25	8	6	83	87
Philippines	6	13,297	0.5	1	36	11	47	74	80	86	0	30	12	22	10	93	94
Poland	2	905	2.0	0	9	-	-	-	-	-	-	69	41	-	-	74	84
Portugal	2	166	4.8	0	8	-	-	-	-	-	76	72	44	-	-	78	91
Qatar	2	45	3.5	0	7	-	-	-	-	-	-	32	13	16	9	86	91
Republic of Korea	2	718	3.8	0	1	-	-	-	-	-	-	64	36	-	-	91	97
Republic of Moldova	4	149	1.2	0	18	4 x	52 x	-	96 x	100 x	35	67	39	-	-	73	78
Romania	3	612	3.3	1	37	-	-	-	-	-	-	69	41	-	-	73	87
Russian Federation	4	5,942	4.2	0	16	-	-	-	-	-	-	45	34	-	-	81	88
Rwanda	10	3,289	6.9	0	32	6 x	87	53	44	98	73	32	13	13 x	10 x	-	-
Saint Kitts and Nevis	7	5	0.3	1 x	46 x	-	-	-	-	-	84	54	27	10 x	8 x	78	86
Saint Lucia	5	13	0.2	1 x	25	-	53 x	-	-	-	62	48	23	12	8	83	86

150 THE STATE OF THE WORLD'S CHILDREN 2023

TABLE 5. ADOLESCENT HEALTH

Countries and areas	Adolescent mortality rate 2021 — Aged 10–19 Total	Adolescent deaths 2021 — Aged 10–19 Total	Annual rate of reduction in the adolescent mortality rate 2000–2021 — Aged 10–19 Total	Adolescent birth rate 2016–2021 — Aged 10–14 Female	Adolescent birth rate 2016–2021 — Aged 15–19 Female	Births by age 18 (%) 2016–2021 — Women aged 20–24 years who gave birth before age 18 Female	Demand for family planning satisfied with modern methods (%) 2016–2021 — Aged 15–19 Female	Informed decisions regarding sexual relations, contraceptive use and reproductive health care (%) 2016–2021 — Aged 15–19 Female	Antenatal care (%) (At least 4 visits) 2016–2021 — Aged 15–19 Female	Skilled birth attendant (%) 2016–2021 — Aged 15–19 Female	Girls vaccinated against HPV (%) 2021 — Aged 15–19 Female	Risk factors (%) Alcohol use 2016 Male	Alcohol use 2016 Female	Tobacco use 2015–2020 Male	Tobacco use 2015–2020 Female	Insufficient physical activity among school going adolescents (aged 11–17) 2016 Male	Insufficient physical activity Female
Saint Vincent and the Grenadines	9	14	-2.7	1	47	-	-	-	-	-	-	44	20	10	9	83	89
Samoa	5	20	1.8	0	55	7	8	-	70	94	-	13	5	23	8	87	87
San Marino	1	0	4.0	0 x	1 x	-	-	-	-	-	23	-	-	7	7	-	-
Sao Tome and Principe	8	39	3.0	0	86	22	54	-	81 x	98	-	30	12	31 x	23 x	-	-
Saudi Arabia	5	2,786	2.5	0 x	8 x	-	-	-	-	-	-	3	2	21 x	9 x	-	-
Senegal	10	3,792	3.7	1	71	16	25	2	50	77	21	18	7	15 x	6 x	85	92
Serbia	2	168	2.6	0	12	3	21 x	-	95 x	98 x	-	61	33	-	-	-	-
Seychelles	6	8	-0.1	1	68	-	-	-	-	-	39	52	26	27	16	79	87
Sierra Leone	26	5,072	1.0	4	102	31	34	22	82	90	-	27	11	15	10	-	-
Singapore	1	63	3.1	0	2	-	-	-	-	-	-	71	43	-	-	70	83
Slovakia	2	128	1.7	0	27	-	-	-	-	-	-	70	42	-	-	66	78
Slovenia	2	30	4.1	0	4	-	-	-	-	-	50	73	46	-	-	75	86
Solomon Islands	6	92	1.4	-	78 x	15 x	13 x	-	-	88 x	-	11	4	30 x	24 x	82	85
Somalia	26	10,376	1.5	87 x	123 x	-	-	-	4 x	31 x	-	1	0	-	-	-	-
South Africa	10	10,356	1.2	1	44	15 x	-	46	77	97	34	27	11	-	-	-	-
South Sudan	24	6,688	2.1	6 x	158 x	28 x	4 x	-	21 x	25 x	-	-	-	-	-	-	-
Spain	1	560	4.8	0	6	-	-	-	-	-	77	70	42	-	-	70	84
Sri Lanka	2	858	5.6	0 x	21 x	3	58	-	-	99	46	26	10	13	3	82	89
State of Palestine	5	579	1.0	0	43	6	37	-	96	99	-	-	-	-	-	-	-
Sudan	13	12,616	2.4	2 x	87 x	22 x	19 x	-	49 x	77 x	-	2	1	15 x	7 x	90	91
Suriname	7	76	-0.2	2	56	-	28	-	66	99	2	39	17	17	7	78	85
Sweden	2	188	1.8	0	3	-	-	-	-	-	83	75	48	-	-	82	87
Switzerland	2	129	2.8	0	2	-	-	-	-	-	71	83	60	-	-	83	89
Syrian Arab Republic	6	3,242	0.2	-	54 x	9 x	31 x	-	-	97 x	-	2	0	32 x	17 x	84	91
Tajikistan	3	530	3.7	0	46	1	18	6	67	96	-	17	6	3	3	-	-
Thailand	8	6,849	0.7	0	32	9	80	-	81	98	-	38	16	22	8	70	85
Timor-Leste	19	604	-0.9	0 x	42 x	7	22	38	74	58	-	19	7	42	21	86	93
Togo	12	2,318	2.4	2	79	17	25	-	47	64	-	22	8	11 x	4 x	-	-
Tokelau	-	-	-	-	-	-	-	-	-	-	-	-	-	-	-	-	-
Tonga	4	9	2.0	0	24 x	3	-	-	90	100	-	12	4	28	8	87	85
Trinidad and Tobago	6	123	-0.1	1 x	32 x	6 x	61 x	-	81 x	99 x	8	58	30	17	11	79	86
Tunisia	5	820	0.6	0	6	1	-	-	-	-	-	4	1	19	5	75	88
Türkiye	3	3,499	4.7	0	15	5	40	-	83 x	99	-	6	2	23	12	77	86
Turkmenistan	6	657	1.5	0	22	1	11	10	96	100	99	26	10	0	0	-	-
Turks and Caicos Islands	3	1	1.7	0	21	12	-	-	-	-	-	-	-	-	-	-	-
Tuvalu	7	1	2.0	0	44	5	-	-	-	100 x	27	12	4	30	14	85	89
Uganda	18	20,789	1.5	1	128	28	46	44	59	80	44	34	14	12	9	84	87
Ukraine	3	1,490	2.9	0	15	4 x	59 x	-	87 x	99 x	-	53	37	-	-	71	83
United Arab Emirates	3	200	1.5	0	4	-	-	-	-	-	-	11	4	18	8	78	87
United Kingdom	2	1,236	2.7	0	11	-	-	-	-	-	59	75	49	-	-	75	85
United Republic of Tanzania	11	16,773	2.5	2	139	22	35	-	48	68	57	34	14	7	2	78	86
United States	4	16,379	0.8	0	17	-	82	-	-	-	48	73	46	-	-	64	80
Uruguay	4	207	0.8	1	33	-	-	-	44 x	100 x	17	71	43	10	14	75	89
Uzbekistan	5	2,808	1.3	0	19	2 x	-	26 x	-	99 x	87	17	6	14 x	14 x	-	-
Vanuatu	7	45	0.6	-	81 x	13 x	-	-	-	93 x	-	11	4	20	15	86	89
Venezuela (Bolivarian Republic of)	13	7,150	-2.1	3	84	24 x	-	-	-	-	-	35	14	16	12	85	93
Viet Nam	4	6,184	1.8	0 x	29	8	60 x	-	55 x	87 x	-	33	13	-	-	82	91
Yemen	11	8,001	0.1	1 x	67 x	17 x	23 x	-	30 x	52 x	-	1	0	24 x	10 x	83	90
Zambia	12	5,620	3.1	3	135	31	63	37	59	84	33	24	9	25 x	26 x	89	89
Zimbabwe	16	5,996	0.4	1	108	24	77 x	48 x	71	89	40	15	5	22 x	16 x	85	89

FOR EVERY CHILD, VACCINATION

TABLE 5. ADOLESCENT HEALTH

Countries and areas	Adolescent mortality rate 2021 — Aged 10–19 Total	Adolescent deaths 2021 — Aged 10–19 Total	Annual rate of reduction in the adolescent mortality rate 2000–2021 — Aged 10–19 Total	Adolescent birth rate 2016–2021 [R] — Aged 10–14 Female	Adolescent birth rate 2016–2021 [R] — Aged 15–19 Female	Births by age 18 (%) 2016–2021 [R] — Women aged 20–24 years who gave birth before age 18 Female	Demand for family planning satisfied with modern methods (%) 2016–2021 [R] — Aged 15–19 Female	Informed decisions regarding sexual relations, contraceptive use and reproductive health care (%) 2016–2021 [R] — Aged 15–19 Female	Antenatal care (%) (At least 4 visits) 2016–2021 [R] — Aged 15–19 Female	Skilled birth attendant (%) 2016–2021 [R] — Aged 15–19 Female	Girls vaccinated against HPV (%) 2021 — Female	Risk factors (%) — Alcohol use 2016 — Male	Alcohol use 2016 — Female	Tobacco use 2015–2020 [R] — Male	Tobacco use 2015–2020 [R] — Female	Insufficient physical activity among school going adolescents (aged 11–17) 2016 — Male	Insufficient physical activity among school going adolescents (aged 11–17) 2016 — Female
SUMMARY																	
East Asia and Pacific	4	110,991	2.5	0	20	-	69	-	69	83	-	44	22	-	-	82	89
Europe and Central Asia	3	27,539	3.6	0	14	-	63	-	-	-	-	53	34	-	-	76	86
Eastern Europe and Central Asia	4	19,592	3.4	-	19	-	56	-	-	-	-	31	19	-	-	74	84
Western Europe	2	7,946	3.4	-	8	-	79	-	-	-	-	75	49	-	-	76	86
Latin America and Caribbean	6	63,793	1.0	2	53	15 j	71	-	86	92 j	-	41	18	12	11	80	88
Middle East and North Africa	6	47,624	1.1	1	35	-	53	-	-	-	-	3	1	-	-	80	90
North America	4	17,309	0.9	0	15	-	83	-	-	-	-	72	45	-	-	65	81
South Asia	6	228,731	3.5	1	29	10	43	25	47	77	-	27	11	-	-	74	79
Sub-Saharan Africa	16	423,740	2.2	5	100	27	41	26	50	61	-	29	12	-	-	-	-
Eastern and Southern Africa	14	186,399	3.0	-	94	26	53	41	52	69	-	23	9	-	-	-	-
West and Central Africa	18	237,341	1.4	-	107	27	24	10	48	55	-	37	15	-	-	-	-
Least developed countries	14	335,546	-	-	94	24	51	38	45	66	-	19	7	-	-	-	-
World	**7**	**919,729**	**1.8**	**2**	**43**	**14**	**52**	**-**	**54**	**70**	**-**	**36**	**17**	**-**	**-**	**78**	**86**

For a complete list of countries and areas in the regions, subregions and country categories, see page on Regional Classifications or visit <data.unicef.org/regionalclassifications>.

It is not advisable to compare data from consecutive editions of *The State of the World's Children* report.

NOTES

- Data not available.

j Excludes Brazil and Mexico.

k Excludes India.

[R] Data refer to the most recent year available during the period specified in the column heading.

x Data refer to years or periods other than those specified in the column heading. Such data are not included in the calculation of regional and global averages. Estimates from data years prior to 2000 are not displayed.

MAIN DATA SOURCES

Adolescent mortality rate – United Nations Inter-agency Group for Child Mortality Estimation (UNICEF, World Health Organization, United Nations Population Division and the World Bank Group). Last update: January 2023.

Adolescent deaths – United Nations Inter-agency Group for Child Mortality Estimation (UNICEF, World Health Organization, United Nations Population Division and the World Bank Group). Last update: January 2023.

Annual rate of reduction in the adolescent mortality rate – United Nations Inter-agency Group for Child Mortality Estimation (UNICEF, World Health Organization, United Nations Population Division and the World Bank Group). Last update: January 2023.

Adolescent birth rate – Global SDG Indicators Database, 2022. Last update: August 2022.

Births by age 18 – DHS, MICS and other national household surveys. Last update: September 2022.

Demand for family planning satisfied with modern methods (adolescent girls and young women 15–19) – United Nations, Department of Economic and Social Affairs, Population Division (2022). World Contraceptive Use 2022. New York: United Nations; based on Demographic and Health Surveys (DHS), Multiple Indicator Cluster Surveys (MICS), Reproductive Health Surveys, other national surveys, and National Health Information Systems (HIS). Last Update: July 2022.

Informed decisions – DHS, MICS and other national household surveys. Last update: September 2022.

Antenatal care (at least four visits) (adolescent girls and young women 15-19) – DHS, MICS and other national household surveys. Last update: September 2022.

Skilled birth attendant (adolescent girls and young women 15-19) – DHS, MICS and other national household surveys. Last update: September 2022.

Girls vaccinated against HPV – WHO/UNICEF estimates of human papillomavirus (HPV) immunization coverage, 2021 revision. Last update: July 2022.

Alcohol use – WHO estimates based on international surveys (WHS, STEPS, GENACIS, and ECAS) as well as national surveys. Last update: January 2022.

Tobacco use – WHO Global Health Observatory, based on School-based surveys, other national surveys and censuses. Last update: January 2022.

Insufficient physical activity – Main data sources included the Global School-based Student Health Survey (GSHS), the Health Behaviour in School-aged Children (HBSC), and some other national surveys; Data host: WHO Global Status Report on NCDs. Last update: January 2022.

DEFINITIONS OF THE INDICATORS

Adolescent mortality rate – The probability of dying among adolescents aged 10–19 years expressed per 1,000 adolescents aged 10.

Adolescent deaths – Number of deaths aged 10–19 years.

Annual rate of reduction in adolescent mortality rate – The annual rate of reduction in adolescent mortality rate (AMR) defined as AMR=100*(ln(AMRt2/AMRt1)/(t1-t2)), where t1=2000 and t2=2021.

Adolescent birth rate – Number of births per 1,000 adolescent girls and young women aged 10–14 and 15–19.

Births by age 18 – Percentage of women aged 20–24 who gave birth before age 18. The indicator refers to women who had a live birth in a recent time period, generally two years for MICS and five years for DHS.

Demand for family planning satisfied with modern methods – Percentage of adolescent girls and young women (aged 15–19) who have their need for family planning satisfied with modern methods.

Informed decisions – Percentage of adolescent girls and young women (aged 15-19) years who make their own informed decisions regarding sexual relations, contraceptive use and reproductive health care.

Antenatal care (at least four visits) – Percentage of adolescent girls and young women (aged 15–19) attended by any provider at least four times.

Skilled birth attendant – Percentage of births from adolescent girls and young women (aged 15–19), attended by skilled heath personnel (typically a doctor, nurse or midwife).

Girls vaccinated against HPV (%) – Percentage of girls who received the last dose of human papillomavirus (HPV) vaccine per national schedule.

Alcohol use – Percentage of adolescents aged 15–19 who had at least one alcoholic drink at any time during the last twelve months.

Tobacco use – Percentage of adolescents aged 13–15 who smoked cigarettes or used smoked or smokeless tobacco products at any time during the last one month.

Insufficient physical activity – Percentage of school going adolescents aged 11–17 not meeting WHO recommendations on physical activity for health, i.e. doing less than 60 minutes of moderate- to vigorous-intensity physical activity daily.

TABLE 6. HIV/AIDS: EPIDEMIOLOGY

Countries and areas	HIV incidence per 1,000 uninfected population				AIDS-related mortality per 100,000 population				Number of children living with HIV			
	Children 0–14	Adolescents 10–19	Adolescent girls 10–19	Adolescent boys 10–19	Children 0–14	Adolescents 10–19	Adolescent girls 10–19	Adolescent boys 10–19	Children 0–9	Adolescents 10–19	Adolescent girls 10–19	Adolescent boys 10–19
Afghanistan	0.02	0.02	0.02	0.02	0.41	0.08	0.08	0.08	<500	<500	<200	<200
Albania	-	-	-	-	-	-	-	-	-	-	-	-
Algeria	0.06	0.01	<0.01	0.01	0.99	0.01	0.03	0.03	1,200	<500	<200	<200
Andorra	-	-	-	-	-	-	-	-	-	-	-	-
Angola	0.64	0.59	1.03	0.15	23.15	10.70	10.56	10.86	25,000	23,000	14,000	9,100
Anguilla	-	-	-	-	-	-	-	-	-	-	-	-
Antigua and Barbuda	-	-	-	-	-	-	-	-	-	-	-	-
Argentina	0.02	0.21	0.17	0.25	0.19	0.20	0.18	0.23	-	-	-	-
Armenia	0.03	0.06	0.09	0.05	0.31	<0.01	<0.01	<0.01	<100	<100	<100	<100
Australia	-	-	-	-	-	-	-	-	-	-	-	-
Austria	-	-	-	-	-	-	-	-	-	-	-	-
Azerbaijan	0.02	0.01	0.02	0.01	0.41	0.21	0.15	0.13	<200	<200	<100	<100
Bahamas	0.55	0.24	0.24	0.23	10.20	1.97	4.04	3.86	<100	<100	<100	<100
Bahrain	-	-	-	-	-	-	-	-	-	-	-	-
Bangladesh	<0.01	<0.01	<0.01	<0.01	0.06	<0.01	<0.01	<0.01	<500	<200	<200	<100
Barbados	-	-	-	-	-	-	-	-	-	-	-	-
Belarus	0.12	0.06	0.08	0.05	2.91	<0.01	<0.01	<0.01	<500	<200	<100	<100
Belgium	-	-	-	-	-	-	-	-	-	-	-	-
Belize	0.27	0.40	0.51	0.30	5.81	1.27	<0.01	<0.01	<100	<200	<100	<100
Benin	0.22	0.14	0.25	0.04	7.69	5.72	5.44	5.92	3,900	5,300	2,800	2,400
Bhutan	-	-	-	-	-	-	-	-	-	-	-	-
Bolivia (Plurinational State of)	0.06	0.04	0.05	0.03	1.29	0.56	0.62	0.51	<500	590	<500	<500
Bosnia and Herzegovina	-	-	-	-	-	-	-	-	-	-	-	-
Botswana	0.90	3.37	5.78	1.03	21.93	33.07	33.78	32.37	3,000	10,000	5,700	4,400
Brazil	-	-	-	-	-	-	-	-	-	-	-	-
British Virgin Islands	-	-	-	-	-	-	-	-	-	-	-	-
Brunei Darussalam	-	-	-	-	-	-	-	-	-	-	-	-
Bulgaria	-	-	-	-	-	-	-	-	-	-	-	-
Burkina Faso	0.13	0.11	0.17	0.05	3.73	4.20	4.04	4.35	3,400	7,000	3,700	3,300
Burundi	0.42	0.09	0.15	0.02	9.48	6.03	5.66	6.32	4,500	7,500	3,900	3,600
Cabo Verde	0.13	0.07	0.11	0.04	1.82	0.92	<0.01	<0.01	<100	<100	<100	<100
Cambodia	0.05	0.18	0.12	0.23	0.87	0.77	0.72	0.82	780	3,900	1,900	2,100
Cameroon	1.04	0.64	1.13	0.16	30.79	14.45	14.15	14.75	20,000	31,000	18,000	13,000
Canada	-	-	-	-	-	-	-	-	-	-	-	-
Central African Republic	0.68	1.09	1.48	0.71	20.08	17.22	16.22	18.36	3,500	7,500	4,100	3,400
Chad	0.32	0.27	0.44	0.11	10.07	5.70	5.58	5.81	6,200	9,000	5,000	3,900
Chile	0.05	0.27	0.06	0.46	-	-	-	-	<200	1,100	<500	890
China	-	-	-	-	-	-	-	-	-	-	-	-
Colombia	0.08	0.21	0.05	0.36	1.87	0.56	0.51	0.61	1,600	4,100	1,200	2,900
Comoros	-	-	-	-	-	-	-	-	-	-	-	-
Congo	2.93	3.11	5.84	0.45	76.46	18.86	21.25	16.50	9,100	9,400	6,800	2,600
Cook Islands	-	-	-	-	-	-	-	-	-	-	-	-
Costa Rica	0.05	0.22	0.10	0.34	1.15	0.42	0.29	0.55	<100	<500	<100	<500
Côte d'Ivoire	0.19	0.16	0.30	0.02	5.68	9.49	8.70	10.25	9,300	23,000	12,000	11,000
Croatia	-	-	-	-	-	-	-	-	-	-	-	-
Cuba	0.03	0.49	0.20	0.77	0.54	0.39	0.16	0.46	<100	940	<500	730
Cyprus	-	-	-	-	-	-	-	-	-	-	-	-
Czechia	-	-	-	-	-	-	-	-	-	-	-	-
Democratic People's Republic of Korea	-	-	-	-	-	-	-	-	-	-	-	-
Democratic Republic of the Congo	0.32	0.13	0.19	0.06	8.05	4.52	4.36	4.68	42,000	43,000	23,000	21,000
Denmark	-	-	-	-	-	-	-	-	-	-	-	-
Djibouti	0.17	0.08	0.11	0.06	5.48	4.23	4.28	4.19	<200	<500	<200	<100
Dominica	-	-	-	-	-	-	-	-	-	-	-	-
Dominican Republic	0.17	0.11	0.14	0.08	4.76	1.50	1.53	1.57	1,300	1,600	820	740
Ecuador	0.08	0.08	0.09	0.07	1.99	0.29	0.26	0.25	790	930	<500	<500
Egypt	-	-	-	-	0.45	0.05	0.06	0.04	930	710	<500	<500
El Salvador	0.09	0.05	0.07	0.03	2.25	0.42	0.51	0.33	<500	<500	<500	<200
Equatorial Guinea	3.67	2.84	4.46	1.28	89.97	20.61	20.19	21.01	2,800	2,100	1,300	790
Eritrea	0.06	0.05	0.08	0.02	1.14	1.07	1.10	1.26	<500	620	<500	<500
Estonia	-	-	-	-	-	-	-	-	-	-	-	-
Eswatini	2.11	7.83	15.15	0.85	35.84	50.47	58.98	42.01	3,600	11,000	6,500	4,000
Ethiopia	0.21	0.12	0.22	0.02	4.57	3.65	3.58	3.71	23,000	45,000	24,000	21,000
Fiji	0.12	0.06	0.10	0.02	1.45	<0.01	<0.01	<0.01	<100	<100	<100	<100
Finland	-	-	-	-	-	-	-	-	-	-	-	-

FOR EVERY CHILD, VACCINATION

153

TABLE 6. HIV/AIDS: EPIDEMIOLOGY

Countries and areas	HIV incidence per 1,000 uninfected population				AIDS-related mortality per 100,000 population				Number of children living with HIV			
	Children 0–14	Adolescents 10–19	Adolescent girls 10–19	Adolescent boys 10–19	Children 0–14	Adolescents 10–19	Adolescent girls 10–19	Adolescent boys 10–19	Children 0–9	Adolescents 10–19	Adolescent girls 10–19	Adolescent boys 10–19
France	<0.01	0.05	0.06	0.05	0.07	0.01	0.02	<0.01	<500	680	<500	<500
Gabon	1.13	0.99	1.86	0.14	34.42	17.06	17.64	16.49	1,600	2,200	1,300	880
Gambia	0.42	0.22	0.39	0.04	11.72	5.24	5.26	5.55	910	950	520	<500
Georgia	0.02	0.03	0.02	0.04	0.37	<0.01	<0.01	<0.01	<100	<100	<100	<100
Germany	<0.01	0.04	0.02	0.06	0.03	<0.01	<0.01	<0.01	<100	<500	<100	<500
Ghana	0.71	0.58	1.06	0.09	22.09	10.77	10.68	10.82	18,000	23,000	14,000	9,000
Greece	-	-	-	-	-	-	-	-	-	-	-	-
Grenada	-	-	-	-	-	-	-	-	-	-	-	-
Guatemala	-	-	-	-	-	-	-	-	-	-	-	-
Guinea	0.58	0.89	1.46	0.32	16.26	8.29	8.33	8.19	7,600	10,000	6,300	3,800
Guinea-Bissau	2.03	0.75	1.15	0.35	47.23	20.83	20.45	21.64	2,500	2,500	1,400	1,100
Guyana	0.53	0.20	0.30	0.10	13.30	3.03	2.48	2.38	<500	<500	<200	<200
Haiti	0.46	0.47	0.81	0.14	6.93	2.09	2.12	2.06	3,700	6,100	3,700	2,400
Holy See	-	-	-	-	-	-	-	-	-	-	-	-
Honduras	0.08	0.01	0.01	0.02	2.41	1.21	1.34	1.19	<500	1,100	530	550
Hungary	-	-	-	-	-	-	-	-	-	-	-	-
Iceland	-	-	-	-	-	-	-	-	-	-	-	-
India	-	-	-	-	-	-	-	-	-	-	-	-
Indonesia	0.14	0.15	0.12	0.17	3.34	0.51	0.50	0.53	15,000	13,000	5,800	7,700
Iran (Islamic Republic of)	0.02	0.01	0.01	0.01	0.49	0.26	0.25	0.26	900	1,000	520	520
Iraq	-	-	-	-	-	-	-	-	-	-	-	-
Ireland	-	-	-	-	-	-	-	-	-	-	-	-
Israel	-	-	-	-	-	-	-	-	-	-	-	-
Italy	-	-	-	-	-	-	-	-	-	-	-	-
Jamaica	0.19	0.96	0.99	0.93	5.75	1.13	0.93	1.33	<500	1,100	530	530
Japan	-	-	-	-	-	-	-	-	-	-	-	-
Jordan	-	-	-	-	-	-	-	-	-	-	-	-
Kazakhstan	0.02	0.03	0.03	0.03	0.33	0.03	0.07	0.06	<500	<500	<500	<500
Kenya	0.74	1.01	1.78	0.24	16.30	13.33	12.84	13.85	48,000	100,000	56,000	44,000
Kiribati	-	-	-	-	-	-	-	-	-	-	-	-
Kuwait	-	-	-	-	-	-	-	-	-	-	-	-
Kyrgyzstan	0.03	0.04	0.05	0.03	0.80	0.17	0.17	0.17	<500	<500	<500	<500
Lao People's Democratic Republic	0.04	0.11	0.11	0.11	1.17	0.27	0.28	0.27	<500	<500	<500	<500
Latvia	0.09	0.09	0.12	0.07	1.63	<0.01	<0.01	<0.01	<100	<100	<100	<100
Lebanon	-	-	-	-	-	-	-	-	-	-	-	-
Lesotho	3.57	4.69	8.24	1.25	91.46	48.64	48.73	48.56	5,000	13,000	7,600	5,600
Liberia	-	-	-	-	8.49	7.24	6.85	7.61	1,500	2,800	1,600	1,200
Libya	0.06	0.05	0.04	0.07	1.18	0.26	0.18	0.33	<500	<200	<100	<200
Liechtenstein	-	-	-	-	-	-	-	-	-	-	-	-
Lithuania	-	-	-	-	-	-	-	-	-	-	-	-
Luxembourg	-	-	-	-	-	-	-	-	-	-	-	-
Madagascar	0.25	0.13	0.22	0.05	5.48	0.44	0.50	0.37	3,200	1,200	900	<500
Malawi	1.03	1.14	2.05	0.17	18.99	21.62	21.97	21.20	30,000	68,000	38,000	30,000
Malaysia	<0.01	0.07	0.03	0.10	0.04	0.04	0.04	0.04	<200	650	<500	<500
Maldives	-	-	-	-	-	-	-	-	-	-	-	-
Mali	0.33	0.08	0.12	0.04	9.04	3.91	3.58	4.23	6,400	6,000	3,100	2,900
Malta	-	-	-	-	-	-	-	-	-	-	-	-
Marshall Islands	-	-	-	-	-	-	-	-	-	-	-	-
Mauritania	0.18	0.04	0.05	0.02	3.92	1.63	1.54	1.72	530	<500	<500	<200
Mauritius	0.09	0.31	0.44	0.21	-	-	-	-	<100	<200	<100	<100
Mexico	0.05	0.20	0.11	0.30	1.04	0.19	0.15	0.23	2,400	8,400	2,700	5,800
Micronesia (Federated States of)	-	-	-	-	-	-	-	-	-	-	-	-
Monaco	-	-	-	-	-	-	-	-	-	-	-	-
Mongolia	-	-	-	-	-	-	-	-	-	-	-	-
Montenegro	-	-	-	-	-	-	-	-	-	-	-	-
Montserrat	-	-	-	-	-	-	-	-	-	-	-	-
Morocco	0.03	<0.01	0.01	<0.01	0.45	0.06	0.07	0.06	690	540	<500	<500
Mozambique	-	-	-	-	-	-	-	-	-	-	-	-
Myanmar	0.35	0.43	0.46	0.39	4.58	0.97	1.16	0.79	6,600	12,000	6,300	5,300
Namibia	1.33	4.30	7.64	1.00	26.72	29.36	31.73	26.97	3,400	12,000	7,000	4,700
Nauru	-	-	-	-	-	-	-	-	-	-	-	-
Nepal	0.02	<0.01	<0.01	<0.01	0.18	0.03	0.03	0.03	660	1,100	540	540
Netherlands (Kingdom of the)	-	-	-	-	-	-	-	-	-	-	-	-
New Zealand	-	-	-	-	-	-	-	-	-	-	-	-
Nicaragua	0.04	0.22	0.15	0.28	0.61	0.32	0.32	0.31	<200	520	<500	<500

154 THE STATE OF THE WORLD'S CHILDREN 2023

TABLE 6. HIV/AIDS: EPIDEMIOLOGY

Countries and areas	HIV incidence per 1,000 uninfected population				AIDS-related mortality per 100,000 population				Number of children living with HIV			
	Children 0–14	Adolescents 10–19	Adolescent girls 10–19	Adolescent boys 10–19	Children 0–14	Adolescents 10–19	Adolescent girls 10–19	Adolescent boys 10–19	Children 0–9	Adolescents 10–19	Adolescent girls 10–19	Adolescent boys 10–19
Niger	0.08	0.01	0.02	<0.01	1.95	1.10	1.00	1.19	1,900	2,100	1,100	1,100
Nigeria	0.71	0.32	0.58	0.06	17.94	6.45	6.64	6.28	130,000	120,000	71,000	50,000
Niue	-	-	-	-	-	-	-	-	-	-	-	-
North Macedonia	-	-	-	-	-	-	-	-	-	-	-	-
Norway	-	-	-	-	-	-	-	-	-	-	-	-
Oman	0.03	0.08	0.06	0.10	0.51	<0.01	<0.01	<0.01	<100	<100	<100	<100
Pakistan					0.66	0.06	0.05	0.06	4,100	3,000	1,300	1,700
Palau	-	-	-	-	-	-	-	-	-	-	-	-
Panama	-	-	-	-	-	-	-	-	-	-	-	-
Papua New Guinea	0.55	0.31	0.49	0.15	9.32	1.13	1.17	1.20	2,500	2,500	1,400	1,100
Paraguay	0.11	0.20	0.15	0.24	2.42	0.37	0.46	0.29	<500	590	<500	<500
Peru	0.07	0.04	0.05	0.03	1.04	0.25	0.22	0.23	1,100	1,000	540	<500
Philippines	0.02	0.33	0.07	0.58	0.25	0.16	0.05	0.25	690	8,000	860	7,100
Poland	-	-	-	-	-	-	-	-	-	-	-	-
Portugal	-	-	-	-	-	-	-	-	-	-	-	-
Qatar	-	-	-	-	-	-	-	-	-	-	-	-
Republic of Korea	-	-	-	-	-	-	-	-	-	-	-	-
Republic of Moldova	0.12	0.16	0.17	0.16	2.86	<0.01	<0.01	<0.01	<200	<200	<100	<100
Romania	0.02	0.01	0.01	<0.01	0.27	<0.01	<0.01	<0.01	<200	<200	<100	<100
Russian Federation	-	-	-	-	-	-	-	-	-	-	-	-
Rwanda	0.42	0.30	0.54	0.05	7.19	6.71	6.43	7.00	5,300	14,000	7,400	6,400
Saint Kitts and Nevis	-	-	-	-	-	-	-	-	-	-	-	-
Saint Lucia	-	-	-	-	-	-	-	-	-	-	-	-
Saint Vincent and the Grenadines	-	-	-	-	-	-	-	-	-	-	-	-
Samoa	-	-	-	-	-	-	-	-	-	-	-	-
San Marino	-	-	-	-	-	-	-	-	-	-	-	-
Sao Tome and Principe	-	-	-	-	-	-	-	-	-	-	-	-
Saudi Arabia	-	-	-	-	-	-	-	-	-	-	-	-
Senegal	0.14	0.03	0.04	0.01	3.77	2.44	2.26	2.62	2,400	3,300	1,700	1,600
Serbia	-	-	-	-	-	-	-	-	-	-	-	-
Seychelles	-	-	-	-	-	-	-	-	-	-	-	-
Sierra Leone	1.43	0.75	1.20	0.31	38.72	15.21	14.39	16.02	7,600	8,000	4,600	3,400
Singapore	-	-	-	-	-	-	-	-	-	-	-	-
Slovakia	-	-	-	-	-	-	-	-	-	-	-	-
Slovenia	-	-	-	-	-	-	-	-	-	-	-	-
Solomon Islands	-	-	-	-	-	-	-	-	-	-	-	-
Somalia	0.02	<0.01	<0.01	<0.01	0.87	0.74	0.72	0.76	500	700	<500	<500
South Africa	1.85	7.19	12.66	1.95	16.82	26.98	30.77	23.23	130,000	320,000	200,000	120,000
South Sudan	1.37	0.99	1.53	0.47	32.15	10.61	10.76	10.47	11,000	10,000	6,000	4,200
Spain	-	-	-	-	-	-	-	-	-	-	-	-
Sri Lanka	-	-	-	-	-	-	-	-	-	-	-	-
State of Palestine	-	-	-	-	-	-	-	-	-	-	-	-
Sudan	0.08	0.04	0.05	0.03	1.96	0.59	0.59	0.58	2,400	2,100	1,100	950
Suriname	0.28	0.21	0.32	0.11	3.96	<0.01	<0.01	<0.01	<100	<200	<100	<100
Sweden	-	-	-	-	-	-	-	-	-	-	-	-
Switzerland	-	-	-	-	-	-	-	-	-	-	-	-
Syrian Arab Republic	-	-	-	-	-	-	-	-	-	-	-	-
Tajikistan	0.06	0.04	0.06	0.02	1.21	0.05	0.10	0.10	640	<500	<500	<200
Thailand	0.01	0.21	0.14	0.29	0.84	0.98	0.96	1.00	640	6,100	2,700	3,400
Timor-Leste	-	-	-	-	-	-	-	-	-	-	-	-
Togo	0.83	0.32	0.58	0.07	20.20	10.66	10.08	11.34	5,300	8,300	4,500	3,800
Tokelau	-	-	-	-	-	-	-	-	-	-	-	-
Tonga	-	-	-	-	-	-	-	-	-	-	-	-
Trinidad and Tobago	-	-	-	-	-	-	-	-	-	-	-	-
Tunisia	0.02	0.01	0.02	<0.01	0.54	0.06	0.12	0.11	<200	<100	<100	<100
Türkiye	-	-	-	-	-	-	-	-	-	-	-	-
Turkmenistan	-	-	-	-	-	-	-	-	-	-	-	-
Turks and Caicos Islands	-	-	-	-	-	-	-	-	-	-	-	-
Tuvalu	-	-	-	-	-	-	-	-	-	-	-	-
Uganda	0.82	1.64	3.02	0.29	19.92	13.99	14.00	13.98	49,000	98,000	59,000	40,000
Ukraine	0.06	0.05	0.06	0.04	0.89	0.24	0.22	0.25	1,300	2,700	1,400	1,400
United Arab Emirates	-	-	-	-	-	-	-	-	-	-	-	-
United Kingdom	-	-	-	-	-	-	-	-	-	-	-	-
United Republic of Tanzania	0.96	1.00	1.60	0.41	23.52	11.99	12.40	11.58	61,000	96,000	54,000	42,000
United States	<0.01	0.05	0.02	0.09	0.14	0.04	0.03	0.05	1,000	5,400	2,000	3,400

FOR EVERY CHILD, VACCINATION

TABLE 6. HIV/AIDS: EPIDEMIOLOGY

Countries and areas	HIV incidence per 1,000 uninfected population				AIDS-related mortality per 100,000 population				Number of children living with HIV			
	Children 0–14	Adolescents 10–19	Adolescent girls 10–19	Adolescent boys 10–19	Children 0–14	Adolescents 10–19	Adolescent girls 10–19	Adolescent boys 10–19	Children 0–9	Adolescents 10–19	Adolescent girls 10–19	Adolescent boys 10–19
Uruguay	0.16	0.09	0.13	0.05	1.53	0.22	<0.01	<0.01	<200	<200	<100	<100
Uzbekistan	0.06	0.05	0.05	0.05	1.91	0.55	0.52	0.53	3,700	4,500	2,300	2,200
Vanuatu	-	-	-	-	-	-	-	-	-	-	-	-
Venezuela (Bolivarian Republic of)	-	-	-	-	5.21	1.58	1.67	1.46	2,700	4,800	2,000	2,800
Viet Nam	0.05	0.03	0.03	0.02	0.60	0.04	0.05	0.03	3,000	3,700	1,800	1,900
Yemen	-	-	-	-	-	-	-	-	-	-	-	-
Zambia	1.25	2.94	5.09	0.84	28.31	26.96	28.73	25.21	40,000	72,000	44,000	28,000
Zimbabwe	1.92	1.77	3.12	0.43	41.30	38.13	37.53	38.79	36,000	77,000	42,000	35,000
SUMMARY												
East Asia and Pacific	0.05	0.09	0.07	0.11	0.90	0.19	0.19	0.18	36,000	59,000	26,000	34,000
Europe and Central Asia	-	-	-	-	-	-	-	-	-	-	-	-
Eastern Europe and Central Asia	-	-	-	-	-	-	-	-	-	-	-	-
Western Europe	-	-	-	-	-	-	-	-	-	-	-	-
Latin America and Caribbean	0.10	0.18	0.12	0.23	1.98	0.59	0.58	0.59	27,000	55,000	24,000	31,000
Middle East and North Africa	0.02	0.02	0.02	0.02	0.44	0.09	0.09	0.08	4,800	4,100	2,100	2,000
North America	-	-	-	-	-	-	-	-	-	-	-	-
South Asia	0.04	0.05	0.04	0.05	0.62	0.14	0.13	0.15	44,000	91,000	42,000	49,000
Sub-Saharan Africa	0.73	0.94	1.62	0.27	16.98	9.92	10.14	9.71	880,000	1,470,000	860,000	610,000
Eastern and Southern Africa	0.93	1.60	2.74	0.47	19.69	13.34	13.81	12.86	600,000	1,140,000	670,000	470,000
West and Central Africa	0.54	0.32	0.55	0.08	14.55	6.72	6.66	6.77	280,000	330,000	190,000	140,000
Least developed countries	-	-	-	-	-	-	-	-	-	-	-	-
World	**0.23**	**0.26**	**0.39**	**0.13**	**4.93**	**2.30**	**2.39**	**2.21**	**1,020,000**	**1,710,000**	**970,000**	**740,000**

For a complete list of countries and areas in the regions, subregions and country categories, see page on Regional Classifications or visit <data.unicef.org/regionalclassifications>.

It is not advisable to compare data from consecutive editions of *The State of the World's Children* report.

NOTES

- Data not available.

Due to rounding of the estimates, disaggregates may not add up to the total.

MAIN DATA SOURCES

HIV incidence per 1,000 uninfected population – UNAIDS 2022 estimates. Last update: July 2022.

AIDS-related mortality per 100,000 population – UNAIDS 2022 estimates. Last update: July 2022.

Number of children living with HIV – UNAIDS 2022 estimates. Last update: July 2022.

DEFINITIONS OF THE INDICATORS

HIV incidence per 1,000 uninfected population – Estimated number of new HIV infections per 1,000 uninfected population at risk of HIV infection.

AIDS-related mortality per 100,000 population – Estimated number of AIDS-related deaths per 100,000 population.

Number of children living with HIV – Estimated number of children living with HIV.

TABLE 7. HIV/AIDS: INTERVENTION COVERAGE

Countries and areas	Percentage of pregnant women living with HIV receiving effective ARVs for PMTCT (%)	Early infant HIV diagnosis (%)	Children living with HIV receiving ART (%)		Comprehensive knowledge of HIV among adolescents age 15-19 (%) 2012–2020 [R]		Condom use among adolescents age 15-19 (%) with multiple partners (%) 2012–2020 [R]		Adolescents age 15-19 tested for HIV in the last 12 months and who have received results (%) 2012–2020 [R]	
			Children 0–14	Adolescents 10–19	Male	Female	Male	Female	Male	Female
Afghanistan	16	6	12	10	4	1	-	-	-	-
Albania	-	-	-	-	20	35	-	-	-	-
Algeria	16	14	82	87	-	8	-	-	-	1
Andorra	-	-	-	-	-	-	-	-	-	-
Angola	76	3	19	19	-	-	-	-	-	-
Anguilla	-	-	-	-	-	-	-	-	-	-
Antigua and Barbuda	-	-	-	-	55 x	40 x	100 x	54 x	-	-
Argentina	-	-	-	-	-	36	-	-	-	-
Armenia	81	86	>95	31	9	15	-	-	-	-
Australia	-	-	-	-	-	-	-	-	-	-
Austria	-	-	-	56	-	-	-	-	-	-
Azerbaijan	59	54	54	39	2 x	3 x	-	-	-	-
Bahamas	68	68	40	48	-	-	-	-	-	-
Bahrain	-	-	-	-	-	-	-	-	-	-
Bangladesh	36	16	48	50	-	11	-	-	-	-
Barbados	-	-	-	-	-	66	-	-	-	10
Belarus	40	41	53	67	53	51	-	-	15	15
Belgium	-	-	-	48	-	-	-	-	-	-
Belize	80	38	41	57	44	40	69	-	7	13
Benin	>95	46	37	57	14	14	43	38	6	7
Bhutan	-	-	-	-	-	22 x	-	-	-	3 x
Bolivia (Plurinational State of)	88	-	46	38	24 x	20 x	-	-	-	-
Bosnia and Herzegovina	-	-	-	45	41	42	-	-	0	0
Botswana	>95	83	69	75	-	-	-	-	-	-
Brazil	-	-	-	49	-	-	-	-	-	-
British Virgin Islands	-	-	-	-	-	-	-	-	-	-
Brunei Darussalam	-	-	-	36	-	-	-	-	-	-
Bulgaria	-	-	-	-	-	-	-	-	-	-
Burkina Faso	>95	23	41	64	31 x	29 x	-	-	-	-
Burundi	50	45	36	69	50	46	-	-	-	-
Cabo Verde	>95	>95	>95	85	-	-	-	-	-	-
Cambodia	80	14	56	75	42	33	-	-	-	-
Cameroon	67	48	35	50	33	37	-	-	-	-
Canada	-	-	-	61	-	-	-	-	-	-
Central African Republic	94	25	65	41	16	12	50	32	2	12
Chad	89	17	35	55	26	17	40	39	7	7
Chile	-	70	43	28	-	-	-	-	-	-
China	-	-	-	59	-	-	-	-	-	-
Colombia	46	35	28	37	26	28	-	-	-	-
Comoros	-	-	-	-	21	18	-	-	-	-
Congo	21	<1	12	13	42	26	55	49	4	7
Cook Islands	-	-	-	-	-	-	-	-	-	-
Costa Rica	78	36	22	29	-	23	-	49	-	3
Côte d'Ivoire	>95	61	54	58	32	24	73	30	8	16
Croatia	-	-	-	-	-	-	-	-	-	-
Cuba	87	87	25	20	46	47	80	75	15	25
Cyprus	-	-	-	-	-	-	-	-	-	-
Czechia	-	-	-	30	-	-	-	-	-	-
Democratic People's Republic of Korea	-	-	-	1	-	-	-	-	-	-
Democratic Republic of the Congo	61	12	38	46	23	18	35	26	5	6
Denmark	-	-	-	-	-	-	-	-	-	-
Djibouti	44	5	33	25	-	-	-	-	-	-
Dominica	-	-	-	-	39 x	49 x	74 x	86 x	-	-
Dominican Republic	72	16	31	35	39	27	-	49	-	16
Ecuador	66	58	60	52	-	-	-	-	-	-
Egypt	18	11	18	21	5	3	-	-	-	-
El Salvador	59	47	25	58	25	25	-	31	-	8
Equatorial Guinea	43	5	39	21	-	-	-	-	-	-
Eritrea	81	46	56	64	32 x	22 x	-	-	-	-
Estonia	-	-	-	71	-	-	-	-	-	-
Eswatini	>95	45	>95	88	44	45	92 x	-	33	48
Ethiopia	78	38	36	68	38	24	-	-	-	-

FOR EVERY CHILD, VACCINATION

TABLE 7. HIV/AIDS: INTERVENTION COVERAGE

Countries and areas	Percentage of pregnant women living with HIV receiving effective ARVs for PMTCT (%)	Early infant HIV diagnosis (%)	Children living with HIV receiving ART (%)		Comprehensive knowledge of HIV among adolescents age 15-19 (%) 2012–2020 [R]		Condom use among adolescents age 15-19 (%) with multiple partners (%) 2012–2020 [R]		Adolescents age 15-19 tested for HIV in the last 12 months and who have received results (%) 2012–2020 [R]	
			Children 0–14	Adolescents 10–19	Male	Female	Male	Female	Male	Female
Fiji	59	70	72	47	-	-	-	-	-	-
Finland	-	-	-	60	-	-	-	-	-	-
France	-	-	-	37	-	-	-	-	-	-
Gabon	71	12	23	32	35	29	-	-	-	-
Gambia	89	15	41	40	15	19	41	0	2	4
Georgia	>95	91	60	73	-	-	-	-	-	2 x
Germany	-	-	-	30	-	-	-	-	-	-
Ghana	87	25	43	45	17	14	50	35	1	7
Greece	-	-	-	-	-	-	-	-	-	-
Grenada	-	-	-	-	67 x	59 x	80 x	92 x	-	-
Guatemala	-	-	-	-	-	-	-	-	-	-
Guinea	82	36	22	26	22	17	-	18	-	5
Guinea-Bissau	39	16	25	24	25	11	53	29	1	4
Guyana	69	94	19	58	33	48	83	-	10	16
Haiti	87	55	63	69	34	36	-	-	-	-
Holy See	-	-	-	-	-	-	-	-	-	-
Honduras	41	55	36	53	35	29	-	-	-	-
Hungary	-	-	-	25	-	-	-	-	-	-
Iceland	-	-	-	-	-	-	-	-	-	-
India	64	-	95	-	26 x	18 x	30	35	-	-
Indonesia	15	5	25	18	4	12	-	-	-	-
Iran (Islamic Republic of)	36	25	33	30	-	-	-	-	-	-
Iraq	-	-	-	7	-	5	-	-	-	1
Ireland	-	-	-	-	-	-	-	-	-	-
Israel	-	-	-	56	-	-	-	-	-	-
Italy	-	-	-	-	-	-	-	-	-	-
Jamaica	66	22	33	39	34	39	75	56	20	35
Japan	-	-	-	17	-	-	-	-	-	-
Jordan	-	-	-	15	8	2	-	-	-	-
Kazakhstan	94	>95	68	74	30 x	20	94 x	-	14 x	11
Kenya	91	65	59	68	58	49	-	-	-	-
Kiribati	-	-	-	-	19	31	20	-	4	1
Kuwait	-	-	-	36	-	-	-	-	-	-
Kyrgyzstan	80	74	50	71	-	17	-	-	-	11
Lao People's Democratic Republic	>95	65	57	48	25	23	57	27	1	1
Latvia	78	75	93	56	-	-	-	-	-	-
Lebanon	-	-	-	-	22	26	-	-	-	-
Lesotho	86	63	65	73	26	28	-	-	44	54
Liberia	>95	20	32	38	-	-	-	-	-	-
Libya	64	49	30	34	-	-	-	-	-	-
Liechtenstein	-	-	-	-	-	-	-	-	-	-
Lithuania	-	-	-	-	-	-	-	-	-	-
Luxembourg	-	-	-	-	-	-	-	-	-	-
Madagascar	15	<1	7	6	26	20	2	7	1	2
Malawi	93	79	74	84	43	39	49	38	17	47
Malaysia	>95	>95	>95	53	-	-	-	-	-	-
Maldives	-	-	-	-	21	27	-	-	-	-
Mali	49	24	42	39	14	13	47	26	2	5
Malta	-	-	-	30	-	-	-	-	-	-
Marshall Islands	-	-	-	-	-	-	-	-	-	-
Mauritania	6	8	21	28	7 x	5 x	-	-	1	2
Mauritius	>95	58	82	24	-	-	-	-	-	-
Mexico	-	-	49	27	-	28	-	36	-	7
Micronesia (Federated States of)	-	-	-	-	-	-	-	-	-	-
Monaco	-	-	-	-	-	-	-	-	-	-
Mongolia	-	-	-	-	17	18	78	-	5	7
Montenegro	-	-	-	-	35	42	64	-	0	0
Montserrat	-	-	-	-	-	-	-	-	-	-
Morocco	44	33	91	86	-	-	-	-	-	-
Mozambique	-	-	-	48	28	27 x	-	-	-	-
Myanmar	18	47	68	56	14	13	-	-	-	-
Namibia	>95	>95	82	80	61	56	-	-	14	28
Nauru	-	-	-	-	-	-	-	-	-	-

TABLE 7. HIV/AIDS: INTERVENTION COVERAGE

Countries and areas	Percentage of pregnant women living with HIV receiving effective ARVs for PMTCT (%)	Early infant HIV diagnosis (%)	Children living with HIV receiving ART (%)		Comprehensive knowledge of HIV among adolescents age 15-19 (%) 2012–2020 [R]		Condom use among adolescents age 15-19 with multiple partners (%) 2012–2020 [R]		Adolescents age 15-19 tested for HIV in the last 12 months and who have received results (%) 2012–2020 [R]	
			Children 0–14	Adolescents 10–19	Male	Female	Male	Female	Male	Female
Nepal	83	6	95	89	23	26	-	-	1	2
Netherlands (Kingdom of the)	-	-	-	-	-	-	-	-	-	-
New Zealand	-	-	-	-	-	-	-	-	-	-
Nicaragua	73	64	40	30	20	11	-	-	-	-
Niger	40	21	53	54	-	-	-	-	-	-
Nigeria	34	15	31	60	29	38	62	43	7	8
Niue	-	-	-	-	-	-	-	-	-	-
North Macedonia	-	-	-	25	-	-	-	-	-	-
Norway	-	-	-	-	-	-	-	-	-	-
Oman	61	44	57	41	-	-	-	-	-	-
Pakistan	23	4	53	14	0	1	-	-	-	-
Palau	-	-	-	-	-	-	-	-	-	-
Panama	-	-	-	19	-	-	-	-	-	-
Papua New Guinea	-	-	58	51	21	21	-	-	-	-
Paraguay	54	47	-	42	-	25	-	61	-	9
Peru	-	47	-	48	-	21 x	-	-	-	-
Philippines	15	7	19	16	15 x	16	-	-	-	-
Poland	-	-	-	62	-	-	-	-	-	-
Portugal	-	-	-	-	-	-	-	-	-	-
Qatar	-	-	-	-	23	10	-	-	-	-
Republic of Korea	-	-	-	22	-	-	-	-	-	-
Republic of Moldova	>95	>95	77	56	26	35	-	-	6	10
Romania	84	77	>95	88	-	-	-	-	-	-
Russian Federation	-	-	-	37	-	-	-	-	-	-
Rwanda	87	80	59	78	55	54	-	-	-	-
Saint Kitts and Nevis	-	-	-	-	55 x	54 x	54 x	50 x	-	-
Saint Lucia	-	-	-	-	-	58	-	-	-	12
Saint Vincent and the Grenadines	-	-	-	-	-	-	-	-	-	-
Samoa	-	-	-	-	-	-	-	-	-	-
San Marino	-	-	-	-	-	-	-	-	-	-
Sao Tome and Principe	-	-	-	-	28	32	76	63	10	18
Saudi Arabia	-	-	-	38	-	-	-	-	-	-
Senegal	68	35	37	59	26	20	-	-	-	-
Serbia	-	-	-	-	43 x	53 x	63 x	-	1 x	1 x
Seychelles	-	-	-	-	-	-	-	-	-	-
Sierra Leone	78	3	13	32	22	27	9	12	3	7
Singapore	-	-	-	-	-	-	-	-	-	-
Slovakia	-	-	-	-	-	-	-	-	-	-
Slovenia	-	-	-	-	-	-	-	-	-	-
Solomon Islands	-	-	-	-	-	-	-	-	-	-
Somalia	42	20	15	21	-	-	-	-	-	-
South Africa	>95	94	48	54	-	-	-	-	-	-
South Sudan	44	15	15	16	-	8 x	-	6 x	-	3 x
Spain	-	-	-	-	-	-	-	-	-	-
Sri Lanka	-	-	-	-	-	-	-	-	-	-
State of Palestine	-	-	-	-	-	3	-	-	-	-
Sudan	4	-	26	29	10 x	8	-	-	-	1
Suriname	79	42	44	71	-	40 x	-	-	-	11 x
Sweden	-	-	-	78	-	-	-	-	-	-
Switzerland	-	-	-	-	-	-	-	-	-	-
Syrian Arab Republic	-	-	-	-	-	-	-	-	-	-
Tajikistan	77	68	89	85	9 x	4	-	-	-	-
Thailand	>95	92	75	59	46	49	-	-	1	3
Timor-Leste	-	-	-	-	13	6	-	-	-	-
Togo	68	26	49	56	32	25	34	49	7	15
Tokelau	-	-	-	-	-	-	-	-	-	-
Tonga	-	-	-	-	8	4	0	-	1	1
Trinidad and Tobago	-	-	-	-	-	55 x	-	-	-	10 x
Tunisia	41	33	33	39	12	13	-	-	-	-
Türkiye	-	-	-	37	-	-	-	-	-	-
Turkmenistan	-	-	-	<0.01	-	19	-	-	-	5
Turks and Caicos Islands	-	-	-	-	-	-	-	-	-	-
Tuvalu	-	-	-	-	-	-	-	-	-	-

FOR EVERY CHILD, VACCINATION

TABLE 7. HIV/AIDS: INTERVENTION COVERAGE

| Countries and areas | Percentage of pregnant women living with HIV receiving effective ARVs for PMTCT (%) | Early infant HIV diagnosis (%) | Children living with HIV receiving ART (%) | | Comprehensive knowledge of HIV among adolescents age 15-19 (%) 2012–2020 [R] | | Condom use among adolescents age 15-19 with multiple partners (%) 2012–2020 [R] | | Adolescents age 15-19 tested for HIV in the last 12 months and who have received results (%) 2012–2020 [R] | |
			Children 0–14	Adolescents 10–19	Male	Female	Male	Female	Male	Female
Uganda	>95	75	68	66	40	41	-	-	19	34
Ukraine	>95	61	>95	86	37	43	90	-	10	7
United Arab Emirates	-	-	-	57	-	-	-	-	-	-
United Kingdom	-	-	-	61	-	-	-	-	-	-
United Republic of Tanzania	80	48	60	76	32	33	-	-	11	24
United States	-	-	92	62	-	-	-	-	-	-
Uruguay	-	75	>95	66	-	36	-	67	-	7
Uzbekistan	51	43	31	74	-	-	-	-	-	-
Vanuatu	-	-	-	-	-	-	-	-	-	-
Venezuela (Bolivarian Republic of)	22	14	28	30	-	-	-	-	-	-
Viet Nam	75	28	82	88	-	51	-	-	-	4
Yemen	-	-	-	-	-	-	-	-	-	-
Zambia	>95	32	67	72	39	41	-	-	15	29
Zimbabwe	88	>95	73	83	41	41	62	-	26	39
SUMMARY										
East Asia and Pacific	41	38	53	45	-	-	-	-	-	-
Europe and Central Asia	-	-	-	-	-	-	-	-	-	-
Eastern Europe and Central Asia	-	-	-	-	-	-	-	-	-	-
Western Europe	-	-	-	-	-	-	-	-	-	-
Latin America and Caribbean	68	46	42	42	-	-	-	-	-	-
Middle East and North Africa	28	15	49	42	-	-	-	-	-	-
North America	-	-	-	-	-	-	-	-	-	-
South Asia	59	-	92	64	-	-	-	-	-	-
Sub-Saharan Africa	83	62	50	60	-	-	-	-	-	-
Eastern and Southern Africa	89	71	56	63	-	-	-	-	-	-
West and Central Africa	60	25	35	51	-	-	-	-	-	-
Least developed countries	-	-	-	-	-	-	-	-	-	-
World	**81**	**62**	**52**	**59**	**-**	**-**	**-**	**-**	**-**	**-**

For a complete list of countries and areas in the regions, subregions and country categories, see page on Regional Classifications or visit <data.unicef.org/regionalclassifications>.

It is not advisable to compare data from consecutive editions of *The State of the World's Children* report.

NOTES

- Data not available.

[R] Data refer to the most recent year available during the period specified in the column heading.

[x] Data refer to years or periods other than those specified in the column heading. Such data are not included in the calculation of regional and global averages. Estimates from data years prior to 2000 are not displayed.

MAIN DATA SOURCES

Pregnant women living with HIV receiving ARVs for PMTCT – Global AIDS Monitoring and UNAIDS 2022 estimates. Last update: July 2022.

Early infant HIV diagnosis – Global AIDS Monitoring and UNAIDS 2022 estimates. Last update: July 2022.

Children living with HIV receiving ART – Global AIDS Monitoring and UNAIDS 2022 estimates. Last update: July 2022.

Comprehensive knowledge of HIV among adolescents age 15–19 – Nationally representative population-based surveys, including MICS, DHS, AIS, and other household surveys 2012–2021. Last update: June 2022.

Condom use among adolescents age 15–19 with multiple partners – Nationally representative population-based surveys, including MICS, DHS, AIS, and other household surveys 2012–2021. Last update: June 2022.

Adolescents age 15–19 tested for HIV in the last 12 months and who have received results – Nationally representative population-based surveys, including MICS, DHS, AIS, and other household surveys 2012–2021. Last update: June 2022.

DEFINITIONS OF THE INDICATORS

Pregnant women living with HIV receiving ARVs for PMTCT – Percentage of the estimated number of pregnant women living with HIV who received effective regimens (excluding single-dose nevirapine) of antiretroviral medicines (ARVs) for prevention of mother-to-child transmission (PMTCT) of HIV.

Early infant HIV diagnosis – Percentage of HIV-exposed infants who received a virologic test for HIV within two months of birth.

Children living with HIV receiving ART – Percentage of children living with HIV who received antiretroviral therapy (ART).

Comprehensive knowledge of HIV among adolescents age 15–19 – Percentage of adolescents aged 15–19 who correctly identify the two ways of preventing the sexual transmission of HIV, who know that a healthy-looking person can be HIV-positive and who reject the two most common misconceptions about HIV transmission.

Condom use among adolescents age 15–19 with multiple partners – Percentage of adolescents aged 15–19 who had more than one sexual partner in the past 12 months reporting the use of a condom during their last sexual intercourse.

Adolescents age 15–19 tested for HIV in the last 12 months and received results – Percentage of adolescents aged 15–19 who have been tested for HIV in the last 12 months and received the result of the last test.

TABLE 8. NUTRITION: NEWBORNS, PRESCHOOL/SCHOOL AGE CHILDREN, WOMEN AND HOUSEHOLDS

Countries and areas	Weight at birth		Malnutrition among preschool-aged children (0–4 years of age)				Vitamin A supplementation, full coveragea (6–59 months of age) (%) 2021 m, &	Malnutrition among school-aged children (5–19 years of age) 2016		Malnutrition among women		Percentage of households consuming iodized salt 2015–2021 R
	Low birthweight (%) 2015 m	Unweighed at birth (%) 2015–2021 m, R	Stunted (%) (2020) Moderate and severe ii,m	Wasted (%) (2015–2022) c,R Severe	Wasted Moderate and severe ^	Overweight (%) (2020) Moderate and severe ii,m		Thinness (%) Thin and severely thin ^	Overweight (%) Overweight and obese ^	Underweight 18+ years (%) (2016) BMI <18.5 kg/m2	Anaemia 15–49 years (%) (2019) Mild, moderate and severe	
Afghanistan	- z	86	35	2	5 k	4	58 f	17	9	16	43	57
Albania	5	3	10	1	2	15	-	1	25	2	25	65
Algeria	7	10	9	1	3	13	-	6	31	4	33	89
Andorra	7	-	- z	-	-	- z	-	1	36	2	12	-
Angola	15	46	38	1	5	3	- f, aa	8	11	11	45	82
Anguilla	-	-	-	-	-	-	-	-	-	-	-	-
Antigua and Barbuda	9	-	- z	-	-	- z	-	3	27	4	17	-
Argentina	7	6	8	<1	2	13	-	1	37	1	12	-
Armenia	9	1	9	2	4	11	-	2	19	4	17	99
Australia	7	1	2	<1 wx	<1 lwx	19	-	1	34	2	9	-
Austria	7	<1	- z	-	-	- z	-	2	26	3	13	-
Azerbaijan	7	1 x	16	1 x	3 x	9	-	3	19	3	35	93 x
Bahamas	13	-	- z	-	-	- z	-	3	36	3	15	-
Bahrain	12	-	5 e	-	-	6 e	-	6	35	4	35	-
Bangladesh	28	49	30	2	10	2	96 f	18	9	23	37	76
Barbados	- z	-	7	2 x	7 x	11	-	4	28	3	17	37 x
Belarus	5	6	4	1 x	2 x	7	-	2	23	2	21	-
Belgium	7	1	2	<1 wx	<1 lwx	5	-	1	24	2	14	-
Belize	9	2	13	1	2	8	-	3	29	3	21	85
Benin	17	40	31	1	5 k	2	80 f	7	11	9	55	85
Bhutan	12	28 x	22	2 x	6 x	5	-	16	10	11	39	98 xy
Bolivia (Plurinational State of)	7	8	13	1	2	9	- f	1	28	2	24	86
Bosnia and Herzegovina	3	2 x	9	2 x	2 x	13	-	2	21	3	24	-
Botswana	16	54 x	23	3 x	7 x	11	64 f	6	18	7	33	83 x
Brazil	8	2	6	<1 x	2 x	7	-	3	28	4	16	98 x
British Virgin Islands	-	-	-	-	-	-	-	-	-	-	-	-
Brunei Darussalam	11	-	13	<1 x	3 x	9	-	6	27	6	17	-
Bulgaria	10	-	6	3 wx	6 wx	6	-	2	29	2	24	92 xy
Burkina Faso	13	36 x	26	1 m	10 m	3	99 f	8	8	13	53	89
Burundi	15	20	58	1 k	6 k	3	81 f	7	10	11	39	89
Cabo Verde	- z	-	10 e	-	-	- z	-	7	12	7	24	92 bx
Cambodia	12	9 x	30	2	10	2	61 f	11	11	14	47	68 x
Cameroon	12	36	27	2	4	10	85 f	6	13	6	41	91
Canada	6	3	- z	-	-	12	-	1	32	2	10	-
Central African Republic	15	37	40	1	5	3	- f	8	11	12	47	76
Chad	- z	88 x	35	2	10 k	3	<1 f	8	9	13	45	65
Chile	6	6	2	-	<1 x	10	-	1	35	1	9	-
China	5	<1 x	5	1 x	2 m	8	-	3	29 k	6	16	97 y
Colombia	10	18	11	<1	2	6	-	2	24	3	21	-
Comoros	24	32 x	23	4 x	11 x	10	- f	7	12	9	34	82 x
Congo	12	10	18	3 x	8 x	5	- f	7	11	11	49	91 x
Cook Islands	3	-	- z	-	-	- z	-	<1	63	<1	27	-
Costa Rica	7	2	9	<1	2	8	-	2	32	2	14	-
Côte d'Ivoire	15	27	18	1	6	3	85 f	6	13	8	51	80
Croatia	5	<1	- z	-	-	- z	-	1	28	2	21	-
Cuba	5	2	7	1	2	10	-	3	30	5	19	90
Cyprus	- z	-	- z	-	-	- z	-	1	33	2	14	-
Czechia	8	<1	3	1 x	5 kx	7	-	2	28	2	21	-
Democratic People's Republic of Korea	- z	<1	18	1	3	2	<1 f	5	23	8	34	38
Democratic Republic of the Congo	11	27	41	2	6	4	56 f	9	10	13	42	85
Denmark	5	<1	- z	-	-	- z	-	1	25	3	12	-

TABLE 8. NUTRITION: NEWBORNS, PRESCHOOL/SCHOOL AGE CHILDREN, WOMEN AND HOUSEHOLDS

Countries and areas	Weight at birth — Low birthweight (%) 2015 [m]	Weight at birth — Unweighed at birth (%) 2015–2021 [m,R]	Malnutrition among preschool-aged children (0–4 years of age) — Stunted (%) (2020) Moderate and severe [g,m]	Wasted (%) (2015–2022) [c,R] Severe	Wasted Moderate and severe ^	Overweight (%) (2020) Moderate and severe [g,m]	Vitamin A supplementation, full coverage (6–59 months of age) (%) 2021 [m,&]	Malnutrition among school-aged children (5–19 years of age) 2016 — Thinness (%) Thin and severely thin ^	Overweight (%) Overweight and obese ^	Malnutrition among women — Underweight 18+ years (%) (2016) BMI <18.5 kg/m2	Anaemia 15–49 years (%) (2019) Mild, moderate and severe	Percentage of households consuming iodized salt 2015–2021 [R]
Djibouti	- z	15 x	34	3 w	10 w	7	- f	6	17	7	32	4 x
Dominica	- z	-	- z	-	-	- z	-	3	33	3	21	-
Dominican Republic	11	4	6	1	2	8	-	3	33	3	26	32 x
Ecuador	11	-	23	1 k	4	10	-	1	28	1	17	-
Egypt	- z	39 x	22	5 x	9 x	18	-	3	37	1	28	93 xy
El Salvador	10	7 x	11	<1 x	2 x	7	-	2	30	2	11	-
Equatorial Guinea	- z	30 x	20	2 x	3 x	9	8 f	8	11	10	45	57 x
Eritrea	- z	65 x	49	4 x	15 x	2	78 f	8	11	17	37	86 x
Estonia	4	6	1	<1 x	2 x	6	-	2	21	2	22	-
Eswatini	10	9 x	23	<1 x	2 x	10	33 f	4	17 l	5	31	90 x
Ethiopia	- z	87	35	1	7 k	3	73 f	10	9	15	24	86
Fiji	- z	1	7	1	5	5	-	4	34	2	32	-
Finland	4	<1	- z	-	-	- z	-	1	27	2	11	-
France	7	<1 x	- z	-	-	- z	-	1	30	3	11	-
Gabon	14	9 x	14	1 x	3 x	7	<1 f	6	16	7	52	89 x
Gambia	17	29	16	1	5	2	27 f	7	12	10	50	67
Georgia	6	<1 x	6	<1 l	1	8	-	3	20	4	28	98 xy
Germany	7	<1	2	<1 w	<1 kw	4	-	1	26	2	12	-
Ghana	14	36	14	1	7	3	35 f	6	11	7	35	69
Greece	9	-	2	<1 lwx	1 wx	14	-	1	37	1	15	-
Grenada	- z	-	- z	-	-	- z	-	4	26	4	19	-
Guatemala	11	6	43	<1	1 k	5	-	1	29	2	7	88 x
Guinea	- z	52	29	4	9	6	96 f	7	10	10	48	53
Guinea-Bissau	21	49	28	2	8	3	<1 f	7	11	9	48	33
Guyana	16	12 x	9	2 x	6 x	7	-	5	25	5	32	43 x
Haiti	- z	68	20	1	4	4	20 f	4	28	5	48	8
Holy See	-	-	-	-	-	-	-	-	-	-	-	-
Honduras	11	12	20	<1	2	6	-	2	27	3	18	88
Hungary	9	<1	- z	-	-	- z	-	2	28	3	20	-
Iceland	4	1	- z	-	-	- z	-	1	28	2	10	-
India	- z	9	31	8 k	19 k	2	- f, aa	27	7	24	53	94
Indonesia	10	6	32	4 k	10	11	-	10	15	13	31	92 bx
Iran (Islamic Republic of)	- z	-	6	1	4	9 e	-	9	26	4	24	94 bx
Iraq	- z	29	12	1	3	9	-	5	32	2	29	68
Ireland	6	2	- z	-	-	- z	-	<1	31	1	12	-
Israel	8	-	- z	-	-	- z	-	1	35	2	13	-
Italy	7	2	- z	-	-	- z	-	1	37	2	14	-
Jamaica	15	4 x	8	1	3	7	-	2	30	3	20	-
Japan	9	<1	5	<1 x	2 x	2	-	2	14	10	19	-
Jordan	14	3	7	<1 l	1	7	-	4	31	1	38	88 bx
Kazakhstan	5	1	7	1	3	9	-	2	20	4	29	94
Kenya	11	35	19	2 w	7 w	4	86 f	8	11	10	29	95 x
Kiribati	- z	25	15	1	4	2	- f	<1	55	1	33	77
Kuwait	10	-	6	1 x	3 m	7	-	4	42	1	24	-
Kyrgyzstan	6	1	11	1	2	6	-	3	16	4	36	99
Lao People's Democratic Republic	17	33	30	3	9	3	- f	9	14	11	40	94
Latvia	5	<1	- z	-	-	- z	-	2	22	2	22	-
Lebanon	9	-	10	<1	1	20	-	5	33	3	28	95 x
Lesotho	15	8	32	1	2	7	- f	5	15 l	5	28	85 x
Liberia	- z	71	28	1	3	5	- f	7	10	8	43	87
Libya	- z	-	44	5 x	10 x	25	-	6	33	2	30	70 bx
Liechtenstein	-	-	-	-	-	-	-	-	-	-	-	-

TABLE 8. NUTRITION: NEWBORNS, PRESCHOOL/SCHOOL AGE CHILDREN, WOMEN AND HOUSEHOLDS

Countries and areas	Weight at birth		Malnutrition among preschool-aged children (0–4 years of age)				Vitamin A supplementation, full coverage (6–59 months of age) (%) 2021	Malnutrition among school-aged children (5–19 years of age) 2016		Malnutrition among women		Percentage of households consuming iodized salt 2015–2021
	Low birthweight (%) 2015	Unweighed at birth (%) 2015–2021	Stunted (%) (2020) Moderate and severe	Wasted (%) (2015–2022) Severe	Wasted Moderate and severe	Overweight (%) (2020) Moderate and severe		Thinness (%) Thin and severely thin	Overweight (%) Overweight and obese	Underweight 18+ years (%) (2016) BMI <18.5 kg/m2	Anaemia 15–49 years (%) (2019) Mild, moderate and severe	
Lithuania	5	15	- z	-	-	- z	-	3	21	2	20	-
Luxembourg	7	2	- z	-	-	- z	-	1	26	2	10	-
Madagascar	17	63 x	40	1 k	7	1	24 f	7	11	15	38	68 x
Malawi	14	6	37	<1 kw	2 kw	5	77 f	6	11	9	31	80
Malaysia	11	-	21	4 k	10	6	-	7	26	7	32	28 xy
Maldives	12	2	14	2	9	5	-	14	17	9	52	97 x
Mali	- z	65	26	2 k	9 k	2	85 f	8	11	10	59	76 y
Malta	6	2	- z	-	-	- z	-	1	37	1	14	-
Marshall Islands	- z	14	32	1	4	4	-	<1	59	1	31	-
Mauritania	- z	84	24	2	10 k	3	- f	8	13	8	43	25 y
Mauritius	17	-	9 e	-	-	8 e	-	7	15	7	24	-
Mexico	8	2	12	<1	2	6	-	2	35	2	15	-
Micronesia (Federated States of)	- z	-	- z	-	-	- z	-	<1	51	1	25	-
Monaco	5	-	- z	-	-	- z	-	-	-	-	12	-
Mongolia	5	1	7	<1	1	10	-	2	18	3	15	75
Montenegro	5	2	8	1	2	10	-	2	25	2	17	-
Montserrat	-	-	-	-	-	-	-	-	-	-	-	-
Morocco	17	3	13	1	3	11	-	6	27	3	30	43 x
Mozambique	14	49 x	38	1	4	6	83 f	4	13	10	48	42 x
Myanmar	12	55	25	1 w	7 w	2	- f, aa	13	12	14	42	85 y
Namibia	16	15 x	18	3 kx	7 kx	5	59 f	8	15	9	25	74 x
Nauru	- z	4 x	15	<1 x	1 x	4	-	<1	65	<1	30	-
Nepal	22	22	30	3	12 k	2	90 f	16	8	17	36	94
Netherlands (Kingdom of the)	6	5	2	<1 x	1 x	5	-	1	25	2	13	-
New Zealand	6	8	- z	-	-	- z	-	<1	40	2	10	-
Nicaragua	11	30 x	14	1 x	2 x	7	-	2	29	2	16	-
Niger	- z	64	47	2	11	2	93 f	10	8	13	50	59 x
Nigeria	- z	77	35	1 k	6 k	3	57 f	10	8	10	55	93
Niue	- z	-	- z	-	-	- z	-	<1	59	1	27	-
North Macedonia	9	<1	4	1	3	10	-	2	26	3	19	-
Norway	4	<1	- z	-	-	- z	-	1	27	2	12	-
Oman	11	-	12	3	9	5	-	7	32	5	29	88 x
Pakistan	- z	89	37	2	7	3	92 f	19	10	15	41	80
Palau	- z	-	- z	-	-	- z	-	<1	64	1	29	-
Panama	10	9 x	15	<1	1	11	-	2	29	3	21	-
Papua New Guinea	- z	51	48	6 x	14 x	9	- f	1	32	3	34	60 x
Paraguay	8	2	5	<1	1	12	-	2	28	2	23	92
Peru	9	3	11	<1	<1	8	-	1	27	2	21	91
Philippines	20	17	29	1	6 m	4	- f	10	13	14	12	57 y
Poland	6	5	2	<1 lx	1 x	7	-	2	26	3	- z	-
Portugal	9	<1	3	<1 w	1 w	9	-	1	32	2	13	-
Qatar	7	-	5 e	-	-	14 e	-	5	39	2	28	99 xy
Republic of Korea	6	8	2	<1	<1	9	-	1	27 k	6	14	-
Republic of Moldova	5	1 x	5	<1 x	2 x	4	-	3	18	3	26	58 x
Romania	8	-	10	1 x	3 x	7	-	3	25	2	23	-
Russian Federation	6	-	- z	-	-	- z	-	2	21	2	21	-
Rwanda	8	6	33	<1	1	5	- f, aa	6	11 l	8	17	90
Saint Kitts and Nevis	- z	-	- z	-	-	- z	-	4	28	3	15	-
Saint Lucia	- z	1 x	3	1 x	4 x	7	-	4	23	4	14	75 x
Saint Vincent and the Grenadines	- z	-	- z	-	-	- z	-	3	29	4	17	-
Samoa	- z	54	7	1	3	7	-	<1	53	1	27	96
San Marino	3	-	- z	-	-	- z	-	-	-	-	13	-

FOR EVERY CHILD, VACCINATION

TABLE 8. NUTRITION: NEWBORNS, PRESCHOOL/SCHOOL AGE CHILDREN, WOMEN AND HOUSEHOLDS

Countries and areas	Weight at birth		Malnutrition among preschool-aged children (0–4 years of age)				Vitamin A supplementation, full coveragea (6–59 months of age) (%) 2021 m,&	Malnutrition among school-aged children (5–19 years of age) 2016		Malnutrition among women		Percentage of households consuming iodized salt 2015–2021 R
	Low birthweight (%) 2015 m	Unweighed at birth (%) 2015–2021 m,R	Stunted (%) (2020) Moderate and severe g,m	Wasted (%) (2015–2022) c,R Severe	Wasted Moderate and severe ^	Overweight (%) (2020) Moderate and severe g,m		Thinness (%) Thin and severely thin ^	Overweight (%) Overweight and obese ^	Underweight 18+ years (%) (2016) BMI <18.5 kg/m2	Anaemia 15–49 years (%) (2019) Mild, moderate and severe	
Sao Tome and Principe	7	3	12	1	4 k	4	- f	5	13	8	44	89
Saudi Arabia	- z	-	4	5 x	12 x	8	-	8	36	2	28	70 xy
Senegal	18	36	17	1	8 k	2	57 f	9	10	11	53	65
Serbia	5	<1	5	1	3	11	-	2	27	3	23	-
Seychelles	12	-	7	1 x	4 x	10	-	6	23	5	25	-
Sierra Leone	14	35	27	2	6	5	66 f	7	11	10	48	82
Singapore	10	-	3	<1 x	4 x	5	-	2	22	8	13	-
Slovakia	8	<1	- z	-	-	- z	-	1	23	3	24	-
Slovenia	6	3	- z	-	-	- z	-	1	27	3	22	-
Solomon Islands	- z	14	29	4	8	4	-	1	23	2	38	88
Somalia	- z	92	27	4 x	14 x	3	- f	7	13	9	43	7 x
South Africa	14	12	23	2 w	3 w	13	42 f	5	25	3	31	91
South Sudan	- z	-	31	10 kx	23 kx	6	90 f	-	-	-	36	60 x
Spain	8	-	- z	-	-	- z	-	1	34	2	13	-
Sri Lanka	16	4	16	3	15	1	-	15	13	13	35	92
State of Palestine	8	1	8	1	1	9	-	-	-	-	-	96
Sudan	- z	90	34	4 x	16 x	3	<1 f	-	-	-	37	34 x
Suriname	15	16	8	1	6	4	-	4	31	3	21	-
Sweden	2	<1	- z	-	-	- z	-	1	24	2	14	-
Switzerland	6	1	- z	-	-	- z	-	<1	22	4	11	-
Syrian Arab Republic	- z	52 x	30	5 x	12 x	18	-	6	28	3	33	72 y
Tajikistan	6	9	15	2	6	3	95 f	4	15	4	35	91
Thailand	11	2	12	3	8	9	-	8	22	8	24	84
Timor-Leste	- z	47	49	1	8 k	3	- f	11	13	18	30	83
Togo	16	30	24	1	6	2	96 f	6	10	9	46	81
Tokelau	-	-	- z	-	-	- z	- z	-	-	-	-	-
Tonga	- z	17	3	<1 k	1	13	-	<1	58	<1	29	53
Trinidad and Tobago	12	10 x	9	2 x	6 x	11	-	6	25	4	18	63 x
Tunisia	7	2	9	1	2	17	-	7	25	3	32	-
Türkiye	11	4	- z	1	2	- z	-	5	29	2	- z	85 x
Turkmenistan	5	1	8	1	4	4	<1 f	3	18	4	27	>99
Turks and Caicos Islands	-	-	-	<1 k	1 k	-	-	-	-	-	-	70
Tuvalu	- z	1	10	1	3	6	-	<1	58	1	28	85
Uganda	- z	34	28	1	4	4	38 f	6	10 l	10	33	91
Ukraine	6	3 x	16	4 x	8 x	17	-	2	21	2	18	36 x
United Arab Emirates	13	-	- z	-	-	- z	-	5	36	2	24	-
United Kingdom	7	2	- z	-	-	- z	-	1	31	2	11	-
United Republic of Tanzania	10	37	32	1 lw	2 w	5	96 f	7	12	10	39	76
United States	8	2	3	<1	<1	9	-	1	42	2	12	-
Uruguay	8	<1	6	<1	1	10	-	2	33	1	15	-
Uzbekistan	5	4	10	<1	2	5	-	3	17	4	25	82 x
Vanuatu	11	10 x	29	1 x	5 x	5	-	2	31	2	29	63 x
Venezuela (Bolivarian Republic of)	9	-	11	-	4 mx	7	-	2	34	2	24	-
Viet Nam	8	3	22	1 m	5 m	6	-	14	10	18	21	61 x
Yemen	- z	92 x	37	5 x	16 kx	3	6 f	14	20	8	62	49 x
Zambia	12	20	32	2	4	6	95 f	6	13	9	32	88 x
Zimbabwe	13	12	23	<1	3	4	16 f	6	15 l	5	29	84
SUMMARY												
East Asia and Pacific	8	7 v	14	1	4	8	-	6	23	8	19	92
Europe and Central Asia	7	2	6	-	-	8	-	2	26	2	19	-

TABLE 8. NUTRITION: NEWBORNS, PRESCHOOL/SCHOOL AGE CHILDREN, WOMEN AND HOUSEHOLDS

Countries and areas	Weight at birth		Malnutrition among preschool-aged children (0–4 years of age)				Vitamin A supplementation, full coveragea (6–59 months of age) (%) 2021 [m, &]	Malnutrition among school-aged children (5–19 years of age) 2016		Malnutrition among women		Percentage of households consuming iodized salt 2015–2021 [R]
	Low birthweight (%) 2015 [m]	Unweighed at birth (%) 2015–2021 [m, R]	Stunted (%) (2020)	Wasted (%) (2015–2022) [c, R]		Overweight (%) (2020)		Thinness (%)	Overweight (%)	Underweight 18+ years (%) (2016)	Anaemia 15–49 years (%) (2019)	
			Moderate and severe [g, m]	Severe	Moderate and severe ^	Moderate and severe [g, m]		Thin and severely thin ^	Overweight and obese ^	BMI <18.5 kg/m2	Mild, moderate and severe	
Eastern Europe and Central Asia	7	3	8	1 q	2 q	9	-	3	23	2	25	-
Western Europe	7	1	3	-	-	7	-	1	30	2	13	-
Latin America and Caribbean	9	7	11	<1	1	7	-	2	30	3	17	-
Middle East and North Africa	11	35	16	3	6	12	-	6	31	3	30	-
North America	8	2	3	<1 d	<1 d	9	-	1	41	2	12	-
South Asia	27	31	32	5	15	2	71	25	8	23	49	90
sub-Saharan Africa	14	52	32	1	6	4	61	7	10	10	41	84
Eastern and Southern Africa	14	51	32	1	5	5	59	7	11	9	33	85
West and Central Africa	14	54	32	2	7	3	63	9	10	10	49	84
Least developed countries	16	53	34	2	7	3	62	10	10	14	39	84
World	**15**	**29** v	**22**	**2**	**7**	**6**	**64**	**11**	**18**	**9**	**30**	**89**

For a complete list of countries and areas in the regions, subregions and country categories, see page 182 or visit <data.unicef.org/regionalclassifications>.

It is not advisable to compare data from consecutive editions of *The State of the World's Children*.

NOTES

– Data not available.

[a] Full coverage with vitamin A supplements is reported as the lower percentage of 2 annual coverage points (i.e., lower point between semester 1 (January–June) and semester 2 (July–December) of 2021. Data are only presented for vitamin A supplementation (VAS) priority countries; thus aggregates are only based on and representative of these priority countries.

[aa] Countries that have not given permission for estimates to be shared externally, as such, results from these countries are not presented in the individual country lines in this table, but are included in the global and regional estimates.

[b] Cannot be confirmed whether the reported value includes households without salt or not.

[c] Global and regional averages for wasting (moderate and severe) and wasting (severe) are estimated using statistical modelling data from the UNICEF-WHO-World Bank Group Joint Child Malnutrition Estimates, May 2021 Edition and thus might not account for all country updates in this table. For more information see <data.unicef.org/malnutrition>.

[d] For wasting and severe wasting estimates, the Northern America regional average is based only on United States data.

[e] The most recent country data point (e.g., from household surveys) used to generate the modelled stunting and overweight estimates is from before the year 2000; interpret with caution.

[f] Identifies countries which are designated 'priority'. Priority countries for national vitamin A supplementation programmes are identified as those having high under-five mortality rates (over 40 per 1,000 live births), and/or evidence of vitamin A deficiency among this age group, and/or a history of vitamin A supplementation programmes.

[g] The collection of household survey data on child height and weight were limited in 2020 due to the physical distancing measures required to prevent the spread of COVID-19. Only four national surveys included in the database were carried out (at least partially) in 2020. The JME estimates are therefore based almost entirely on data collected before 2020 and do not take into account the impact of the COVID-19 pandemic.

[k] Statistically significant gender differences disadvantaging boys observed.

[l] Statistically significantly gender differences disadvantaging girls observed.

[m] Gender assessment not possible

[p] Based on small denominators (typically 25–49 unweighted cases). No data based on fewer than 25 unweighted cases are displayed.

[q] Regional estimates for Eastern Europe and Central Asia exclude the Russian Federation.

[R] Data refer to the most recent year available during the period specified in the column heading

[v] Aggregated estimates for East Asia and Pacific and the World include estimates for China from the year 2013, which is outside of the year range 2015-2021.

[w] Reduced age range.

[x] Data refer to years or periods other than those specified in the column heading. Such data are not included in the calculation of regional and global averages. Estimates from data years prior to 2000 are not displayed.

[y] Data differ from the standard definition; if they fall within the noted reference period, such data are included in the calculation of regional and global averages.

[z] Country modeled estimates not presented but has been used for regional and global aggregates. For more details please consult the databases at https://data.unicef.org/topic/nutrition/child-nutrition/

[^] In the majority of countries, no statistically significant gender differences are observed, thus sex-disaggregated data are not presented

[&] The vitamin A supplementation coverage estimates for 2021 were not finalized at the time of publication for some priority countries and may be available in the coming months. For the latest data please visit <data.unicef.org /topic/nutrition/vitamin-a-deficiency/>

MAIN DATA SOURCES

Low birthweight – Modelled estimates from UNICEF and WHO. Last update: May 2019.

Unweighed at birth – Demographic and Health Surveys (DHS), Multiple Indicator Cluster Surveys (MICS), other national household surveys, data from routine reporting systems. Last update: December 2022

Stunting, overweight (preschoolers) – Modeled estimates from UNICEF and WHO. Last update: May 2021

Wasting and severe wasting (preschoolers) – DHS, MICS, and other national household surveys. Last update: December 2022 for country data and May 2021 for regional and global aggregates.

Vitamin A supplementation – UNICEF. Last Update: January 2023

Thinness and overweight (school age children), and underweight (women 18+) – NCD Risk Factor Collaboration (NCD-RisC), based on Worldwide trends in body-mass index, underweight, overweight and obesity from 1975 to 2016: a pooled analysis of 2416 population-based measurement studies in 128.9 million children, adolescents, and adults. The Lancet 2017, 390 (10113): 2627–2642. Last update: August 2019.

Anaemia (women 15–49 years) – Global Health Observatory, WHO. Last update: April 2021

Iodized salt consumption – DHS, MICS, other national household surveys, and school-based surveys. Last update: December 2022.

DEFINITIONS OF THE INDICATORS

Low birthweight – Percentage of infants weighing less than 2,500 grams at birth.

Unweighed at birth – Percentage of births without a birthweight in the data source; Note that (i) estimates from household surveys include live births among women age 15–49 years in the survey reference period (e.g. last 2 years) for which a birthweight was not available from an official document (e.g. health card) or could not be recalled by the respondent at the time of interview and may have been recalculated to count birthweights <250g and >5500g as missing and (ii) estimates from administrative sources (e.g. Medical Birth Registries) were calculated using numerator data from the country administrative source and denominator data were the number of annual births according to the *2022 Revision of World Population Prospects*. These estimates include unweighed births and weighed births not recorded in the system.

Stunting (preschoolers) – Moderate and severe: Percentage of children aged 0–59 months who are below minus two standard deviations from median height-for-age of the WHO Child Growth Standards.

Wasting (preschoolers) – Moderate and severe: Percentage of children aged 0–59 months who are below minus two standard deviations from median weight-for-height of the WHO Child Growth Standards.

Wasting (preschoolers) – Severe: Percentage of children aged 0–59 months who are below minus three standard deviations from median weight-for-height of the WHO Child Growth Standards.

Overweight (preschoolers) – Moderate and severe: Percentage of children aged 0–59 months who are above two standard deviations from median weight-for-height of the WHO Child Growth Standards (includes severe overweight).

Vitamin A supplementation, full coverage – The estimated percentage of children aged 6–59 months reached with 2 doses of vitamin A supplements approximately 4–6 months apart in a given calendar year.

Thinness (school age children) – Percentage of children aged 5–19 years with BMI < -2 SD of the median according to the WHO growth reference for school-age children and adolescents.

Overweight (school age children) – Percentage of children aged 5–19 years with BMI > 1 SD of the median according to the WHO growth reference for school-age children and adolescents.

Underweight (women 18+) – Percentage of women 18+ years of age with a body mass index (BMI) less than 18.5 kg/m2.

Anaemia (women 15–49 years) – Percentage of women aged 15–49 years with a haemoglobin concentration less than 120 g/L for non-pregnant women and lactating women, and less than 110 g/L for pregnant women, adjusted for altitude and smoking.

Households consuming salt with iodine – Percentage of households consuming salt with any iodine (>0 ppm).

FOR EVERY CHILD, VACCINATION

165

TABLE 9. NUTRITION: BREASTFEEDING AND DIETS

Countries and areas	Infant and Young Child Feeding (0–23 months) 2015–2021 [R, ∧]											
	Early initiation of breastfeeding (%)	Exclusive breastfeeding (<6 months) (%)	Introduction to solid, semi-sold or soft foods (6–8 months)	Continued breastfeeding (12–23 months) (%)			Percentage of children consuming (6–23 months) (%)			Minimum meal frequency (6–23 months) (%)	Minimum acceptable diet (6–23 months) (%)	Zero vegetable or fruit consumption (6–23 months) (%)
				All children	Poorest 20%	Richest 20%	<=2 food groups (severe food poverty)	3–4 food groups (moderate food poverty)	At least 5 food groups (minimum dietary diversity)			
Afghanistan	63 m	58 m	61	74	80	70	40	38	22	49	15	59
Albania	57	37	89	43	38	37	18	29	52	45	27	26
Algeria	33	29	88	37	36	43	17	44	39	46	19	26
Andorra	–	–	–	–	–	–	–	–	–	–	–	–
Angola	48	37	79 k	67	74	53	30	41	29	31	12	36
Anguilla	–	–	–	–	–	–	–	–	–	–	–	–
Antigua and Barbuda	–	–	–	–	–	–	–	–	–	–	–	–
Argentina	57 m	32 x	97 x	39 x	49 x	33 x	–	–	–	64 x	–	–
Armenia	41	44	90	29	32	24	14	49	36	62	22	22
Australia	–	–	–	20 m	–	–	–	–	–	–	–	–
Austria	–	–	–	–	–	–	–	–	–	–	–	–
Azerbaijan	20 mx	12 mx	77 x	26 x	24 x	15 x	24 x	41 x	35 x	–	–	38 x
Bahamas	–	–	–	–	–	–	–	–	–	–	–	–
Bahrain	–	–	–	–	–	–	–	–	–	–	–	–
Bangladesh	47	63	75	90	91	86	20	46	34	65	27	45
Barbados	40 mx	20 mx	90 mx	41 x	– px	– px	–	–	–	58 x	–	–
Belarus	24	22	96	17	10	20	1	29	70	93	57	3
Belgium	–	–	–	–	–	–	–	–	–	–	–	–
Belize	68 m	33	79	47	59	37	10	32	58	64 x	–	30
Benin	54	41	56	69	77	52	44	30	26	44	15	54
Bhutan	77	53	93	77	91	– p	47	37	16	63 x	–	61
Bolivia (Plurinational State of)	63	56	83	61	74 rx	53 rx	7	23	70	–	–	16
Bosnia and Herzegovina	42 mx	18 x	76 mx	12 x	16 x	10 x	–	–	–	71 x	–	–
Botswana	53	30	73	15	–	–	–	–	–	–	–	–
Brazil	62	46	86	44	50	32	–	–	57	–	–	21
British Virgin Islands	–	–	–	–	–	–	–	–	–	–	–	–
Brunei Darussalam	–	–	–	–	–	–	–	–	–	–	–	–
Bulgaria	–	–	–	–	–	–	–	–	–	–	–	–
Burkina Faso	59	58	61	92	93 rx	77 rx	23	42	36	65	27	26
Burundi	87 m	72 m	83 m	87	92 r	84 r	18	64	10	39	10	9
Cabo Verde	71 m	42 m	98 m	42 m	–	–	–	–	–	–	–	–
Cambodia	54 m	51 m	82 x	58 x	65 x	39 x	16 x	44 x	51 m	72 x	30 x	35 x
Cameroon	48	39	76	43	65	12	28	53	20	44	10	32
Canada	–	–	–	–	–	–	–	–	–	–	–	–
Central African Republic	49	36	77	73	74 r	52 r	19 x	54 x	27 x	26	9 x	22 x
Chad	16	16	71	73	73	64	40	36	23	34	11	48
Chile	–	–	–	–	–	–	–	–	–	–	–	–
China	29 mx	34 m	83 mx	–	–	–	–	–	37 x	63 x	25 x	29 x
Colombia	69	37	90 l	42	49	36	7	24	69	60	42	15
Comoros	34 x	11 x	80 x	65 x	68 x	69 x	31 kx	47 x	22 x	28 x	5 x	52 kx
Congo	25 mx	33 x	84 x	32 x	54 x	20 x	35 lx	52 kx	14 x	29 x	4 x	51 x
Cook Islands	–	–	–	–	–	–	–	–	–	–	–	–
Costa Rica	53 m	25	99	46	47	40	3	21	76	76 x	–	10
Côte d'Ivoire	43 m	34 m	65	63	76	36	29	48	28 m	48	14	44
Croatia	–	–	–	–	–	–	–	–	–	–	–	–
Cuba	64 m	41	94	25	35	23	9	33	58	76 x	54 x	22
Cyprus	–	–	–	–	–	–	–	–	–	–	–	–
Czechia	–	–	–	–	–	–	–	–	–	–	–	–
Democratic People's Republic of Korea	43 m	71 m	78 m	–	–	–	–	–	47 m	–	–	–
Democratic Republic of the Congo	47	54	82	70	79	50	33	52	15	34	8	28
Denmark	–	–	–	–	–	–	–	–	–	–	–	–
Djibouti	52 mx	12 mx	–	–	–	–	–	–	–	–	–	–
Dominica	–	–	–	–	–	–	–	–	–	–	–	–
Dominican Republic	42	16	90	22	30	14	8	26	66	77 x	42 x	19
Ecuador	72	40 mx	63	53	–	–	23	24	53	48	29	27
Egypt	27 x	40 x	75 x	50 x	58 x	43 x	26 x	39 x	35 x	56 x	23 x	45 x
El Salvador	42 mx	47 x	90 x	67 x	71 x	57 x	5 x	22 x	73 x	87 x	64 x	16 x
Equatorial Guinea	–	7 mx	–	31 mx	47 rx	34 rx	–	–	–	–	–	–
Eritrea	93 mxy	69 mx	44 mx	86 mx	–	–	–	–	–	–	–	–
Estonia	–	–	–	–	–	–	–	–	–	–	–	–
Eswatini	48 mx	64 x	90 x	28 x	29 x	19 x	11 x	41 x	48 x	81 x	37 x	21 x
Ethiopia	72	59	69	81	69	77	46	40	13	55	11	69

166
THE STATE OF THE WORLD'S CHILDREN 2023

TABLE 9. NUTRITION:BREASTFEEDING AND DIETS

Countries and areas	Infant and Young Child Feeding (0–23 months) 2015–2021 [R, ^]											
	Early initiation of breastfeeding (%)	Exclusive breastfeeding (<6 months) (%)	Introduction to solid, semi-sold or soft foods (6–8 months)	Continued breastfeeding (12–23 months) (%)			Percentage of children consuming (6–23 months) (%)			Minimum meal frequency (6–23 months) (%)	Minimum acceptable diet (6–23 months) (%)	Zero vegetable or fruit consumption (6–23 months) (%)
				All children	Poorest 20%	Richest 20%	<=2 food groups (severe food poverty)	3–4 food groups (moderate food poverty)	At least 5 food groups (minimum dietary diversity)			
Fiji	63	43	95	46	52	32	8	33	59	69	41	12
Finland	–	–	–	–	–	–	–	–	–	–	–	–
France	–	–	–	–	–	–	–	–	–	–	–	–
Gabon	32 x	5 x	82 x	23 x	34 x	19 x	35 x	47 x	18 x	–	–	52 x
Gambia	35	54	76	74	76	68	33	44	23	51	15	57
Georgia	33 m	20	90	25	29	20	8	40	53	65	28	9
Germany	–	–	–	–	–	–	–	–	–	–	–	–
Ghana	52	43	79	66	79	58	31	43	26	41	13	43
Greece	–	–	–	–	–	–	–	–	–	–	–	–
Grenada	–	–	–	–	–	–	–	–	–	–	–	–
Guatemala	63	53	80	72	85	48	9	31	59	82	52	27
Guinea	43	33	52	78	84	57	54	32	14	22	4	63
Guinea-Bissau	46 m	59	64	75	80	55	53 k	39 l	8	35	3	69
Guyana	49 mx	21 x	81 x	46 x	64 x	25 x	11 x	36 x	52 x	61 x	36 x	17 x
Haiti	47	40	91	52	59	43	32 k	49	19	39	11	55
Holy See	–	–	–	–	–	–	–	–	–	–	–	–
Honduras	51	30	92	51	63	37	10	33	57	85 x	55 x	37
Hungary	–	–	–	–	–	–	–	–	–	–	–	–
Iceland	–	–	–	–	–	–	–	–	–	–	–	–
India	41	64	49	80 l	87	71	40	36	24	35	11	52
Indonesia	58 m	51	86	67	74	56	12	34	54	71	40	18
Iran (Islamic Republic of)	81 m	47 m	76 mx	–	–	–	–	–	–	–	–	–
Iraq	32	26	85	35	47	32	14	41	45	74	34	25
Ireland	–	–	–	–	–	–	–	–	–	–	–	–
Israel	–	–	–	–	–	–	–	–	–	–	–	–
Italy	–	–	–	–	–	–	–	–	–	–	–	–
Jamaica	65 mx	24 x	64 x	38 x	39 x	29 x	–	–	–	37 x	–	–
Japan	–	–	–	–	–	–	–	–	–	–	–	–
Jordan	47	18	83 m	34	50	–	19	42	38	58	25	44
Kazakhstan	83 m	38	66 l	41	40	45	11	40	49	73	37	21
Kenya	62 x	61 x	80 x	75 x	79 x	69 x	19 x	45 x	36 x	50 x	22 x	29 x
Kiribati	46	64	90	61	70	53	34	56	9	74	8	51
Kuwait	–	–	–	–	–	–	–	–	–	–	–	–
Kyrgyzstan	81	46	91	47	53	36	9	31	60	75	43	14
Lao People's Democratic Republic	50	44	87 l	43	66	19	21	43	36	69	26	36
Latvia	–	–	–	–	–	–	–	–	–	–	–	–
Lebanon	41 mxy	–	–	14 mx	–	–	–	–	–	–	–	–
Lesotho	56	59	91	34	55	14	28	55	17	68	10	35
Liberia	66	55	45	68	73	52	43	49	9	22	3	56
Libya	29 mx	–	–	–	–	–	–	–	–	–	–	–
Liechtenstein	–	–	–	–	–	–	–	–	–	–	–	–
Lithuania	–	–	–	–	–	–	–	–	–	–	–	–
Luxembourg	–	–	–	–	–	–	–	–	–	–	–	–
Madagascar	60	54	90	79	79	81	24	50	26	65	20	29
Malawi	60	64	88	83	88	67	26	57	17	37	9	26
Malaysia	–	40	–	–	–	–	–	–	–	–	–	–
Maldives	66	63	97	73	79	– p	6	23	71	68	50	15
Mali	60	48	61	73	82 r	73 r	30	44	26	29	8	44
Malta	–	–	–	–	–	–	–	–	–	–	–	–
Marshall Islands	61	43	64 m	36	25	– p	29	36	34	50	15	46
Mauritania	56	41	55	67	74	64	38	42	20	23	8	55
Mauritius	–	–	–	–	–	–	–	–	–	–	–	–
Mexico	39 m	36 m	93 m	48 m	52 r	16 r	9	32	59	57 m	48	18
Micronesia (Federated States of)	–	–	–	–	–	–	–	–	–	–	–	–
Monaco	–	–	–	–	–	–	–	–	–	–	–	–
Mongolia	70	58 m	88	64 k	65	51	10	51	45 m	66	28	45
Montenegro	24 m	20	87	25	55	20	8	26	66	76	48	11
Montserrat	–	–	–	–	–	–	–	–	–	–	–	–
Morocco	43 m	35 m	84 x	35 x	45 x	19 x	–	–	–	–	–	–
Mozambique	69 mx	41 mx	95 mx	75 x	80 x	53 x	29 x	43 x	28 x	41 x	13 x	36 x
Myanmar	67	51 k	75	78	84	66	35	44	21	57	16	56
Namibia	71 x	48 x	80 x	47 x	55 x	27 x	40 x	35 x	25 x	38 x	12 x	52 x
Nauru	76 mxy	67 mx	–	67 mx	–	–	–	–	–	–	–	–

FOR EVERY CHILD, VACCINATION

TABLE 9. NUTRITION:BREASTFEEDING AND DIETS

Countries and areas	Early initiation of breastfeeding (%)		Exclusive breastfeeding (<6 months) (%)		Introduction to solid, semi-sold or soft foods (6–8 months)		Infant and Young Child Feeding (0–23 months) 2015–2021 [R, ^]																		
							Continued breastfeeding (12–23 months) (%)						Percentage of children consuming (6–23 months) (%)						Minimum meal frequency (6–23 months) (%)		Minimum acceptable diet (6–23 months) (%)		Zero vegetable or fruit consumption (6–23 months) (%)	
							All children		Poorest 20%		Richest 20%		<=2 food groups (severe food poverty)		3–4 food groups (moderate food poverty)		At least 5 food groups (minimum dietary diversity)							
Nepal	42		62		86		91		94		84		17		43		40		69		30		38	
Netherlands (Kingdom of the)	–		–		–		–		–		–		–		–		–		–		–		–	
New Zealand	–		–		–		–		–		–		–		–		–		–		–		–	
Nicaragua	54	mxy	32	mx	89	x	52	x	64	x	28	x	–		–		–		–		–		–	
Niger	57		26		88		72		85	rx	71	rx	26		57		17		71		15		43	
Nigeria	42		29		74		61		82		32		33		44		23		41		10		53	
Niue	–		–		–		–		–		–		–		–		–		–		–		–	
North Macedonia	10		28		96	k	30		37		33		11		35		54		80		43		13	
Norway	–		–		–		–		–		–		–		–		–		–		–		–	
Oman	82	m	23	m	95	m	–		–		–		–		–		–		–		–		–	
Pakistan	20		48		65		63		75		52		38		47		15		61		13		61	
Palau	–		–		–		–		–		–		–		–		–		–		–		–	
Panama	55	y	21	x	83		41	x	57	x	18	x	–		–		–		60	x	–		–	
Papua New Guinea	55		60		79		79		79		64		26		42		32		44		18		13	
Paraguay	50	m	30		87		33		41		43		6		42		52		71		38		16	
Peru	49		64		94		72		75		67		3		13		84		–		–		6	
Philippines	57		55	m	89	x	60		68		49		12	x	34	x	54	x	–		–		22	x
Poland	–		–		–		–		–		–		–		–		–		–		–		–	
Portugal	–		–		–		–		–		–		–		–		–		–		–		–	
Qatar	34	mx	29	x	74	x	47	x	–		–		–		–		–		40	x	–		–	
Republic of Korea	–		–		–		–		–		–		–		–		–		–		–		–	
Republic of Moldova	61	mx	36	x	75	x	27	x	44	x	22	x	6	x	24	x	70	x	46	x	–		10	x
Romania	58	mx	16	mx	–		–		–		–		–		–		–		–		–		–	
Russian Federation	25	mx	–		–		–		–		–		–		–		–		–		–		–	
Rwanda	85		81		81		90		95		81		12		53		34		45		21		16	
Saint Kitts and Nevis	–		–		–		–		–		–		–		–		–		–		–		–	
Saint Lucia	50	mx	3	mx	–	mpx	29	mx	–		–	px	–		–		–		43	x	–		–	
Saint Vincent and the Grenadines	–		–		–		–		–		–		–		–		–		–		–		–	
Samoa	53		52		83		50		58		36		23		57		20		46		12		25	
San Marino	–		–		–		–		–		–		–		–		–		–		–		–	
Sao Tome and Principe	36		63		80		46		51		39		22		45		32		58	x	22	x	32	
Saudi Arabia	–		–		–		–		–		–		–		–		–		–		–		–	
Senegal	32		41		64		72		78		57		37		43		19		37		9		52	
Serbia	8		24		96		16		28		18		2		13		86		95		74		2	
Seychelles	–		–		–		–		–		–		–		–		–		–		–		–	
Sierra Leone	88		51		99		54	k	67	r	51	r	46		29		24		32		9		54	
Singapore	–		–		–		–		–		–		–		–		–		–		–		–	
Slovakia	–		–		–		–		–		–		–		–		–		–		–		–	
Slovenia	–		–		–		–		–		–		–		–		–		–		–		–	
Solomon Islands	79	m	76	m	–		71	m	–		–		–		–		–		–		–		–	
Somalia	60	m	34	m	41	m	45	m	61	rx	23	rx	63		24		13		–		–		65	
South Africa	67		32		83		34		47		25		23		37		40		43		19		37	
South Sudan	50	x	45	x	42	x	62	x	67	x	58	x	–		–		–		10	x	–		–	
Spain	–		–		–		–		–		–		–		–		–		–		–		–	
Sri Lanka	90		81		94		90	l	90		81		5		17		78		–		–		11	
State of Palestine	41		39		90		29		29		28		13		42		45		71		31		28	
Sudan	69	mx	55	x	61	x	73	x	72	x	74	x	34	x	42	x	24	x	41	x	14	x	67	x
Suriname	52		9		81		23		27		21		23		48		28		52		16		29	
Sweden	–		–		–		–		–		–		–		–		–		–		–		–	
Switzerland	–		–		–		–		–		–		–		–		–		–		–		–	
Syrian Arab Republic	36	m	29		75	m	45	x	57	x	42	x	–		–		–		–		–		–	
Tajikistan	62		36		63		57		63		53		34		44		23		36		8		58	
Thailand	34	m	14		92		19		27		16		6		24		69		86		61		14	
Timor-Leste	47		65		73		49		61	r	44	r	30		30		40		56		25		34	
Togo	48		64		76		80		90		72		30		51		19		61		13		48	
Tokelau	–		–		–		–		–		–		–		–		–		–		–		–	
Tonga	38		40		91		35		47		16		13		34		53		49		27		10	
Trinidad and Tobago	46	mx	21	x	56	x	34	x	45	x	–	px	–		–		–		61	x	–		–	
Tunisia	32		14		97		30		39		28		8		28		63		85		54		20	
Türkiye	71	m	41	m	85	m	53	m	–		–		–		–		–		–		–		–	
Turkmenistan	68		56		91		45		49		38		4		27		69		97		64		12	
Turks and Caicos Islands	49		–	mp	–	mp	16	m	–		–		21		22		56		68		29		35	
Tuvalu	39		44		97	m	29		–		–		14		57		29		–		18		44	

168   THE STATE OF THE WORLD'S CHILDREN 2023

TABLE 9. NUTRITION:BREASTFEEDING AND DIETS

Countries and areas	Infant and Young Child Feeding (0–23 months) 2015–2021 [R, ^]											
	Early initiation of breastfeeding (%)	Exclusive breastfeeding (<6 months) (%)	Introduction to solid, semi-sold or soft foods (6–8 months)	Continued breastfeeding (12–23 months) (%)			Percentage of children consuming (6–23 months) (%)			Minimum meal frequency (6–23 months) (%)	Minimum acceptable diet (6–23 months) (%)	Zero vegetable or fruit consumption (6–23 months) (%)
				All children	Poorest 20%	Richest 20%	<=2 food groups (severe food poverty)	3–4 food groups (moderate food poverty)	At least 5 food groups (minimum dietary diversity)			
Uganda	72 m	65	89 m	60 m	77 r	53 r	24 m	62 m	14 m	51 m	10 m	54 m
Ukraine	66 mx	20 x	75 x	31 x	31 x	30 x	–	–	–	55 x	–	–
United Arab Emirates	–	–	–	–	–	–	–	–	–	–	–	–
United Kingdom	–	–	–	–	–	–	–	–	–	–	–	–
United Republic of Tanzania	54 m	58 m	87 m	72	75	70	19	59	21	39	9	29
United States	–	26 m	–	12 m	–	–	–	–	–	–	–	–
Uruguay	61	58	92	45	–	–	6	24	70	–	–	6
Uzbekistan	86	49	57	63	63	56	35	42	23	24	6	42
Vanuatu	85 mxy	73 mx	72 mx	58 mx	69 rx	40 rx	–	–	–	–	–	–
Venezuela (Bolivarian Republic of)	–	–	–	–	–	–	–	–	–	–	–	–
Viet Nam	23	45	86	44	44	43	9	36	56	77	46	17
Yemen	53 x	10 x	69 x	63 x	73 x	56 x	30 x	49 x	21 x	57 x	15 x	66 x
Zambia	75	70	94	63	74	51	24	53	23	41	12	29
Zimbabwe	59	42	90	50	61	33	25	58	17	68	11	28
SUMMARY												
East Asia and Pacific	41 v	42	84 v	59 q	66 q	50 q	14 q	35 q	42 v	66 v	30 v	27 v
Europe and Central Asia	–	–	–	–	–	–	–	–	–	–	–	–
Eastern Europe and Central Asia	72	42	75	51	51	46	–	–	–	–	–	–
Western Europe	–	–	–	–	–	–	–	–	–	–	–	–
Latin America and Caribbean	55	43	88	48	54	32	10	29	60	59 q	43 q	20
Middle East and North Africa	47	32	–	–	–	–	–	–	–	–	–	–
North America	–	26	–	12	–	–	–	–	–	–	–	–
South Asia	39	61	56	78	85	69	37	39	24	43	13	53
sub-Saharan Africa	54	45	76	67	76	52	32	47	21	44	11	44
Eastern and Southern Africa	65	55	79	68	72	63	31	48	21	47	12	45
West and Central Africa	46	38	74	66	79	43	33	46	21	41	11	44
Least developed countries (LDCs)	57	54	76	75	79	66	32	47	22	48	14	44
World	**47** v	**48**	**72** v	**65**	**75**	**56**	**30**	**41**	**31** v	**50** v	**18** v	**41** v

For a complete list of countries and areas in the regions, subregions and country categories, see page 182 or visit <data.unicef.org/regionalclassifications>.

It is not advisable to compare data from consecutive editions of *The State of the World's Children*.

NOTES

– Data not available.

[k] Statistically significant gender differences disadvantaging boys observed.

[l] Statistically significantly gender differences disadvantaging girls observed.

[m] Gender assessment not possible

[p] Based on small denominators (typically 25–49 unweighted cases). No data based on fewer than 25 unweighted cases are displayed.

[q] Regional estimates for East Asia and Pacific exclude China, Latin America and the Caribbean exclude Brazil, Eastern Europe and Central Asia exclude the Russian Federation.

[r] Disaggregated data are from different sources than the data presented for all children for the same indicator.

[R] Data refer to the most recent year available during the period specified in the column heading.

[v] Aggregated estimates for East Asia and Pacific and the World include estimates for China from the year 2013, which is outside of the year range 2015-2021.

[x] Data refer to years or periods other than those specified in the column heading. Such data are not included in the calculation of regional and global averages. Estimates from data years prior to 2000 are not displayed.

[y] Data differ from the standard definition or refer to only part of a country. If they fall within the noted reference period, such data are included in the calculation of regional and global averages.

[^] In the majority of countries, no statistically significant gender differences are observed, thus sex-disaggregated data are not presented.

MAIN DATA SOURCES

Infant and young child feeding (0–23 months) – DHS, MICS and other national household surveys. Last update: October 2022.

DEFINITIONS OF THE INDICATORS

Early initiation of breastfeeding – Percentage of children born in the last 24 months who were put to the breast within one hour of birth.

Exclusive breastfeeding (<6 months) – Percentage of infants 0–5 months of age who were fed exclusively with breastmilk during the previous day.

Continued breastfeeding (12–23 months) – Percentage of children 12–23 months of age who were fed with breastmilk during the previous day.

Introduction of solid, semi-solid or soft foods (6–8 months) – Percentage of infants 6–8 months of age who were fed with solid, semi-solid or soft food during the previous day.

Severe food poverty (6–23 months) – Percentage of children 6–23 months of age who received foods from zero, one or two out of 8 defined food groups during the previous day.

Moderate food poverty (6–23 months) – Percentage of children 6–23 months of age who received foods from three or four out of 8 defined food groups during the previous day.

Minimum Diet Diversity (6–23 months) – Percentage of children 6–23 months of age who received foods from at least 5 out of 8 defined food groups during the previous day.

Minimum Meal Frequency (6–23 months) – Percentage of children 6–23 months of age who received solid, semi-solid, or soft foods (but also including milk feeds for non-breastfed children) the minimum number of times or more during the previous day.

Minimum Acceptable Diet (6–23 months) – Percentage of children 6–23 months of age who received a minimum acceptable diet during the previous day.

Zero vegetable or fruit consumption (6–23 months) – Percentage of children 6–23 months of age who did not consume any vegetables or fruits during the previous day.

TABLE 10. EARLY CHILDHOOD DEVELOPMENT

Countries and areas	Attendance in early childhood education (%) 2013–2021 [R]					Early stimulation and responsive care by adults (%) [H] 2013–2021 [R]					Learning materials at home (%) 2013–2021 [R]		Children with inadequate supervision (%) 2013–2021 [R]					Children developmentally on track (%) 2013–2021 [R]				
	Total	Male	Female	Poorest 20%	Richest 20%	Total	Male	Female	Poorest 20%	Richest 20%	Children's books (Total)	Play-things (Total) [H]	Total	Male	Female	Poorest 20%	Richest 20%	Total	Male	Female	Poorest 20%	Richest 20%
Afghanistan	1 x	1 x	1 x	0 x	4 x	73 x,y	74 x,y	73 x,y	72 x,y	80 x,y	2 x	53 x	40 x	42 x	39 x	43 x	27 x	-	-	-	-	-
Albania	73	73	73	62	88	78 y	75 y	80 y	57 y	88 y	32 x	53 x	7	7	6	9	3	-	-	-	-	-
Algeria	14	14	15	6	26	61	60	62	48	77	8	49	13	13	12	13	13	77	74	79	70	85
Andorra	-	-	-	-	-	-	-	-	-	-	-	-	-	-	-	-	-	-	-	-	-	-
Angola	11 y	10 y	11 y	7 y	20 y	-	-	-	-	-	-	-	-	-	-	-	-	-	-	-	-	-
Anguilla	-	-	-	-	-	-	-	-	-	-	-	-	-	-	-	-	-	-	-	-	-	-
Antigua and Barbuda	-	-	-	-	-	-	-	-	-	-	-	-	-	-	-	-	-	-	-	-	-	-
Argentina	64 y	63 y	66 y	59 y	84 y	85 y	83 y	88 y	77 y	94 y	48 y	88 y	6 y	6 y	6 y	7 y	3 y	86 y	85 y	87 y	83 y	88 y
Armenia	-	-	-	-	-	-	-	-	-	-	-	-	-	-	-	-	-	-	-	-	-	-
Australia	-	-	-	-	-	-	-	-	-	-	-	-	-	-	-	-	-	-	-	-	-	-
Austria	-	-	-	-	-	-	-	-	-	-	-	-	-	-	-	-	-	-	-	-	-	-
Azerbaijan	11 x	12 x	11 x	5 x	20 x	-	-	-	-	-	-	-	-	-	-	-	-	-	-	-	-	-
Bahamas	-	-	-	-	-	-	-	-	-	-	-	-	-	-	-	-	-	-	-	-	-	-
Bahrain	-	-	-	-	-	-	-	-	-	-	-	-	-	-	-	-	-	-	-	-	-	-
Bangladesh	19	19	19	15	26	63	63	63	47	79	6	67	11	11	11	17	6	75	71	78	68	84
Barbados	90 x	88 x	91 x	90 x,p	97 x,p	97 x,y	97 x,y	97 x,y	100 x,p,y	100 x,p,y	85 x	76 x	1 x	2 x	1 x	0 x	3 x	97 x	95 x	99 x	100 x,p	100 x,p
Belarus	91	91	91	80	95	97	96	98	92	99	91	81	2	2	2	3	3	87	84	89	82	87
Belgium	-	-	-	-	-	-	-	-	-	-	-	-	-	-	-	-	-	-	-	-	-	-
Belize	55	52	58	29	72	88 y	89 y	86 y	80 y	94 y	44	68	13	15	11	15	11	83	80	85	76	91
Benin	19 y	18 y	20 y	5 y	49 y	39 y	39 y	39 y	32 y	56 y	2 y	55 y	29 y	28 y	30 y	36 y	22 y	54 y	52 y	56 y	45 y	65 y
Bhutan	10 x	10 x	10 x	3 x	27 x	54 x,y	52 x,y	57 x,y	40 x,y	73 x,y	6 x	52 x	14 x	13 x	15 x	17 x	7 x	72 x	68 x	75 x	67 x	80 x
Bolivia (Plurinational State of)	21	19	23	-	-	-	-	-	-	-	-	-	-	-	-	-	-	-	-	-	-	-
Bosnia and Herzegovina	13 x	12 x	14 x	2 x	31 x	95 x,y	95 x,y	96 x,y	87 x,y	100 x,y	56 x	56 x	2 x	2 x	2 x	3 x	1 x	96 x	95 x	98 x	95 x	94 x
Botswana	24	-	-	-	-	-	-	-	-	-	-	-	-	-	-	-	-	-	-	-	-	-
Brazil	93 y	-	-	-	-	-	-	-	-	-	-	-	-	-	-	-	-	-	-	-	-	-
British Virgin Islands	-	-	-	-	-	-	-	-	-	-	-	-	-	-	-	-	-	-	-	-	-	-
Brunei Darussalam	-	-	-	-	-	-	-	-	-	-	-	-	-	-	-	-	-	-	-	-	-	-
Bulgaria	-	-	-	-	-	-	-	-	-	-	-	-	-	-	-	-	-	-	-	-	-	-
Burkina Faso	3 y	3 y	3 y	-	-	14 x,y	14 x,y	14 x,y	12 x,y	26 x,y	-	-	-	-	-	-	-	-	-	-	-	-
Burundi	7 y	7 y	7 y	1 y	31 y	58 y	58 y	59 y	56 y	67 y	0 y	35 y	42 y	42 y	42 y	43 y	30 y	40 y	34 y	46 y	33 y	54 y
Cabo Verde	88 y	87 y	88 y	-	-	-	-	-	-	-	-	-	-	-	-	-	-	-	-	-	-	-
Cambodia	15 y	12 y	17 y	7 y	38 y	45 y	42 y	48 y	33 y	60 y	4 y	34 y	10 y	10 y	10 y	16 y	4 y	73 y	74 y	73 y	67 y	82 y
Cameroon	28	27	29	2	66	44 y	45 y	44 y	50 y	52 y	4	53	34	34	35	52	23	61	59	63	56	73
Canada	-	-	-	-	-	-	-	-	-	-	-	-	-	-	-	-	-	-	-	-	-	-
Central African Republic	6	6	7	2	27	27	28	26	24	39	0	56	49	49	49	50	47	36	34	39	35	46
Chad	1	1	1	0	4	55	54	55	53	56	1	58	64	64	64	63	63	45	43	47	42	48
Chile	-	-	-	-	-	93 y	93 y	94 y	91 y	96 y	-	98 y	1	1	1	1	0	-	-	-	-	-
China	-	-	-	-	-	-	-	-	-	-	-	-	-	-	-	-	-	-	-	-	-	-
Colombia	36 y	-	-	-	-	-	-	-	-	-	-	-	-	-	-	-	-	-	-	-	-	-
Comoros	14 x	13 x	15 x	10 x	28 x	-	-	-	-	-	-	-	-	-	-	-	-	-	-	-	-	-
Congo	36	36	37	7	77	59 y	59 y	58 y	47 y	77 y	3	51	42	42	41	54	30	61	57	65	46	72
Cook Islands	-	-	-	-	-	-	-	-	-	-	-	-	-	-	-	-	-	-	-	-	-	-
Costa Rica	44	41	47	41	52	76	75	77	66	87	39	82	7	7	7	7	6	86	82	90	79	94
Côte d'Ivoire	14	14	15	2	51	29 y	29 y	29 y	18 y	61 y	1	45	20	20	19	20	18	63	61	65	63	72
Croatia	82 y	81 y	82 y	-	-	-	-	-	-	-	-	-	-	-	-	-	-	-	-	-	-	-
Cuba	50	47	53	-	-	90	89	91	-	-	42	86	2	2	2	-	-	95	94	95	-	-
Cyprus	-	-	-	-	-	-	-	-	-	-	-	-	-	-	-	-	-	-	-	-	-	-
Czechia	-	-	-	-	-	-	-	-	-	-	-	-	-	-	-	-	-	-	-	-	-	-
Democratic People's Republic of Korea	73	73	73	-	-	95	94	95	-	-	50	59	16	17	16	-	-	88	86	89	-	-
Democratic Republic of the Congo	5	6	5	1	20	44	44	44	39	58	1	39	47	47	46	53	29	57	56	57	44	72
Denmark	-	-	-	-	-	-	-	-	-	-	-	-	-	-	-	-	-	-	-	-	-	-
Djibouti	14 x	12 x	16 x	-	-	37 x,y	38 x,y	35 x,y	-	-	15 x	24 x	8 x	8 x	8 x	-	-	-	-	-	-	-
Dominica	-	-	-	-	-	-	-	-	-	-	-	-	-	-	-	-	-	-	-	-	-	-
Dominican Republic	48	46	50	33	63	63	61	65	47	82	9	68	8	8	7	9	5	87	85	89	81	90
Ecuador	-	-	-	-	-	78 y	76 y	81 y	-	-	28 y	48 y	5 y	5 y	5 y	-	-	-	-	-	-	-
Egypt	47 y	48 y	47 y	34 y	50 y	-	-	-	-	-	-	-	4	4	4	7	2	-	-	-	-	-
El Salvador	25	24	26	19	44	59 y	57 y	62 y	45 y	78 y	18	62	4	4	3	4	4	81	79	83	79	86
Equatorial Guinea	-	-	-	-	-	-	-	-	-	-	-	-	-	-	-	-	-	-	-	-	-	-
Eritrea	-	-	-	-	-	-	-	-	-	-	-	-	-	-	-	-	-	-	-	-	-	-
Estonia	-	-	-	-	-	-	-	-	-	-	-	-	-	-	-	-	-	-	-	-	-	-

170   THE STATE OF THE WORLD'S CHILDREN 2023

TABLE 10. EARLY CHILDHOOD DEVELOPMENT

Countries and areas	Attendance in early childhood education (%) 2013–2021 R					Early stimulation and responsive care by adults (%) H 2013–2021 R					Learning materials at home (%) 2013–2021 R		Children with inadequate supervision (%) 2013–2021 R					Children developmentally on track (%) 2013–2021 R				
	Total	Male	Fe-male	Poor-est 20%	Richest 20%	Total	Male	Female	Poorest 20%	Richest 20%	Chil-dren's books (Total)	Play-things H (Total)	Total	Male	Fe-male	Poor-est 20%	Rich-est 20%	Total	Male	Fe-male	Poorest 20%	Richest 20%
Eswatini	30	26	33	28	48	39 y	33 y	44 y	25 y	59 y	6	67	17	16	17	18	15	65	64	66	61	77
Ethiopia	-	-	-	-	-	-	-	-	-	-	-	-	-	-	-	-	-	-	-	-	-	-
Fiji	22	23	20	23	25	97	97	97	95	99	24	75	13	15	12	14	9	-	-	-	-	-
Finland	-	-	-	-	-	-	-	-	-	-	-	-	-	-	-	-	-	-	-	-	-	-
France	-	-	-	-	-	-	-	-	-	-	-	-	-	-	-	-	-	-	-	-	-	-
Gabon	-	-	-	-	-	-	-	-	-	-	-	-	-	-	-	-	-	-	-	-	-	-
Gambia	24	23	25	19	40	16	15	18	11	31	1	49	16	17	16	18	16	67	65	69	63	78
Georgia	78	77	79	61	87	78	78	77	68	85	57	66	4	3	5	4	3	90	91	89	88	92
Germany	-	-	-	-	-	-	-	-	-	-	-	-	-	-	-	-	-	-	-	-	-	-
Ghana	71	71	70	46	94	34	35	33	20	60	7	50	30	30	30	39	21	68	65	72	54	87
Greece	-	-	-	-	-	-	-	-	-	-	-	-	-	-	-	-	-	-	-	-	-	-
Grenada	-	-	-	-	-	-	-	-	-	-	-	-	-	-	-	-	-	-	-	-	-	-
Guatemala	-	-	-	-	-	-	-	-	-	-	-	-	-	-	-	-	-	-	-	-	-	-
Guinea	9	9	9	3	32	31 y	33 y	30 y	22 y	51 y	0	32	34	36	33	38	36	49	48	50	45	51
Guinea-Bissau	14	12	17	5	54	43	42	44	31	72	1	44	70	71	70	68	73	73	72	75	70	75
Guyana	61	63	59	45	76	87	85	90	82	94	47	69	5	5	5	10	1	86	85	87	78	90
Haiti	63 y	63 y	63 y	31 y	84 y	54 y	52 y	57 y	34 y	79 y	8 y	48 y	22 y	23 y	22 y	28 y	15 y	65 y	62 y	69 y	61 y	77 y
Holy See	-	-	-	-	-	-	-	-	-	-	-	-	-	-	-	-	-	-	-	-	-	-
Honduras	14	14	13	15	18	36	35	37	21	60	7	70	6	6	6	8	4	75	75	74	70	81
Hungary	-	-	-	-	-	-	-	-	-	-	-	-	-	-	-	-	-	-	-	-	-	-
Iceland	-	-	-	-	-	-	-	-	-	-	-	-	-	-	-	-	-	-	-	-	-	-
India	14 y	-	-	-	-	-	-	-	-	-	-	-	-	-	-	-	-	-	-	-	-	-
Indonesia	18	17	18	-	-	-	-	-	-	-	-	-	-	-	-	-	-	88	-	-	-	-
Iran (Islamic Republic of)	18	-	-	-	-	70 x,y	69 x,y	70 x,y	-	-	36	83 y	13	-	-	-	-	-	-	-	-	-
Iraq	2	2	3	1	5	44	44	45	31	53	3	47	10	10	10	12	12	79	78	80	71	89
Ireland	-	-	-	-	-	-	-	-	-	-	-	-	-	-	-	-	-	-	-	-	-	-
Israel	-	-	-	-	-	-	-	-	-	-	-	-	-	-	-	-	-	-	-	-	-	-
Italy	-	-	-	-	-	-	-	-	-	-	-	-	-	-	-	-	-	-	-	-	-	-
Jamaica	92 x	92 x	91 x	88 x	100 x	88 x,y	86 x,y	90 x,y	76 x,y	86 x,y	55 x	61 x	2 x	2 x	2 x	2 x	1 x	89 x	86 x	93 x	79 x	97 x
Japan	-	-	-	-	-	-	-	-	-	-	-	-	-	-	-	-	-	-	-	-	-	-
Jordan	13 y	12 y	14 y	5 y	35 y	92 y	92 y	91 y	85 y	99 y	16 y	71 y	16 y	17 y	16 y	16 y	21 y	71 y	66 y	76 y	66 y	76 y
Kazakhstan	55	53	58	45	70	86 y	84 y	87 y	83 y	95 y	51	60	5	4	6	8	3	86	85	86	87	88
Kenya	16 x	14 x	17 x	-	-	-	-	-	-	-	-	-	-	-	-	-	-	-	-	-	-	-
Kiribati	72	69	75	76	76	77	76	79	71	84	4	60	31	31	30	35	31	80	78	82	70	89
Kuwait	-	-	-	-	-	-	-	-	-	-	-	-	-	-	-	-	-	-	-	-	-	-
Kyrgyzstan	39	40	38	25	57	87	88	86	88	88	21	72	8	7	8	11	5	72	68	75	73	78
Lao People's Democratic Republic	32	30	34	13	69	30	29	30	21	49	4	61	12	13	12	17	6	89	88	91	85	94
Latvia	-	-	-	-	-	-	-	-	-	-	-	-	-	-	-	-	-	-	-	-	-	-
Lebanon	62 x	63 x	60 x	-	-	56 x,y	58 x,y	54 x,y	-	-	29 x	16 x,y	9 x	8 x	10 x	-	-	-	-	-	-	-
Lesotho	46	45	46	20	83	28	27	29	16	45	3	57	17	17	17	27	9	73	68	78	66	77
Liberia	-	-	-	-	-	-	-	-	-	-	-	-	-	-	-	-	-	-	-	-	-	-
Libya	6 x	-	-	-	-	-	-	-	-	-	-	-	-	-	-	-	-	-	-	-	-	-
Liechtenstein	-	-	-	-	-	-	-	-	-	-	-	-	-	-	-	-	-	-	-	-	-	-
Lithuania	-	-	-	-	-	-	-	-	-	-	-	-	-	-	-	-	-	-	-	-	-	-
Luxembourg	-	-	-	-	-	-	-	-	-	-	-	-	-	-	-	-	-	-	-	-	-	-
Madagascar	15	15	15	7	42	25	25	26	17	44	1	52	34	33	34	36	25	67	65	68	64	81
Malawi	34	31	36	21	55	35	34	37	27	48	1	37	44	45	43	47	33	60	56	64	52	70
Malaysia	53	52	55	-	-	25 y	25 y	24 y	-	-	56	62	3	3	3	-	-	-	-	-	-	-
Maldives	78 y	78 y	79 y	69 y	82 y,p	96 y	96 y	97 y	97 y	-	59 y	48 y	12 y	10 y	14 y	11 y	22 y	93 y	91 y	95 y	92 y	-
Mali	5	6	5	1	21	55 y	55 y	55 y	53 y	65 y	0	52	32	32	32	31	27	62	60	63	54	67
Malta	-	-	-	-	-	-	-	-	-	-	-	-	-	-	-	-	-	-	-	-	-	-
Marshall Islands	5	5	5	4	11	72 y	72 y	73 y	71 y	83 y	19	71	9	9	10	10	9	79	80	78	84	82
Mauritania	12	12	12	3	30	44 y	46 y	42 y	30 y	65 y	1	33	34	35	34	39	26	60	58	62	52	68
Mauritius	-	-	-	-	-	-	-	-	-	-	-	-	-	-	-	-	-	-	-	-	-	-
Mexico	65	61	70	-	-	71	71	71	-	-	29	75	6	7	5	-	-	80	81	79	-	-
Micronesia (Federated States of)	-	-	-	-	-	-	-	-	-	-	-	-	-	-	-	-	-	-	-	-	-	-
Monaco	-	-	-	-	-	-	-	-	-	-	-	-	-	-	-	-	-	-	-	-	-	-
Mongolia	74	72	76	34	89	58	57	59	39	76	29	65	13	12	13	16	9	76	72	80	78	76
Montenegro	53	51	56	18	65	91	91	91	69	100	58	64	5	4	5	5	2	90	90	91	76	92
Montserrat	-	-	-	-	-	-	-	-	-	-	-	-	-	-	-	-	-	-	-	-	-	-
Morocco	39 x	36 x	41 x	6 x	78 x	36 y	36 y	36 y	26 y	47 y	21 x,y	14 x,y	7	-	-	-	-	-	-	-	-	-

FOR EVERY CHILD, VACCINATION 171

TABLE 10. EARLY CHILDHOOD DEVELOPMENT

Countries and areas	Attendance in early childhood education (%) 2013–2021 [R]					Early stimulation and responsive care by adults (%) [H] 2013–2021 [R]					Learning materials at home (%) 2013–2021 [R]		Children with inadequate supervision (%) 2013–2021 [R]					Children developmentally on track (%) 2013–2021 [R]				
	Total	Male	Female	Poorest 20%	Richest 20%	Total	Male	Female	Poorest 20%	Richest 20%	Children's books	Playthings [H]	Total	Male	Female	Poorest 20%	Richest 20%	Total	Male	Female	Poorest 20%	Richest 20%
Mozambique	-	-	-	-	-	47 x,y	45 x,y	48 x,y	48 x,y	50 x,y	3 x	-	33 x	33 x	32 x	-	-	-	-	-	-	-
Myanmar	23 y	22 y	25 y	11 y	42 y	52 y	51 y	53 y	41 y	73 y	5 y	72 y	13 y	14 y	13 y	21 y	5 y	-	-	-	-	-
Namibia	-	-	-	-	-	-	-	-	-	-	-	-	-	-	-	-	-	-	-	-	-	-
Nauru	-	-	-	-	-	-	-	-	-	-	-	-	-	-	-	-	-	-	-	-	-	-
Nepal	62	64	60	52	87	73	74	73	61	91	3	66	25	26	24	40	13	65	65	66	53	82
Netherlands (Kingdom of the)	-	-	-	-	-	-	-	-	-	-	-	-	-	-	-	-	-	-	-	-	-	-
New Zealand	-	-	-	-	-	-	-	-	-	-	-	-	-	-	-	-	-	-	-	-	-	-
Nicaragua	-	-	-	-	-	-	-	-	-	-	-	-	-	-	-	-	-	-	-	-	-	-
Niger	3 x	3 x	2 x	0 x	9 x	-	-	-	-	-	-	-	-	-	-	-	-	-	-	-	-	-
Nigeria	36	36	35	8	78	63 y	62 y	63 y	46 y	87 y	6	46	32	32	31	31	30	61	60	62	47	85
Niue	-	-	-	-	-	-	-	-	-	-	-	-	-	-	-	-	-	-	-	-	-	-
North Macedonia	37	41	32	7	67	88	86	91	70	99	55	62	6	7	5	11	1	82	76	89	67	91
Norway	-	-	-	-	-	-	-	-	-	-	-	-	-	-	-	-	-	-	-	-	-	-
Oman	29	28	31	-	-	81 y	78 y	84 y	-	-	25	75	45	44	45	-	-	68	65	72	-	-
Pakistan	-	-	-	-	-	-	-	-	-	-	-	-	-	-	-	-	-	-	-	-	-	-
Palau	-	-	-	-	-	-	-	-	-	-	-	-	-	-	-	-	-	-	-	-	-	-
Panama	37	38	35	28	67	74 y	73 y	74 y	55 y	89 y	26	69	3	3	2	6	1	80	80	81	77	95
Papua New Guinea	-	-	-	-	-	-	-	-	-	-	-	-	-	-	-	-	-	-	-	-	-	-
Paraguay	31	30	32	10	61	64 y	62 y	65 y	40 y	90 y	23	60	3	2	3	4	2	82	80	84	76	91
Peru	77 y	76 y	79 y	70 y	90 y	-	-	-	-	-	-	-	-	-	-	-	-	-	-	-	-	-
Philippines	29 x	26 x	33 x	17 x	58 x	-	-	-	-	-	-	-	-	-	-	-	-	-	-	-	-	-
Poland	-	-	-	-	-	-	-	-	-	-	-	-	-	-	-	-	-	-	-	-	-	-
Portugal	-	-	-	-	-	-	-	-	-	-	-	-	-	-	-	-	-	-	-	-	-	-
Qatar	41 x	41 x	41 x	-	-	88 x,y	89 x,y	88 x,y	-	-	40 x	55 x	12 x	12 x	11 x	-	-	84 x	83 x	85 x	-	-
Republic of Korea	-	-	-	-	-	-	-	-	-	-	-	-	-	-	-	-	-	-	-	-	-	-
Republic of Moldova	71 x	74 x	67 x	50 x	88 x	89 x,y	86 x,y	92 x,y	81 x,y	95 x,y	68 x	68 x	6 x	6 x	6 x	9 x	5 x	84 x	83 x	84 x	75 x	87 x
Romania	81 y	80 y	81 y	-	-	-	-	-	-	-	-	-	-	-	-	-	-	-	-	-	-	-
Russian Federation	-	-	-	-	-	-	-	-	-	-	-	-	-	-	-	-	-	-	-	-	-	-
Rwanda	34 y	33 y	36 y	24 y	64 y	47 y	46 y	49 y	35 y	62 y	2 y	37 y	28 y	30 y	26 y	35 y	13 y	82 y	80 y	84 y	76 y	91 y
Saint Kitts and Nevis	-	-	-	-	-	-	-	-	-	-	-	-	-	-	-	-	-	-	-	-	-	-
Saint Lucia	85 x	87 x	84 x	-	-	93 x,y	89 x,y	96 x,y	-	-	68 x	59 x	5 x	5 x	5 x	-	-	91 x	91 x	92 x	-	-
Saint Vincent and the Grenadines	-	-	-	-	-	-	-	-	-	-	-	-	-	-	-	-	-	-	-	-	-	-
Samoa	26	23	29	18	36	87	86	88	83	92	9	51	16	18	13	16	16	73	70	77	65	75
San Marino	-	-	-	-	-	-	-	-	-	-	-	-	-	-	-	-	-	-	-	-	-	-
Sao Tome and Principe	35	36	34	19	57	43	42	44	37	68	6	71	21	21	22	29	17	63	59	67	61	75
Saudi Arabia	-	-	-	-	-	-	-	-	-	-	-	-	-	-	-	-	-	-	-	-	-	-
Senegal	21 y	21 y	21 y	6 y	51 y	20 y	18 y	21 y	15 y	33 y	1 y	29 y	39 y	39 y	38 y	30 y	54 y	67 y	66 y	68 y	59 y	71 y
Serbia	61	58	63	11	80	96	95	97	93	97	78	83	4	3	4	7	2	97	96	99	99	97
Seychelles	-	-	-	-	-	-	-	-	-	-	-	-	-	-	-	-	-	-	-	-	-	-
Sierra Leone	12	11	12	1	41	19	19	19	13	31	2	41	30	30	30	32	25	51	48	55	43	72
Singapore	-	-	-	-	-	-	-	-	-	-	-	-	-	-	-	-	-	-	-	-	-	-
Slovakia	-	-	-	-	-	-	-	-	-	-	-	-	-	-	-	-	-	-	-	-	-	-
Slovenia	-	-	-	-	-	-	-	-	-	-	-	-	-	-	-	-	-	-	-	-	-	-
Solomon Islands	-	-	-	-	-	-	-	-	-	-	-	-	-	-	-	-	-	-	-	-	-	-
Somalia	2 x	2 x	2 x	1 x	6 x	79 x,y	80 x,y	79 x,y	76 x,y	85 x,y	-	-	-	-	-	-	-	-	-	-	-	-
South Africa	48 y	-	-	-	-	-	-	-	-	-	-	-	-	-	-	-	-	-	-	-	-	-
South Sudan	6 x	6 x	6 x	2 x	13 x	-	-	-	-	-	-	-	-	-	-	-	-	-	-	-	-	-
Spain	-	-	-	-	-	-	-	-	-	-	-	-	-	-	-	-	-	-	-	-	-	-
Sri Lanka	60	-	-	52	73	95 y	94 y	96 y	-	-	47	85	-	-	-	-	-	-	-	-	-	-
State of Palestine	34	36	33	26	45	76	75	77	66	87	12	73	14	14	14	17	12	84	82	86	81	90
Sudan	22	22	23	7	59	-	-	-	-	-	2	46	-	-	-	-	-	-	-	-	-	-
Suriname	46	43	49	32	67	66	63	70	46	80	26	65	6	6	6	8	3	77	72	83	65	94
Sweden	-	-	-	-	-	-	-	-	-	-	-	-	-	-	-	-	-	-	-	-	-	-
Switzerland	-	-	-	-	-	-	-	-	-	-	-	-	-	-	-	-	-	-	-	-	-	-
Syrian Arab Republic	8 x	8 x	7 x	4 x	18 x	70 x,y	70 x,y	69 x,y	52 x,y	84 x,y	30 x	52 x	17 x	17 x	17 x	22 x	15 x	-	-	-	-	-
Tajikistan	6 x	-	-	-	-	74 x,y	73 x,y	74 x,y	56 x,y	86 x,y	17 x	46 x	13 x	13 x	12 x	15 x	11 x	-	-	-	-	-
Thailand	86	85	88	85	88	92	90	94	85	98	34	80	5	6	4	5	3	93	91	95	90	96
Timor-Leste	14 y	13 y	16 y	9 y	16 y	81 y	83 y	79 y	72 y	89 y	4 y	40 y	29 y	29 y	30 y	33 y	26 y	53 y	51 y	56 y	34 y	74 y
Togo	20	21	20	10	40	19	18	19	16	26	1	38	29	29	29	38	21	52	50	55	48	61
Tokelau	-	-	-	-	-	-	-	-	-	-	-	-	-	-	-	-	-	-	-	-	-	-
Tonga	35	30	41	29	37	88	87	88	86	92	24	63	9	10	7	14	6	79	79	79	75	82

TABLE 10. EARLY CHILDHOOD DEVELOPMENT

Countries and areas	Attendance in early childhood education (%) 2013–2021 [R]					Early stimulation and responsive care by adults (%) [H] 2013–2021 [R]					Learning materials at home (%) 2013–2021 [R]		Children with inadequate supervision (%) 2013–2021 [R]					Children developmentally on track (%) 2013–2021 [R]				
	Total	Male	Female	Poorest 20%	Richest 20%	Total	Male	Female	Poorest 20%	Richest 20%	Children's books Total	Playthings [H] Total	Total	Male	Female	Poorest 20%	Richest 20%	Total	Male	Female	Poorest 20%	Richest 20%
Trinidad and Tobago	85 x	85 x	84 x	72 x	93 x	96 x,y	95 x,y	96 x,y	94 x,y	100 x,y	76 x	76 x	2 x	2 x	1 x	3 x	1 x	91 x	89 x	93 x	90 x	93 x
Tunisia	51	52	49	17	71	73	73	74	44	91	24	62	13	13	12	18	8	82	83	82	75	91
Türkiye	-	-	-	-	-	65	66	65	42	88	29	76	6	6	7	9	5	74	70	78	62	85
Turkmenistan	41	40	42	17	77	90	90	90	88	93	32	75	2	3	2	2	2	95	95	95	90	97
Turks and Caicos Islands	93	95	92	-	100 p	87	86	88	57 p	97	55	74	1	1	0	0	0	91	93	88	-	95 p
Tuvalu	73	75	70	70 p	79 p	87	87	88	83	91 p	24	66	17	19	14	31	7	69	70	67	65 p	76 p
Uganda	37 y	34 y	39 y	15 y	66 y	53 y	51 y	55 y	38 y	74 y	2 y	50 y	37 y	37 y	37 y	49 y	21 y	65 y	64 y	66 y	56 y	82 y
Ukraine	52 x	54 x	50 x	30 x	68 x	98 x,y	97 x,y	98 x,y	95 x,y	99 x,y	91 x	52 x	7 x	6 x	7 x	11 x	5 x	89 x	89 x	89 x	88 x	91 x
United Arab Emirates	-	-	-	-	-	-	-	-	-	-	-	-	-	-	-	-	-	-	-	-	-	-
United Kingdom	-	-	-	-	-	-	-	-	-	-	-	-	-	-	-	-	-	-	-	-	-	-
United Republic of Tanzania	-	-	-	-	-	-	-	-	-	-	-	-	-	-	-	-	-	-	-	-	-	-
United States	-	-	-	-	-	-	-	-	-	-	-	-	-	-	-	-	-	-	-	-	-	-
Uruguay	85	84	85	-	-	93 y	94 y	91 y	88 y	98 y	59	75	3	3	3	3	4	87	89	84	79	97
Uzbekistan	51 y	51 y	51 y	-	-	91 x,y	91 x,y	90 x,y	83 x,y	95 x,y	43 x	67 x	5 x	5 x	5 x	6 x	7 x	-	-	-	-	-
Vanuatu	-	-	-	-	-	-	-	-	-	-	-	-	-	-	-	-	-	-	-	-	-	-
Venezuela (Bolivarian Republic of)	66 x,y	-	-	-	-	-	-	-	-	-	-	-	-	-	-	-	-	-	-	-	-	-
Viet Nam	71	74	69	53	86	76 y	76 y	76 y	52 y	96 y	27	46	7	7	6	13	4	89	88	89	81	92
Yemen	3 x	3 x	3 x	0 x	8 x	33 x,y	34 x,y	32 x,y	16 x,y	57 x,y	10 x	49 x	34 x	36 x	33 x	46 x	22 x	-	-	-	-	-
Zambia	-	-	-	-	-	-	-	-	-	-	-	-	-	-	-	-	-	-	-	-	-	-
Zimbabwe	28	28	29	16	53	37	37	37	29	54	3	69	20	21	20	28	12	71	68	74	66	77

SUMMARY

East Asia and Pacific	-	-	-	-	-	-	-	-	-	-	-	-	-	-	-	-	-	-	-	-	-	-
Europe and Central Asia	-	-	-	-	-	-	-	-	-	-	-	-	-	-	-	-	-	-	-	-	-	-
Eastern Europe and Central Asia	-	-	-	-	-	-	-	-	-	-	-	-	-	-	-	-	-	-	-	-	-	-
Western Europe	-	-	-	-	-	-	-	-	-	-	-	-	-	-	-	-	-	-	-	-	-	-
Latin America and Caribbean	68	-	-	-	-	-	-	-	-	-	-	-	-	-	-	-	-	-	-	-	-	-
Middle East and North Africa	27	30	30	19	36	-	-	-	-	-	-	-	9	9	9	10	8	-	-	-	-	-
North America	-	-	-	-	-	-	-	-	-	-	-	-	-	-	-	-	-	-	-	-	-	-
South Asia	16	-	-	-	-	-	-	-	-	-	-	-	-	-	-	-	-	-	-	-	-	-
Sub-Saharan Africa	25	24	24	8	54	48	48	48	38	67	3	46	36	36	35	39	29	60	59	62	50	77
Eastern and Southern Africa	-	-	-	-	-	-	-	-	-	-	-	-	-	-	-	-	-	-	-	-	-	-
West and Central Africa	24	24	24	7	55	49	49	49	39	69	3	45	36	36	36	38	30	59	58	61	48	76
Least developed countries	18	18	19	10	38	48	47	48	38	63	2	50	32	32	32	37	23	-	-	-	-	-
World	**29**	-	-	-	-	-	-	-	-	-	-	-	-	-	-	-	-	-	-	-	-	-

For a complete list of countries and areas in the regions, subregions and country categories, see page on Regional Classifications or visit <data.unicef.org/regionalclassifications>.

It is not advisable to compare data from consecutive editions of *The State of the World's Children* report.

NOTES

- Data not available.

[y] Data differ from the standard definition or refer to only part of a country. If they fall within the noted reference period, such data are included in the calculation of regional and global averages.

[p] Based on small denominators (typically 25–49 unweighted cases). No data based on fewer than 25 unweighted cases are displayed.

[x] Data refer to years or periods other than those specified in the column heading. Such data are not included in the calculation of regional and global averages. Estimates from data years prior to 2000 are not displayed.

[H] A more detailed explanation of the methodology and the changes in calculating these estimates can be found in the section titled, General note on the data.

[R] Data refer to the most recent year available during the period specified in the column heading.

MAIN DATA SOURCES

Attendance in early childhood education – Demographic and Health Surveys (DHS), Multiple Indicator Cluster Surveys (MICS), and other national surveys. Last update: March 2022.

Early stimulation and responsive care by adults – DHS, MICS and other national surveys. Last update: March 2022.

Learning materials at home: Children's books – DHS, MICS and other national surveys. Last update: March 2022.

Learning materials at home: Playthings – DHS, MICS and other national surveys. Last update: March 2022.

Children with inadequate supervision – DHS, MICS and other national surveys. Last update: March 2022.

Children developmentally on track – DHS, MICS and other national surveys. Last update: March 2022.

DEFINITIONS OF THE INDICATORS

Attendance in early childhood education – Percentage of children 36–59 months old who are attending an early childhood education programme.

Early stimulation and responsive care by adults – Percentage of children 24–59 months old with whom an adult has engaged in four or more of the following activities to provide early stimulation and responsive care in the past three days: a) reading books to the child, b) telling stories to the child, c) singing songs to the child, d) taking the child outside the home, e) playing with the child, and f) spending time with the child naming, counting or drawing things.

Learning materials at home: Children's books – Percentage of children 0–59 months old who have three or more children's books at home.

Learning materials at home: Playthings – Percentage of children 0–59 months old with two or more of the following playthings at home: household objects or objects found outside (sticks, rocks, animals, shells, leaves etc.), homemade toys or toys that came from a store.

Children with inadequate supervision – Percentage of children 0–59 months old left alone or in the care of another child younger than 10 years of age for more than one hour at least once in the past week.

Children developmentally on track – Children 36–59 months old who are developmentally on track in at least three of the following domains: literacy-numeracy, physical development, social-emotional development and learning.

TABLE 11. EDUCATION

	Equitable access								Completion						Learning							
	Out-of-school rate 2013–2022 [R]								Completion rate 2013–2022 [R]						Learning outcomes 2013–2022 [R]						Literacy rate 2013–2022	
	One year before primary entry age		Primary education		Lower secondary education		Upper secondary education		Primary education		Lower secondary education		Upper secondary education		Proportion of children in grade 2 or 3 achieving minimum proficiency level		Proportion of children at the end of primary achieving a minimum proficiency level		Proportion of children at the end of lower secondary achieving a minimum proficiency level		Youth (15–24 years) literacy rate (%)	
Countries and areas	Male	Fe-male	Male	Fe-male	Male	Fe-male	Male	Fe-male	Male	Female	Male	Female	Male	Female	Read-ing	Math	Read-ing	Math	Read-ing	Math	Male	Fe-male
Afghanistan	-	-	-	-	-	-	44	69	67	40	49	26	32	14	-	-	-	-	-	-	71	42
Albania	4	2	6	2	5	1	22	15	94	96	98	97	76	80	-	-	-	62	48	58	99	100
Algeria	-	-	-	-	-	-	-	-	93	96	60	78	35	59	-	-	-	-	21	19	98	97
Andorra	-	-	-	-	-	-	-	-	-	-	-	-	-	-	-	-	-	-	-	-	-	-
Angola	31	39	-	-	-	-	-	-	63	57	42	32	24	15	-	-	-	-	-	-	-	-
Anguilla	14	0	-	-	-	-	-	-	-	-	-	-	-	-	-	-	-	-	-	-	-	-
Antigua and Barbuda	14	4	2	2	2	3	12	13	-	-	-	-	-	-	-	-	-	-	-	-	-	-
Argentina	1	0	-	-	1	1	15	7	96	98	74	85	54	66	-	-	-	-	48	31	99	100
Armenia	36	38	11	10	11	9	13	1	99	99	95	99	69	79	-	-	-	64	-	50	100	100
Australia	18	18	1	2	2	2	9	6	-	-	-	-	-	-	94	70	-	68	80	78	-	-
Austria	2	1	0	0	1	0	11	9	-	-	-	-	-	-	-	-	98	84	76	79	-	-
Azerbaijan	16	17	12	9	1	0	0	0	-	-	-	-	-	-	-	-	81	72	-	-	100	100
Bahamas	64	60	-	-	-	-	-	-	-	-	-	-	-	-	-	-	-	-	-	-	-	-
Bahrain	31	28	2	3	7	0	18	6	-	-	-	-	-	-	-	-	69	54	-	55	-	-
Bangladesh	-	-	-	-	40	25	40	33	76	89	59	71	32	27	-	-	-	-	-	-	93	96
Barbados	13	12	2	3	4	4	8	4	99 x	99 x	98 x	98 x	91 x	97 x	-	-	-	-	-	-	-	-
Belarus	0	4	5	6	1	1	8	5	100	100	99	99	98	98	82	73	-	-	77	71	100	100
Belgium	4	3	1	0	0	0	2	2	-	-	-	-	-	-	-	-	97	80	79	80	-	-
Belize	15	16	1	2	14	16	35	28	95	96	55	66	48	51	-	-	-	-	-	-	-	-
Benin	15	16	4	10	38	46	59	69	51	44	25	13	12	5	38	62	46	19	-	-	70	52
Bhutan	58	59	5	2	18	6	33	22	67 x	71 x	41 x	38 x	25 x	18 x	-	-	-	-	-	-	-	-
Bolivia (Plurinational State of)	7	7	5	5	12	11	22	22	91	93	84	82	66	65	48	38	15	8	-	-	100	100
Bosnia and Herzegovina	70	71	13	13	5	7	20	17	99 x	100 x	97 x	97 x	92 x	92 x	-	-	-	-	40	46	-	-
Botswana	79	78	10	8	11	9	21	18	95	98	92	92	55	66	-	-	-	-	-	-	-	-
Brazil	0	1	1	1	3	1	16	14	95	97	81	89	65	75	-	-	-	-	50	32	99	99
British Virgin Islands	6	0	-	-	-	-	24	16	-	-	-	-	-	-	-	-	-	-	-	-	-	-
Brunei Darussalam	5	6	2	2	-	-	19	14	-	-	-	-	-	-	-	-	-	-	48	52	100	100
Bulgaria	16	17	15	15	14	15	14	18	-	-	-	-	-	-	-	-	95	71	53	56	-	-
Burkina Faso	79	79	24	25	49	44	68	66	32 x	29 x	13 x	6 x	6 x	2 x	34	61	33	25	-	-	64	54
Burundi	52	50	12	8	33	26	65	59	46	54	26	19	4	3	79	99	5	18	-	-	-	-
Cabo Verde	19	18	7	8	12	13	29	24	-	-	-	-	-	-	-	-	-	-	-	-	-	-
Cambodia	30	29	11	11	17	12	54	56	68	79	41	39	20	20	-	-	11	19	8	10	-	-
Cameroon	56	57	4	13	33	40	50	58	75	74	52	43	26	21	39	58	30	11	-	-	88	82
Canada	2	2	-	-	0	0	12	12	-	-	-	-	-	-	-	-	96	69	86	84	-	-
Central African Republic	-	-	-	-	43	61	76	86	30	24	15	10	8	5	-	-	-	-	-	-	48	29
Chad	85	87	17	35	55	70	71	85	30	23	18	9	7	3	34	65	8	2	-	-	-	-
Chile	4	5	0	1	3	4	5	5	96	97	94	97	83	88	-	-	-	-	68	33	-	-
China	-	-	-	-	-	-	-	-	97	97	93	93	63	67	82	85	-	-	80	79	100	100
Colombia	1	0	2	1	2	0	18	16	91	95	74	81	69	78	-	-	-	-	50	35	99	99
Comoros	71	70	18	18	20	18	52	48	75 x	77 x	47 x	45 x	24 x	32 x	-	-	-	-	-	-	78	78
Congo	71	70	15	16	-	-	-	-	78	82	56	45	28	19	63	86	34	8	-	-	85	79
Cook Islands	14	0	2	2	1	1	34	22	-	-	-	-	-	-	-	-	-	-	-	-	-	-
Costa Rica	2	1	3	3	4	4	9	7	98	99	70	76	56	60	-	-	-	-	58	40	99	100
Côte d'Ivoire	78	72	0	7	40	44	53	63	60	53	36	22	17	15	33	68	22	3	-	-	93	76
Croatia	4	5	-	-	-	-	14	10	-	-	-	-	-	-	-	-	-	70	78	69	-	-
Cuba	6	3	1	1	13	12	16	12	100	100	93	95	54	63	97	97	100	100	100	100	-	-
Cyprus	0	3	0	1	2	2	6	9	-	-	-	-	-	-	-	-	-	77	56	63	-	-
Czechia	7	8	1	0	0	0	4	4	-	-	-	-	-	-	-	-	97	78	79	80	-	-
Democratic People's Republic of Korea	-	-	-	-	-	-	-	-	100	100	100	100	100	100	94	83	-	-	-	-	-	-

TABLE 11. EDUCATION

	Equitable access								Completion						Learning						Literacy rate 2013–2022	
	Out-of-school rate 2013–2022 [R]								Completion rate 2013–2022 [R]						Learning outcomes 2013–2022 [R]							
	One year before primary entry age		Primary education		Lower secondary education		Upper secondary education		Primary education		Lower secondary education		Upper secondary education		Proportion of children in grade 2 or 3 achieving minimum proficiency level		Proportion of children at the end of primary achieving a minimum proficiency level		Proportion of children at the end of lower secondary achieving a minimum proficiency level		Youth (15–24 years) literacy rate (%)	
Countries and areas	Male	Female	Male	Female	Male	Female	Male	Female	Male	Female	Male	Female	Male	Female	Reading	Math	Reading	Math	Reading	Math	Male	Female
Democratic Republic of the Congo	-	-	-	-	-	-	-	-	67	66	58	52	36	27	42	77	9	3	-	-	-	-
Denmark	4	3	1	0	0	1	10	9	-	-	-	-	-	-	97	75	-	-	84	85	-	-
Djibouti	84	87	31	36	40	39	52	53	-	-	-	-	-	-	-	-	-	-	-	-	-	-
Dominica	7	0	1	1	3	1	14	27	-	-	-	-	-	-	-	-	-	-	-	-	-	-
Dominican Republic	2	1	5	4	10	8	28	25	88	93	70	83	51	71	-	-	-	-	21	9	-	-
Ecuador	18	15	-	-	5	2	22	20	98	98	89	92	78	79	-	-	-	-	49	29	98	99
Egypt	63	63	-	-	3	2	23	24	91	92	79	81	43	41	-	-	-	27	-	21	-	-
El Salvador	15	12	7	7	-	-	42	41	84	89	73	74	34	36	-	-	-	-	-	-	98	99
Equatorial Guinea	57	55	56	55																		
Eritrea	73	73	45	50	32	40	45	53	-	-	-	-	-	-	-	-	-	-	-	-	94	93
Estonia	7	7	3	2	2	1	2	2	-	-	-	-	-	-	-	-	-	-	89	90	-	-
Eswatini	-	-	15	16	3	3	14	18	64	77	47	54	31	33	-	-	-	-	-	-	94	97
Ethiopia	55	59	9	17	45	49	73	75	47	48	19	22	11	14	-	-	55	73	29	18	-	-
Fiji	11	15	1	1	-	-	24	9	-	-	-	-	-	-	-	-	-	-	-	-	-	-
Finland	0	2	2	2	1	0	3	5	-	-	-	-	-	-	-	-	98	78	86	85	-	-
France	0	0	0	0	0	1	5	4	-	-	-	-	-	-	-	-	94	57	79	79	-	-
Gabon	-	-	24	23	32	29	44	40	66 x	75 x	32 x	33 x	14 x	14 x	66	89	76	23	-	-	88	91
Gambia	42	37	19	8	22	7	48	37	64	60	50	48	33	28	5	4	-	-	-	-	-	-
Georgia	-	-	1	0	2	1	6	4	100	100	98	98	79	83	-	-	86	56	36	39	100	100
Germany	3	3	2	0	5	3	14	15	-	-	-	-	-	-	-	-	95	75	79	79	-	-
Ghana	8	6	7	5	9	6	25	25	69	73	45	50	12	9	6	8	-	-	-	-	93	92
Greece	4	3	1	1	3	4	4	6	-	-	-	-	-	-	-	-	-	-	69	64	99	99
Grenada	15	16	4	3	-	-	12	11	-	-	-	-	-	-	-	-	-	-	-	-	-	-
Guatemala	18	17	11	10	33	37	62	64	80	76	52	45	27	25	-	-	-	-	30	11	95	94
Guinea	51	55	8	21	46	62	63	78	52	39	33	20	22	13	23	60	22	7	-	-	70	43
Guinea-Bissau	-	-	-	-	-	-	-	-	29	25	18	16	14	8	-	-	-	-	-	-	-	-
Guyana	-	-	-	-	-	-	-	-	-	-	-	-	-	-	-	-	-	-	-	-	-	-
Haiti	-	-	-	-	-	-	-	-	49	58	32	38	17	16	-	-	-	-	-	-	-	-
Holy See	0	0	0	0	0	0	0	0	-	-	-	-	-	-	-	-	-	-	-	-	-	-
Honduras	25	23	16	15	41	38	60	55	85	89	50	58	29	37	-	-	-	-	30	15	95	97
Hungary	6	8	5	6	3	3	13	11	-	-	-	-	-	-	-	-	97	74	75	68	-	-
Iceland	8	2	0	1	1	0	17	14	-	-	-	-	-	-	-	-	-	-	74	79	-	-
India	15	14	6	4	17	13	43	41	92	91	82	79	46	40	47	53	46	44	38	40	93	90
Indonesia	8	0	3	8	19	14	23	22	96	98	86	90	64	63	-	-	-	18	30	28	100	100
Iran (Islamic Republic of)	37	35	-	-	1	3	17	18	-	-	-	-	-	-	-	-	-	-	-	-	-	-
Iraq	-	-	-	-	-	-	-	-	78	73	46	47	45	43	-	-	-	-	-	-	-	-
Ireland	0	0	-	-	-	-	2	1	-	-	-	-	-	-	98	84	-	-	88	84	-	-
Israel	0	0	-	-	-	-	-	-	-	-	-	-	-	-	91	-	-	-	69	66	-	-
Italy	8	9	3	4	2	3	6	5	-	-	-	-	-	-	-	-	98	73	77	62	100	100
Jamaica	-	-	37	29	-	-	57	33	99 x	100 x	97 x	97 x	80 x	83 x	85	67	-	-	-	-	-	-
Japan	-	-	-	-	-	-	-	-	-	-	-	-	-	-	-	-	-	-	-	-	-	-
Jordan	51	50	20	21	28	28	46	41	96	97	86	88	49	63	-	-	-	-	59	41	99	99
Kazakhstan	22	23	10	9	-	-	-	-	100	100	100	100	95	96	-	-	98	71	36	51	100	100
Kenya	-	-	-	-	-	-	-	-	77	82	61	69	44	38	53	42	44	29	-	-	88	88
Kiribati	4	0	-	-	-	-	-	-	92	96	69	88	13	20	-	-	-	-	-	-	-	-
Kuwait	33	28	4	1	9	4	20	17	-	-	-	-	-	-	-	-	-	21	-	21	99	100
Kyrgyzstan	14	12	-	-	0	1	30	25	99	100	99	99	89	85	39	30	40	40	49	35	100	100
Lao People's Democratic Republic	30	29	8	9	30	31	45	49	84	83	54	53	32	31	-	-	2	8	-	-	-	-
Latvia	3	1	2	1	2	1	6	4	-	-	-	-	-	-	-	-	99	85	78	83	100	100

FOR EVERY CHILD, VACCINATION

TABLE 11. EDUCATION

Countries and areas	Equitable access — Out-of-school rate 2013–2022 [R]								Completion — Completion rate 2013–2022 [R]						Learning — Learning outcomes 2013–2022 [R]						Literacy rate 2013–2022	
	One year before primary entry age		Primary education		Lower secondary education		Upper secondary education		Primary education		Lower secondary education		Upper secondary education		Proportion of children in grade 2 or 3 achieving minimum proficiency level		Proportion of children at the end of primary achieving a minimum proficiency level		Proportion of children at the end of lower secondary achieving a minimum proficiency level		Youth (15–24 years) literacy rate (%)	
	Male	Female	Male	Female	Male	Female	Male	Female	Male	Female	Male	Female	Male	Female	Reading	Math	Reading	Math	Reading	Math	Male	Female
Lebanon	-	-	-	-	-	-	-	-	-	-	-	-	-	-	-	-	-	27	32	35	100	100
Lesotho	58	57	8	6	18	11	38	29	69	92	33	55	27	37	13	1	-	-	-	-	-	-
Liberia	21	21	22	21	17	26	20	31	36	33	29	23	18	9	-	-	-	-	-	-	-	-
Libya	-	-	-	-	-	-	-	-	-	-	-	-	-	-	-	-	-	-	-	-	-	-
Liechtenstein	0	6	3	2	1	7	2	16	-	-	-	-	-	-	-	-	-	-	-	-	-	-
Lithuania	4	4	-	-	-	-	4	2	-	-	-	-	-	-	-	-	97	81	76	74	-	-
Luxembourg	0	0	1	1	1	4	21	17	-	-	-	-	-	-	-	-	-	-	71	73	-	-
Madagascar	43	38	-	-	31	29	63	64	52	60	26	27	16	15	13	4	6	6	-	-	81	79
Malawi	-	-	-	-	19	18	62	76	43	52	23	21	15	13	-	-	-	-	-	-	-	-
Malaysia	10	9	2	1	13	10	42	37	-	-	-	-	-	-	-	-	58	64	54	59	97	97
Maldives	8	5	3	1	3	15	55	44	-	-	-	-	-	-	-	-	-	-	-	-	-	-
Mali	53	57	38	44	49	56	71	79	50	41	36	25	23	12	-	-	-	-	-	-	55	38
Malta	0	5	-	-	2	1	10	7	-	-	-	-	-	-	-	-	73	69	64	62	99	100
Marshall Islands	38	41	29	30	30	26	46	41	-	-	-	-	-	-	-	-	-	-	-	-	-	-
Mauritania	-	-	25	21	31	25	63	59	68	58	53	40	31	23	-	-	-	-	-	-	-	-
Mauritius	7	12	-	-	5	2	26	17	-	-	-	-	-	-	-	-	-	-	-	-	-	-
Mexico	2	0	-	-	9	6	29	25	98	98	87	90	56	60	-	-	-	-	55	44	99	99
Micronesia (Federated States of)	30	34	17	16	15	10	-	-	-	-	-	-	-	-	-	-	-	-	-	-	-	-
Monaco	-	-	-	-	-	-	-	-	-	-	-	-	-	-	-	-	-	-	-	-	-	-
Mongolia	3	5	2	3	8	7	15	9	96	98	87	93	60	73	44	-	-	-	-	-	99	99
Montenegro	15	17	3	3	6	6	13	10	95	98	93	97	83	90	-	-	-	43	56	54	99	99
Montserrat	19	0	15	15	-	-	-	-	-	-	-	-	-	-	-	-	-	-	-	-	-	-
Morocco	24	30	2	3	6	9	24	27	-	-	-	-	-	-	-	-	36	18	27	12	98	97
Mozambique	-	-	1	4	35	41	57	66	44 x	39 x	15 x	11 x	8 x	5 x	-	-	-	-	-	-	-	-
Myanmar	88	88	-	-	22	20	47	38	82	84	45	45	14	19	-	-	11	12	-	-	95	96
Namibia	33	30	-	-	3	0	22	23	75	86	48	62	33	39	-	-	-	-	-	-	94	96
Nauru	8	0	6	3	12	4	52	60	-	-	-	-	-	-	-	-	-	-	-	-	-	-
Nepal	6	15	-	-	7	3	26	13	81	83	71	75	27	28	-	-	-	-	-	-	94	91
Netherlands (Kingdom of the)	3	2	1	1	3	2	1	0	-	-	-	-	-	-	-	-	99	84	76	84	-	-
New Zealand	8	9	1	1	0	0	4	1	-	-	-	-	-	-	-	-	90	56	81	78	-	-
Nicaragua	-	-	-	-	-	-	-	-	-	-	-	-	-	-	-	-	-	-	-	-	-	-
Niger	76	76	37	45	61	69	84	89	35 x	24 x	10 x	4 x	4 x	1 x	44	67	14	8	-	-	51	36
Nigeria	-	-	-	-	-	-	-	-	71	71	66	59	57	44	17	11	-	-	-	-	82	68
Niue	0	38	-	-	-	-	-	-	-	-	-	-	-	-	-	-	-	-	-	-	-	-
North Macedonia	51	51	1	1	-	-	-	-	97	100	93	95	86	79	-	-	-	52	45	39	-	-
Norway	4	4	0	0	0	1	8	8	-	-	-	-	-	-	99	82	-	65	81	81	-	-
Oman	13	14	-	-	2	3	8	17	-	-	-	-	-	-	-	-	59	33	-	27	98	99
Pakistan	0	12	-	-	-	-	-	-	64	55	55	45	24	23	-	-	-	-	-	-	80	65
Palau	20	0	-	-	-	-	-	-	-	-	-	-	-	-	-	-	-	-	-	-	-	-
Panama	88	88	10	11	13	12	35	31	95	96	75	81	57	68	-	-	-	-	36	19	99	99
Papua New Guinea	28	29	4	10	24	32	50	60	-	-	-	-	-	-	-	-	-	-	-	-	-	-
Paraguay	23	23	-	-	-	-	32	28	93	96	81	79	60	67	-	-	-	-	32	8	99	99
Peru	0	1	-	-	3	3	15	21	95 x	95 x	83 x	83 x	78 x	72 x	-	-	-	-	-	-	100	99
Philippines	36	33	3	4	12	7	24	17	89	95	75	88	74	83	-	-	10	17	19	-	98	99
Poland	1	2	1	1	2	4	2	2	-	-	-	-	-	-	-	-	98	73	85	85	-	-
Portugal	8	6	0	1	0	0	-	-	-	-	-	-	-	-	-	-	97	74	80	77	100	100
Qatar	6	5	3	0	4	10	-	-	-	-	-	-	-	-	-	-	66	40	49	37	-	-
Republic of Korea	11	10	1	1	5	5	7	8	-	-	-	-	-	-	-	-	-	95	85	85	-	-
Republic of Moldova	0	1	-	-	-	-	13	12	99 x	99 x	95 x	98 x	63 x	71 x	-	-	-	-	57	50	-	-

176 — THE STATE OF THE WORLD'S CHILDREN 2023

TABLE 11. EDUCATION

Equitable access — Out-of-school rate 2013–2022 [R] · **Completion — Completion rate 2013–2022 [R]** · **Learning — Learning outcomes 2013–2022 [R]** · **Literacy rate 2013–2022**

Countries and areas	One year before primary entry age – Male	– Female	Primary education – Male	– Female	Lower secondary – Male	– Female	Upper secondary – Male	– Female	Completion Primary – Male	– Female	Completion Lower secondary – Male	– Female	Completion Upper secondary – Male	– Female	Grade 2/3 Reading	Grade 2/3 Math	End of primary Reading	End of primary Math	End of lower secondary Reading	End of lower secondary Math	Youth (15–24) literacy Male	Youth (15–24) literacy Female
Romania	15	16	13	13	11	12	21	19	-	-	-	-	-	-	-	-	-	-	59	53	99	99
Russian Federation	7	7	1	0	2	1	3	2	-	-	-	-	-	-	-	-	99	91	78	78	100	100
Rwanda	48	47	6	6	6	2	50	49	48	61	25	30	19	16	-	-	-	-	-	-	84	89
Saint Kitts and Nevis	0	21	-	-	-	-	4	5	-	-	-	-	-	-	-	-	-	-	-	-	-	-
Saint Lucia	2	0	6	1	9	10	14	19	99 x	99 x	85 x	98 x	70 x	90 x	-	-	-	-	-	-	-	-
Saint Vincent and the Grenadines	1	42	-	-	6	0	18	17	-	-	-	-	-	-	-	-	-	-	-	-	-	-
Samoa	65	65	-	-	-	-	21	11	96	99	95	99	48	66	-	-	-	-	-	-	99	99
San Marino	16	0	2	5	9	8	53	62	-	-	-	-	-	-	-	-	-	-	-	-	-	-
Sao Tome and Principe	49	46	6	6	12	7	19	16	82	92	60	60	26	31	-	-	-	-	-	-	98	98
Saudi Arabia	49	45	5	5	0	3	3	9	-	-	-	-	-	-	-	-	63	23	48	15	100	99
Senegal	85	83	30	19	64	57	81	79	44	50	27	30	11	10	48	79	41	27	9	8	-	-
Serbia	8	7	3	3	3	3	16	13	100	100	100	99	96	92	-	-	68	62	60	-	100	100
Seychelles	4	2	2	14	9	7	20	9	-	-	-	-	-	-	-	-	-	-	-	-	99	100
Sierra Leone	60	57	2	2	49	49	64	67	63	65	47	42	27	18	6	6	-	-	-	-	71	63
Singapore	-	-	0	0	0	0	0	0	-	-	-	-	-	-	-	-	97	96	89	92	100	100
Slovakia	15	15	3	3	4	5	11	11	-	-	-	-	-	-	-	-	93	71	69	75	-	-
Slovenia	9	8	1	0	2	1	1	1	-	-	-	-	-	-	-	-	96	75	82	84	-	-
Solomon Islands	36	33	9	4	-	-	-	-	-	-	-	-	-	-	-	-	-	-	-	-	-	-
Somalia	-	-	-	-	-	-	-	-	-	-	-	-	-	-	-	-	-	-	-	-	-	-
South Africa	29	27	12	10	11	10	21	20	95	98	85	91	45	52	22	16	-	-	-	-	98	99
South Sudan	78	81	58	67	49	63	57	72	31 x	18 x	22 x	10 x	12 x	4 x	-	-	-	-	-	-	48	47
Spain	5	5	3	3	1	1	2	1	-	-	-	-	-	-	-	-	97	65	84	75	99	100
Sri Lanka	-	-	2	3	0	0	18	13	99	99	94	96	32	43	-	-	-	-	-	-	99	99
State of Palestine	33	30	5	5	5	1	31	16	99	100	78	94	51	74	-	-	-	-	-	-	99	99
Sudan	60	60	31	35	33	35	53	50	66	64	49	52	33	28	-	-	-	-	-	-	73	73
Suriname	10	6	13	10	19	11	42	34	80	90	41	58	18	26	30	12	-	-	-	-	99	98
Sweden	0	0	-	-	-	-	1	3	-	-	-	-	-	-	-	-	98	74	82	81	-	-
Switzerland	0	1	-	-	0	1	17	20	-	-	-	-	-	-	-	-	-	-	76	83	-	-
Syrian Arab Republic	-	-	-	-	-	-	-	-	-	-	-	-	-	-	-	-	-	-	-	-	-	-
Tajikistan	87	88	1	2	-	-	19	27	99	98	95	93	80	63	-	-	-	-	-	-	-	-
Thailand	0	0	-	-	-	-	21	21	98	99	81	92	59	72	-	-	-	-	40	47	98	99
Timor-Leste	51	48	7	3	12	9	27	22	77	85	63	70	49	55	-	-	-	-	-	-	82	85
Togo	1	0	2	4	15	28	47	66	83	76	55	39	31	12	25	47	19	16	-	-	92	84
Tokelau	0	6	-	-	-	-	31	29	-	-	-	-	-	-	-	-	-	-	-	-	-	-
Tonga	0	11	-	-	17	4	49	33	98	99	65	76	45	56	-	-	-	-	-	-	99	100
Trinidad and Tobago	21	20	-	-	-	-	27	25	-	-	-	-	-	-	-	-	80	-	58	48	-	-
Tunisia	-	-	-	-	-	-	-	-	94	97	68	80	40	57	47	-	-	-	28	25	-	-
Türkiye	23	25	5	5	3	4	17	19	99	98	96	92	51	44	-	-	70	-	74	56	100	100
Turkmenistan	-	-	-	-	-	-	-	-	100	100	99	99	97	97	71	53	-	-	-	-	-	-
Turks and Caicos Islands	8	0	9	9	9	15	48	41	98	100	98	100	100	96	-	-	-	-	-	-	-	-
Tuvalu	10	0	18	16	31	36	68	61	98	100	74	91	45	60	-	-	-	-	-	-	-	-
Uganda	-	-	16	12	49	49	72	78	39	43	27	23	18	15	33	21	52	53	49	42	89	90
Ukraine	-	-	9	7	4	3	7	4	100 x	99 x	100 x	100 x	97 x	97 x	-	-	-	-	74	-	-	-
United Arab Emirates	0	0	-	-	2	3	3	2	-	-	-	-	-	-	-	-	68	53	57	50	95	98
United Kingdom	0	0	1	1	2	2	4	3	-	-	-	-	-	-	-	-	97	83	83	81	-	-
United Republic of Tanzania	45	42	18	15	66	64	84	88	75	84	31	27	32	27	56	35	-	-	-	-	-	-
United States	10	10	1	1	-	-	3	5	-	-	-	-	-	-	-	-	96	77	81	73	-	-
Uruguay	9	0	1	0	1	0	13	8	96	98	66	73	48	29	-	-	-	-	58	49	99	99
Uzbekistan	37	38	0	2	0	2	14	15	-	-	-	-	-	-	-	-	-	-	-	-	100	100

TABLE 11. EDUCATION

	Equitable access								Completion						Learning						Literacy rate 2013–2022
	Out-of-school rate 2013–2022 [R]								Completion rate 2013–2022 [R]						Learning outcomes 2013–2022 [R]						
	One year before primary entry age		Primary education		Lower secondary education		Upper secondary education		Primary education		Lower secondary education		Upper secondary education		Proportion of children in grade 2 or 3 achieving minimum proficiency level		Proportion of children at the end of primary achieving a minimum proficiency level		Proportion of children at the end of lower secondary achieving a minimum proficiency level		Youth (15–24 years) literacy rate (%)
Countries and areas	Male	Fe-male	Male	Fe-male	Male	Fe-male	Male	Fe-male	Male	Female	Male	Female	Male	Female	Read-ing	Math	Read-ing	Math	Read-ing	Math	Male	Fe-male
Vanuatu	4	0	3	4	27	24	58	52	-	-	-	-	-	-	-	-	-	-	-	-	96	97
Venezuela (Bolivarian Republic of)	14	14	10	10	15	13	28	19	-	-	-	-	-	-	-	-	-	-	-	-	-	-
Viet Nam	0	0	-	-	-	-	-	-	96	97	81	87	50	61	-	-	82	92	86	81	99	99
Yemen	96	96	10	21	23	34	46	68	70	55	55	39	37	23	-	-	-	-	-	-	-	-
Zambia	-	-	17	13	-	-	-	-	71	73	54	50	33	27	-	-	-	-	5	2	93	92
Zimbabwe	-	-	15	13	-	-	40	45	86	92	45	53	17	14	20	5	-	-	-	-	-	-

SUMMARY

East Asia and Pacific	17	15	3	4	10	8	23	15	95	96	86	89	62	66	-	-	-	-	-	-	99	99
Europe and Central Asia	13	13	2	2	2	2	9	9	-	-	-	-	-	-	-	-	-	-	-	-	100	100
Eastern Europe and Central Asia	20	21	4	4	2	2	13	14	99	99	97	96	66	60	-	-	-	-	-	-	100	100
Western Europe	4	4	1	1	2	2	6	6	-	-	-	-	-	-	-	-	-	-	-	-	-	-
Latin America and Caribbean	5	5	3	2	7	6	23	20	93	95	79	84	59	66	-	-	-	-	-	-	98	99
Middle East and North Africa	51	51	4	6	8	12	28	33	86	84	66	70	42	44	-	-	-	-	-	-	92	88
North America	9	8	1	0	0	0	3	6	-	-	-	-	-	-	-	-	-	-	-	-	-	-
South Asia	12	13	9	9	18	15	43	42	85	84	76	72	41	36	-	-	-	-	-	-	92	89
Sub-Saharan Africa	51	51	18	22	35	38	55	61	61	62	40	37	31	25	-	-	-	-	-	-	79	74
Eastern and Southern Africa	49	49	16	18	34	37	56	60	61	63	33	33	26	23	-	-	-	-	-	-	80	80
West and Central Africa	53	53	21	27	37	39	54	62	62	60	47	40	35	25	-	-	-	-	-	-	78	68
Least developed countries	48	47	15	19	33	35	54	58	58	58	36	34	24	19	-	-	-	-	-	-	81	77
World	**25**	**25**	**8**	**10**	**16**	**16**	**34**	**33**	**82**	**82**	**70**	**69**	**46**	**44**	**-**	**-**	**-**	**-**	**-**	**-**	**93**	**91**

For a complete list of countries and areas in the regions, subregions and country categories, see page on Regional Classifications or visit <data.unicef.org/regionalclassifications>.

It is not advisable to compare data from consecutive editions of *The State of the World's Children* report.

The database on foundational learning skills based on the MICS6 provides disaggregation by sex, place of residence, wealth, and age group. For more information, please click here <https://data.unicef.org/resources/dataset/learning-and-skills/>.

NOTES

- Data not available.

[R] Data refer to the most recent year available during the period specified in the column heading.

[x] Data refer to years or periods other than those specified in the column heading. Such data are not included in the calculation of regional and global averages. Estimates from data years prior to 2000 are not displayed.

MAIN DATA SOURCES

Out of school rate – UNESCO Institute for Statistics (UIS). Last update: June 2022.

Completion rate – UNICEF Global Database based on Demographic and Health Surveys (DHS), Multiple Indicator Cluster Surveys (MICS), and other national household surveys. Last update: June 2022.

Proportion of children and young people (a) in grade 2/3; (b) at the end of primary education; and (c) at the end of lower secondary education achieving at least a minimum proficiency in (i) reading and (ii) mathematics – United Nations Statistics Division database. Last update: June 2022.

Youth literacy rate – UNESCO Institute for Statistics (UIS). Last update: June 2022.

DEFINITIONS OF THE INDICATORS

Out-of-school rate for children one year before the official primary entry age – Number of children aged one year younger than the primary entry age who are not enrolled in pre-primary or primary schools, expressed as a percentage of the population of one year before the official primary entry age.

Out-of-school rate for children of primary school age – Number of children of official primary school age who are not enrolled in pre-primary, primary or secondary school, expressed as a percentage of the population of official primary school age.

Out-of-school rate for children of lower secondary school age – Number of children of lower secondary school age who are not enrolled in primary or secondary school, expressed as a percentage of the population of official lower secondary school age.

Out-of-school rate for children of upper secondary school age – Number of children of upper secondary school age who are not enrolled in primary or secondary school or higher education, expressed as a percentage of the population of official upper secondary school age.

Completion rate for primary education – Number of children or young people aged 3–5 years above the intended age for the last grade of primary education who have completed the last grade of primary school.

Completion rate for lower secondary education – Number of children or young people aged 3–5 years above the intended age for the last grade of lower secondary education who have completed the last grade of lower secondary.

Completion rate for upper secondary education – Number of children or young people aged 3–5 years above the intended age for the last grade of upper secondary education who have completed the last grade of upper secondary.

Proportion of children and young people (a) in grade 2/3; (b) at the end of primary education; and (c) at the end of lower secondary education achieving at least a minimum proficiency in (i) reading and (ii) mathematics – Percentage of children and young people in Grade 2 or 3 of primary education, at the end of primary education and the end of lower secondary education achieving at least a minimum proficiency level in (a) reading and (b) mathematics. This indicator is SDG4 global indicator 4.1.1.

Youth literacy rate – Number of literate persons aged 15–24 years, expressed as a percentage of the total population in that group.

TABLE 12. CHILD PROTECTION

Countries and areas	Child labour (%) [H] 2013–2021 [R] Total	Male	Female	Child marriage (%) [H] 2015–2021 [R] Married by 18 Female	Male	Birth registration (%) [H] 2012–2021 [R] Children under 1 Total	Children under 5 Total	Male	Female	Female genital mutilation (%) [H] 2012–2020 [R] Prevalence Women (Fa)	Girls (Fb)	Attitudes Want the practice to stop (Fc)	Justification of wife-beating among adolescents (%) 2015–2021 [R] Male	Female	Violent discipline (%) [H] 2013–2021 [R] Total	Male	Female	Sexual violence in childhood (%) 2013–2020 [R] Male	Female	Children in residential care [H] 2010–2021 [R] Total per 100,000	Children in detention [H] 2008–2021 [R] Total per 100,000
Afghanistan	13	14	12	28	7	51	42	43	42	-	-	-	71 y	78 y	74 x,y	75 x,y	74 x,y	-	1 y	15	40 y
Albania	3 x,y	4 x,y	3 x,y	12	1	98	98	99	98	-	-	-	11	5	48 y	49 y	45 y	-	-	95	14
Algeria	3	3	2	4	-	99	100	100	100	-	-	-	-	25	84	85	83	-	-	-	18
Andorra	-	-	-	-	-	100 v	100 v	100 v	100 v	-	-	-	-	-	-	-	-	-	-	-	0
Angola	19	17	20	30	6	12	25	25	25	-	-	-	24	25	-	-	-	-	5	-	-
Anguilla	-	-	-	-	-	-	-	-	-	-	-	-	-	-	-	-	-	-	-	140	156
Antigua and Barbuda	-	-	-	-	-	-	-	-	-	-	-	-	-	-	-	-	-	-	-	35	49
Argentina	-	-	-	15 y	-	99 y	100 y	100 y	99 y	-	-	-	-	4 y	59 y	60 y	58 y	-	-	74 y	41
Armenia	4	5	3	5	0	100	99	99	99	-	-	-	25	9	69	71	67	-	-	128	7
Australia	-	-	-	-	-	100 v	100 v	100 v	100 v	-	-	-	-	-	-	-	-	-	-	55	25 y
Austria	-	-	-	-	-	100 v	100 v	100 v	100 v	-	-	-	-	-	-	-	-	-	-	409	42
Azerbaijan	-	-	-	11 x	0 x	88 x	94 x	93 x	94 x	-	-	-	63 x	24 x	77 x,y	80 x,y	74 x,y	-	0 x	478	12
Bahamas	-	-	-	-	-	-	-	-	-	-	-	-	-	-	-	-	-	-	-	-	67
Bahrain	-	-	-	-	-	-	100	100	100	-	-	-	-	-	-	-	-	-	-	-	2
Bangladesh	7	9	5	51	4 x	40	56	56	56	-	-	-	-	17	89	89	89	-	3 y	26	4
Barbados	1 x,y	2 x,y	1 x,y	29 x,y	-	94	99	99	99	-	-	-	-	5 x	75 x,y	78 x,y	72 x,y	-	-	168 y	71
Belarus	4	5	3	5	2	-	100 y	100 y	100 y	-	-	-	0	1	57	59	55	-	-	309	25
Belgium	-	-	-	0 y	-	100 v	100 v	100 v	100 v	-	-	-	-	-	-	-	-	-	-	-	2
Belize	3	4	3	34 y	22 y	90	96	95	96	-	-	-	8	6	65	67	63	-	-	86 y	77 y
Benin	25	24	26	31	5	87	86	85	86	9	0	86	17	29	91	91	91	-	5	-	9
Bhutan	4 x,y	3 x,y	4 x,y	26 x	-	100 x	100 x	100 x	100 x	-	-	-	-	70 x	-	-	-	-	-	1,249	91
Bolivia (Plurinational State of)	14	14	13	20	5	-	92 y	-	-	-	-	-	-	34 y	-	-	-	-	-	135	256
Bosnia and Herzegovina	-	-	-	3 x	0 x	98 x	100 x	100 x	99 x	-	-	-	5 x	1 x	55 x,y	60 x,y	50 x,y	-	-	136 y	43
Botswana	-	-	-	-	-	79 y	88 y	87 y	88 y	-	-	-	-	-	-	-	-	-	-	214	264
Brazil	5	5	5	26 x	-	-	96	-	-	-	-	-	-	-	-	-	-	-	-	63	61 y
British Virgin Islands	-	-	-	-	-	-	-	-	-	-	-	-	-	-	-	-	-	-	-	12 y	0
Brunei Darussalam	-	-	-	-	-	-	100 y	-	-	-	-	-	-	-	-	-	-	-	-	-	-
Bulgaria	-	-	-	-	-	100 v	100 v	100 v	100 v	-	-	-	-	-	-	-	-	-	-	192	11
Burkina Faso	42 x,y	44 x,y	40 x,y	52	4 x	73 x	77 x	77 x	77 x	76 x	13 x	90 x	40 x	39 x	83 x,y	84 x,y	82 x,y	-	-	33	33
Burundi	31	30	32	19	1	73	84	84	83	-	-	-	48	63	90	91	89	0	4	118	25
Cabo Verde	-	-	-	8	2	-	91 x	-	-	-	-	-	6	7	-	-	-	-	-	204	97
Cambodia	13 x	12 x	14 x	19 x	4 x	64	73	74	73	-	-	-	26 x,y	46 x,y	-	-	-	-	2	158	110
Cameroon	39	40	38	30	3	56	62	62	62	1 x	-	84 x	34	28	85	85	85	2	7	36	19
Canada	-	-	-	-	-	100 v	100 v	100 v	100 v	-	-	-	-	-	-	-	-	-	-	-	31 y
Central African Republic	27	25	29	61	17	41	45	46	44	22	1	69	38	61	90	90	90	-	-	-	20
Chad	39	39	40	61	8	22	26	26	26	34	7	53	54	74	85	85	86	-	2	-	20
Chile	6 x	7 x	5 x	-	-	-	99 x,y	-	-	-	-	-	-	-	-	-	-	-	-	159	183
China	-	-	-	-	-	-	-	-	-	-	-	-	-	-	-	-	-	-	-	19	20
Colombia	7	7	7	23	7	94	97	97	97	-	-	-	5	4	-	-	-	0	2 y	73	112
Comoros	28 x,y	25 x,y	32 x,y	32 x	12 x	87	87	87	87	-	-	-	29 x	43 x	-	-	-	-	3 x	-	19
Congo	14	13	15	27	6 x	94	96	96	96	-	-	-	45	56	83	83	82	-	-	-	19
Cook Islands	-	-	-	-	-	100 y	100 y	100 y	100 y	-	-	-	-	-	-	-	-	-	-	-	6,592 y
Costa Rica	4	4	3	17	-	-	100 y	100 y	100 y	-	-	-	-	3	49	50	49	-	-	316	17
Côte d'Ivoire	22	22	23	27	4	66	72	75	71	37	10	79	29	43	87	88	85	-	-	29	16
Croatia	-	-	-	-	-	100 v	100 v	100 v	100 v	-	-	-	-	-	-	-	-	-	-	177	4
Cuba	-	-	-	29	6	99	100	100	100	-	-	-	1	3	42	43	40	-	-	19	0
Cyprus	-	-	-	-	-	100 v	100 v	100 v	100 v	-	-	-	-	-	-	-	-	-	-	-	44
Czechia	-	-	-	-	-	100 v	100 v	100 v	100 v	-	-	-	-	-	-	-	-	-	-	-	411
Democratic People's Republic of Korea	4	5	4	0	0	100 x	100 x	100 x	100 x	-	-	-	4	4	59	63	55	-	-	-	-
Democratic Republic of the Congo	15	13	17	29	6	38	40	40	40	-	-	-	52	60	89	90	88	-	13	-	-
Denmark	-	-	-	1 y	-	100 y	100 y	100 y	100 y	-	-	-	-	-	-	-	-	-	-	556 y	96
Djibouti	-	-	-	5 x	-	91 x	92 x	93 x	91 x	94	43	51 x	-	-	72 x,y	73 x,y	71 x,y	-	-	-	-
Dominica	-	-	-	-	-	-	-	-	-	-	-	-	-	-	-	-	-	-	-	117	0
Dominican Republic	4	5	3	31	8 x	89	92	92	93	-	-	-	14 x	3	63	65	62	-	1	85	59
Ecuador	-	-	-	22	-	-	87 y	-	-	-	-	-	-	-	-	-	-	-	-	28	9
Egypt	5	6	4	17 x,y	0 x	98	99	100	99	87	14 y	38	-	46 x,y	93	93	93	-	-	31	-
El Salvador	7	6	7	26 x	-	-	91 y	91 y	91 y	-	-	-	-	10 x	52	55	50	-	-	28	77 y
Equatorial Guinea	-	-	-	30 x	4 x	-	54 x	53 x	54 x	-	-	-	56 x	57 x	-	-	-	-	-	-	14
Eritrea	-	-	-	41 x	2 x	-	-	-	-	83 x	33 x	82 x	60 x	51 x	-	-	-	-	-	23	-
Estonia	-	-	-	-	-	100 v	100 v	100 v	100 v	-	-	-	-	-	-	-	-	-	-	-	28
Eswatini	8 x,y	8 x,y	7 x,y	5 x	1 x	38	54	51	50	-	-	-	29 x	32 x	88	89	88	-	-	343	188
Ethiopia	45 y	51 y	39 y	40	5	2	3	3	3	65	16	79	33	60	-	-	-	-	5	-	-
Fiji	17	20	13	4	2	71	87	87	86	-	-	-	19	20	81	82	79	-	-	44	-

TABLE 12. CHILD PROTECTION

Countries and areas	Child labour (%)[H] 2013–2021[R]			Child marriage (%)[H] 2015–2021[R] Married by 18		Birth registration (%)[H] 2012–2021[R] Children under 1	Children under 5			Female genital mutilation (%)[H] 2012–2020[R] Prevalence		Attitudes Want the practice to stop (Fc)	Justification of wife-beating among adolescents (%) 2015–2021[R]		Violent discipline (%)[H] 2013–2021[R]			Sexual violence in childhood (%) 2013–2020[R]		Children in residential care[H] 2010–2021[R]	Children in detention[H] 2008–2021[R]
	Total	Male	Female	Female	Male	Total	Total	Male	Female	Women (Fa)	Girls (Fb)		Male	Female	Total	Male	Female	Male	Female	Total per 100,000	Total per 100,000
Finland	-	-	-	0 y	-	100 v	100 v	100 v	100 v	-	-	-	-	-	-	-	-	-	-	-	41
France	-	-	-	-	-	100 v	100 v	100 v	100 v	-	-	-	-	-	-	-	-	-	-	-	20
Gabon	20 x,y	19 x,y	17 x,y	22 x	5 x	88	90	91	88	-	-	-	47 x	58 x	-	-	-	-	9 x	50	1,373
Gambia	17	17	17	23	0	41	59	60	58	73	46	46	50	57	89	90	88	-	5	-	4
Georgia	2	2	1	14	1	98	99	99	99	-	-	-	-	5 x	69	71	67	-	-	53 y	31
Germany	-	-	-	-	-	100 v	100 y	100 y	100 y	-	-	-	-	-	-	-	-	-	-	429	16
Ghana	20	19	22	19	4	57	71	72	69	2	0	94	22	37	94	94	94	-	10 x	27	5
Greece	-	-	-	-	-	100 v	100 v	100 v	100 v	-	-	-	-	-	-	-	-	-	-	88	10
Grenada	-	-	-	-	-	-	-	-	-	-	-	-	-	-	-	-	-	-	14 y	283	265
Guatemala	-	-	-	29	10	89 y	96 y	-	-	-	-	-	12	14	-	-	-	1	4	71	251
Guinea	24	24	25	47	2	57	62	62	62	95	39	26	57	65	89	90	89	-	-	18	10
Guinea-Bissau	17	18	16	26	2	36	46	47	45	52	30	76	30	34	76	75	76	-	-	42	0 y
Guyana	11	10	12	30 x,y	9 x,y	68	89	88	89	-	-	-	14 x	10 x	70	74	65	-	-	305	18
Haiti	36 x,y	44 x,y	26 x,y	15	2	57	85	84	85	-	-	-	15	23	83	84	82	-	5	589	20
Holy See	-	-	-	-	-	-	-	-	-	-	-	-	-	-	-	-	-	-	-	-	-
Honduras	15	18	13	34	10	87	97	97	97	-	-	-	7	7	63	64	61	-	5	178	10 y
Hungary	-	-	-	-	-	100 v	100 v	100 v	100 v	-	-	-	-	-	-	-	-	-	-	383	166
Iceland	-	-	-	-	-	100 v	100 v	100 v	100 v	-	-	-	-	-	-	-	-	-	-	-	0
India	-	-	-	27	4	79	80	79	80	-	-	-	35	41	-	-	-	-	1	83	29
Indonesia	-	-	-	16	5 x,y	-	77 y	-	-	-	49 y	-	32 y,p	40	-	-	-	-	-	604	14
Iran (Islamic Republic of)	-	-	-	17 x	-	-	99 x,y	99 x,y	99 x,y	-	-	-	-	-	-	-	-	-	-	44	-
Iraq	5	5	4	28	-	98	99	99	99	7	1	94	-	31	81	82	80	-	-	3	26
Ireland	-	-	-	-	-	100 v	100 v	100 v	100 v	-	-	-	-	-	-	-	-	-	-	52	4
Israel	-	-	-	-	-	100 v	100 v	100 v	100 v	-	-	-	-	-	-	-	-	-	-	-	52
Italy	-	-	-	-	-	100 v	100 v	100 v	100 v	-	-	-	-	-	-	-	-	-	-	-	64
Jamaica	3	3	2	8 x	-	97	98	-	-	-	-	-	28 x,y	17	85 x,y	87 x,y	82 x,y	-	2 y	159	73
Japan	-	-	-	-	-	100 v	100 v	100 v	100 v	-	-	-	-	-	-	-	-	-	-	166	128
Jordan	2	2	1	10	0	97	98	98	98	-	-	-	64 y	63 y	82	83	80	-	-	21	107 y
Kazakhstan	-	-	-	7	0 x	99	100	100	100	-	-	-	14 x	8	53	55	50	-	-	93	12
Kenya	-	-	-	23 x	3 x	68	67	67	66	21	3	93	37 x	45 x	-	-	-	2	4	220	5
Kiribati	17	19	15	18	9	85	92	93	90	-	-	-	63	64	92	92	92	-	6	-	181
Kuwait	-	-	-	-	-	-	-	-	-	-	-	-	-	-	-	-	-	-	-	27	-
Kyrgyzstan	22	25	19	13	0 x	97	99	100	98	-	-	-	40 x	24	74	76	73	-	-	874	81
Lao People's Democratic Republic	28	27	29	33	11	60 y	73 y	73 y	73 y	-	-	-	17	30	69	70	68	-	-	-	-
Latvia	-	-	-	-	-	100 v	100 v	100 v	100 v	-	-	-	-	-	-	-	-	-	-	-	50
Lebanon	-	-	-	6 y	-	98 y	99 y	100 y	98 y	-	-	-	-	7 y	57 y	60 y	54 y	-	-	-	15
Lesotho	14	15	13	16	2	28	45	46	44	-	-	-	27	30	76	77	75	-	-	-	7 y
Liberia	32	29	34	25	8	64	66	67	65	32	-	64	39	45	85 y	85 y	85 y	-	6	184	2
Libya	-	-	-	-	-	-	-	-	-	-	-	-	-	-	-	-	-	-	-	-	-
Liechtenstein	-	-	-	-	-	100 v	100 v	100 v	100 v	-	-	-	-	-	-	-	-	-	-	-	0
Lithuania	-	-	-	0 y	-	100 v	100 y	100 y	100 y	-	-	-	-	-	-	-	-	-	-	753	99
Luxembourg	-	-	-	-	-	100 v	100 v	100 v	100 v	-	-	-	-	-	-	-	-	-	-	-	0
Madagascar	37	38	35	40	12	74	79	79	78	-	-	-	30	41	86	87	85	-	-	-	26
Malawi	14	14	14	42	7	7 y	6 y	6 y	5 y	-	-	-	19	24	72	73	72	-	4	71	-
Malaysia	-	-	-	-	-	-	-	-	-	-	-	-	-	-	71 y	74 y	67 y	-	-	80	27 y
Maldives	-	-	-	2	2	96	99	99	99	13	1	66	33 y	35 y	-	-	-	-	0	180	-
Mali	13 y	15 y	12 y	54 y	2 y	87 y	87 y	88 y	86 y	89 y	73 y	18 y	50	74	73	73	73	-	7 y	7	10
Malta	-	-	-	-	-	100 v	100 v	100 v	100 v	-	-	-	-	-	-	-	-	-	-	283	118
Marshall Islands	-	-	-	26 x	12 x	80	84	85	82	-	-	-	71 x	47 x	-	-	-	-	-	-	-
Mauritania	14	15	13	37	2	45 y	66 y	66 y	66 y	67	51	50	18	26	80	80	80	-	-	8	-
Mauritius	-	-	-	-	-	-	-	-	-	-	-	-	-	-	-	-	-	-	-	-	101
Mexico	6	3	5	21	-	89 y	97 y	97 y	97 y	-	-	-	-	6	53 y	55 y	51 y	-	-	55	16
Micronesia (Federated States of)	-	-	-	-	-	-	-	-	-	-	-	-	-	-	-	-	-	-	-	-	-
Monaco	-	-	-	-	-	100 v	100 v	100 v	100 v	-	-	-	-	-	-	-	-	-	-	-	-
Mongolia	15	16	13	12	2	98	100	100	100	-	-	-	3	8	49	53	45	-	-	93 y	114
Montenegro	8	9	7	6	3	98	99	100	99	-	-	-	14	2	66	66	66	-	-	103 y	32
Montserrat	-	-	-	-	-	100 v	100 v	100 v	100 v	-	-	-	-	-	-	-	-	-	-	0	0
Morocco	-	-	-	14	-	-	97 y	97 y	97 y	-	-	-	-	64 x	-	-	-	-	-	965 y	79
Mozambique	-	-	-	53	10	46	55	54	56	-	-	-	21	14	-	-	-	0	2	65	508
Myanmar	10	10	10	16	5	78	81	82	81	-	-	-	57	53	77 y	80 y	75 y	-	1	2 y	19 y
Namibia	-	-	-	7 x	1 x	65 y	78 y	-	-	-	-	-	30 x	28 x	-	-	-	-	1	90	7
Nauru	-	-	-	27 x	12 x	-	96	-	-	-	-	-	-	-	-	-	-	-	-	-	-
Nepal	22	20	23	33	9	59	77	76	78	-	-	-	25	22	82	83	81	-	3	112	14 y

180 THE STATE OF THE WORLD'S CHILDREN 2023

TABLE 12. CHILD PROTECTION

Countries and areas	Child labour (%) [H] 2013–2021 [R]			Child marriage (%) [H] 2015–2021 [R] Married by 18		Birth registration (%) [H] 2012–2021 [R] Children under 1	Children under 5			Female genital mutilation (%) [H] 2012–2020 [R] Prevalence		Attitudes	Justification of wife-beating among adolescents (%) [R] 2015–2021		Violent discipline (%) [H] 2013–2021 [R]			Sexual violence in childhood (%) 2013–2020 [R]		Children in residential care [H] 2010–2021 [R]	Children in detention [H] 2008–2021 [R]
	Total	Male	Female	Female	Male	Total	Total	Male	Female	Women (Fa)	Girls (Fb)	Want the practice to stop (Fc)	Male	Female	Total	Male	Female	Male	Female	Total per 100,000	Total per 100,000
Netherlands (Kingdom of the)	-	-	-	-	-	100 v	100 v	100 v	100 v	-	-	-	-	-	-	-	-	-	-	-	36
New Zealand	-	-	-	-	-	100 v	100 v	100 v	100 v	-	-	-	-	-	-	-	-	-	-	92	10
Nicaragua	-	-	-	35 x	19 x	-	85	-	-	-	-	-	-	8 x,y	-	-	-	-	-	105	-
Niger	34 x,y	34 x,y	34 x,y	76 x	6 x	67	64	65	62	2	-	82	41 x	54 x	82 x,y	82 x,y	81 x,y	-	-	17	-
Nigeria	31	32	31	43	3	35	43	43	42	20	19	67	26	30	85	86	84	-	5	-	-
Niue	-	-	-	-	-	-	-	-	-	-	-	-	-	-	-	-	-	-	-	-	-
North Macedonia	3	4	2	8	-	99	100	100	100	-	-	-	-	11	73	76	70	-	-	26	16
Norway	-	-	-	0 y	-	100 v	100 v	100 v	100 v	-	-	-	-	-	-	-	-	-	-	-	3
Oman	-	-	-	4 x	-	-	100 y	100 y	100 y	-	-	-	-	10 x	-	-	-	-	-	13	-
Pakistan	11 y	13 y	10 y	18 y	5 y	35 y	42 y	43 y	42 y	-	-	-	58 y,p	51 y	-	-	-	-	1 y	-	3
Palau	-	-	-	-	-	-	-	-	-	-	-	-	-	-	-	-	-	-	-	-	-
Panama	2	3	1	26 x	-	-	97	97	97	-	-	-	23 y	23 y	45	47	43	-	3	79	86
Papua New Guinea	-	-	-	27	4	13	13	13	14	-	-	-	72	69	-	-	-	-	7	-	12
Paraguay	18	20	13	22	-	57	71	71	71	-	-	-	-	7	52	55	49	-	-	68	28
Peru	15	14	15	14	-	-	96	-	-	-	-	-	-	-	-	-	-	-	-	85	101
Philippines	-	-	-	17	3 x	88	92	92	91	-	-	-	-	12	-	-	-	-	2	11	1
Poland	-	-	-	-	-	100 y	100 y	100 y	100 y	-	-	-	-	-	-	-	-	-	-	-	179
Portugal	-	-	-	-	-	100 v	100 v	100 v	100 v	-	-	-	-	-	-	-	-	-	-	-	145
Qatar	-	-	-	4 x	1 x	-	100 y	100 y	100 y	-	-	-	22 x	5 x	50 x,y	53 x,y	46 x,y	-	-	-	-
Republic of Korea	-	-	-	-	-	-	-	-	-	-	-	-	-	-	-	-	-	-	-	-	393
Republic of Moldova	-	-	-	12 x	1 x	98	100	99	100	-	-	-	14 x	13 x	76 x,y	77 x,y	74 x,y	-	5 x	118	34
Romania	-	-	-	-	-	-	100 y	100 y	100 y	-	-	-	-	-	-	-	-	-	-	325	31
Russian Federation	-	-	-	6	-	100 v	100 v	100 v	100 v	-	-	-	-	-	-	-	-	-	-	1,410	85
Rwanda	19 y	17 y	21 y	6	0	77	86	86	85	-	-	-	24	53	-	-	-	3	12	47	36
Saint Kitts and Nevis	-	-	-	-	-	-	-	-	-	-	-	-	-	-	-	-	-	-	-	39	137
Saint Lucia	3 x,y	5 x,y	2 x,y	24 x,y	-	78	92	91	93	-	-	-	-	15 x	68 x,y	71 x,y	64 x,y	-	-	78	65
Saint Vincent and the Grenadines	-	-	-	-	-	-	-	-	-	-	-	-	-	-	-	-	-	-	-	120	20
Samoa	14	16	11	7	2	41	67	67	67	-	-	-	22	26	91	92	89	-	5	-	-
San Marino	-	-	-	-	-	100 v	100 v	100 v	100 v	-	-	-	-	-	-	-	-	-	-	-	0
Sao Tome and Principe	11	9	12	28	3	99	99	99	98	-	-	-	10	17	84	84	82	-	3 x	-	-
Saudi Arabia	-	-	-	-	-	-	99 y	100 y	99 y	-	-	-	-	-	-	-	-	-	-	-	-
Senegal	23	27	19	31	1	77	79	80	77	25	16	79	40	42	-	-	-	-	0	114	10
Serbia	10	11	8	6	1 x	100	100	100	100	-	-	-	6 x,y	2	45	46	43	-	-	39	22
Seychelles	-	-	-	-	-	-	-	-	-	-	-	-	-	-	-	-	-	-	-	-	0
Sierra Leone	25	26	25	30	4	93	90	90	91	83	8	34	29	44	87	87	86	0	3	59	10
Singapore	-	-	-	0 y	-	-	100	-	-	-	-	-	-	-	-	-	-	-	-	-	-
Slovakia	-	-	-	-	-	100 y	100	100	100	-	-	-	-	-	-	-	-	-	-	-	40
Slovenia	-	-	-	-	-	100 v	100 v	100 v	100 v	-	-	-	-	-	-	-	-	-	-	-	37
Solomon Islands	18 y	17 y	19 y	21	4	-	88	87	89	-	-	-	60	78	86 y	86 y	85 y	-	-	-	-
Somalia	-	-	-	45 x	-	3 x	3 x	3 x	3 x	99 y	-	19 y	-	75 x,y	-	-	-	-	-	-	-
South Africa	4 y	4 y	3 y	4	1	-	89 y	-	-	-	-	-	14	7	-	-	-	-	1 y	72	4
South Sudan	-	-	-	52 x	-	34 x	35 x	35 x	36 x	-	-	-	72 x	-	-	-	-	-	-	-	45
Spain	-	-	-	-	-	100 v	100 v	100 v	100 v	-	-	-	-	-	-	-	-	-	-	-	45
Sri Lanka	1	1	1	10	-	-	97 x	97 x	97 x	-	-	-	-	22	-	-	-	-	-	165	132
State of Palestine	7	10	5	13	-	97	99	99	99	-	-	-	-	18	90	92	88	4 y	2 y	163	150
Sudan	18	20	16	34 x	-	62	67	69	66	87	30	53	-	36 x	64	65	63	-	-	3	3
Suriname	4	5	4	36 y	20 y	98 y	98 y	98 y	99 y	-	-	-	8	6	87	89	86	-	-	861	83 y
Sweden	-	-	-	-	-	100 v	100 v	100 v	100 v	-	-	-	-	-	-	-	-	4 y	13 x,y	-	7
Switzerland	-	-	-	-	-	100 v	100 v	100 v	100 v	-	-	-	-	-	-	-	-	-	-	-	2
Syrian Arab Republic	-	-	-	13 x	-	89 x	96 x	96 x	96 x	-	-	-	-	-	89 x,y	90 x,y	88 x,y	-	-	-	-
Tajikistan	-	-	-	9	-	90	96	96	96	-	-	-	-	44	69	70	68	-	0	200	9
Thailand	-	-	-	20	10	100	100	100	100	-	-	-	8	8	58	61	55	-	-	189	48 y
Timor-Leste	9	9	10	15	1	38	60	60	61	-	-	-	48	69	-	-	-	-	3	255	-
Togo	39	38	39	25	3	79	83	84	82	3	0	95	22	25	92	92	91	-	4	120 y	5
Tokelau	-	-	-	-	-	-	-	-	-	-	-	-	-	-	-	-	-	-	-	-	-
Tonga	26	33	19	10	3	93	98	97	98	-	-	-	-	22	87	89	84	-	0	-	-
Trinidad and Tobago	1 x,y	1 x,y	1 x,y	11 x,y	-	85 x	97 x	97 x	97 x	-	-	-	-	8 x	77 x,y	79 x,y	75 x,y	-	25	164	12
Tunisia	2 x,y	3 x,y	1 x,y	1	0	100	100	100	100	-	-	-	22	14	88	89	87	-	-	101	53 y
Türkiye	4	4	4	15	-	-	98 y	98 y	99 y	-	-	-	-	6	-	-	-	-	-	56 y	21 y
Turkmenistan	0	0	0	6	-	99	100	100	100	-	-	-	-	46	69	70	67	-	-	241	19
Turks and Caicos Islands	6	9	3	23	5 p	97 p	99	99	99	-	-	-	4 p	0	79	81	78	-	1	108	0
Tuvalu	4	3	5	2	2	81	87	85	89	-	-	-	51	37	80	81	78	-	0	-	-
Uganda	18	17	19	34	6	26	32	32	32	0	1 x	83 x	53	58	85	85	85	1	5	227	21

FOR EVERY CHILD, VACCINATION

TABLE 12. CHILD PROTECTION

Countries and areas	Child labour (%) 2013–2021 [R]			Child marriage (%) 2015–2021 [H][R]		Birth registration (%) 2012–2021 [H][R]				Female genital mutilation (%) 2012–2020 [R]			Justification of wife-beating among adolescents (%) 2015–2021 [R]		Violent discipline (%) 2013–2021 [R]			Sexual violence in childhood (%) 2013–2020 [R]		Children in residential care [H] 2010–2021 [R]	Children in detention [H] 2008–2021 [R]
				Married by 18		Children under 1	Children under 5			Prevalence		Attitudes									
	Total	Male	Female	Female	Male	Total	Total	Male	Female	Women (Fa)	Girls (Fb)	Want the practice to stop (Fc)	Male	Female	Total	Male	Female	Male	Female	Total per 100,000	Total per 100,000
Ukraine	3 x,y	3 x,y	3 x,y	9 x	4 x	99	100	100	100	-	-	-	2 x	2 x	61 x,y	68 x,y	55 x,y	-	2 x	632	16
United Arab Emirates	-	-	-	-	-	-	100 y	100 y	100 y	-	-	-	-	-	-	-	-	-	-	-	25
United Kingdom	-	-	-	0 y	-	100 v	100 v	100 v	100 v	-	-	-	-	-	-	-	-	1 y	7 y	66	17
United Republic of Tanzania	25	26	24	31	4	23	26	28	25	10	0	95	50	59	-	-	-	-	7	49	-
United States	-	-	-	-	-	100 v	100 v	100 v	100 v	-	-	-	-	-	-	-	-	-	-	77	144
Uruguay	4 x	5 x	3 x	25 x	-	99	100	100	100	-	-	-	-	3 x	55 y	58 y	51 y	-	-	352	95
Uzbekistan	-	-	-	7 x	*1* x	100 x	100 x	100 x	100 x	-	-	-	-	63 x	-	-	-	-	-	281	-
Vanuatu	16 y	15 y	16 y	21 x	5 x	-	43 y	44 y	43 y	-	-	-	63 x	56 x	84 y	83 y	84 y	-	-	-	-
Venezuela (Bolivarian Republic of)	-	-	-	-	-	-	81 y	-	-	-	-	-	-	-	-	-	-	-	-	31	404
Viet Nam	7	6	8	11 x	*3* x	88	96	96	96	-	-	-	-	28 x	68	72	65	-	-	-	13
Yemen	-	-	-	32 x	-	27	31	31	30	19	*15*	75	-	49 x	79 y	81 y	77 y	-	-	-	1
Zambia	23 x	23 x	23 x	29	3	13	14	14	14	-	-	-	32	47	-	-	-	-	3	66	237
Zimbabwe	28	33	22	34	2	30	49	48	49	-	-	-	49	54	64	65	63	-	2	-	6
SUMMARY																					
East Asia and Pacific	-	-	-	7	-	-	-	-	-	-	-	-	-	-	-	-	-	-	-	131	32
Europe and Central Asia	-	-	-	-	-	99	100	100	100	-	-	-	-	-	-	-	-	-	-	503	36
Eastern Europe and Central Asia	-	-	-	10	-	99	99	99	99	-	-	-	-	-	-	-	-	-	-	585	30
Western Europe	-	-	-	-	-	100	100	100	100	-	-	-	-	-	-	-	-	-	-	-	41
Latin America and Caribbean	7	6	6	21	-	-	95	-	-	-	-	-	-	-	8	-	-	-	-	85	75
Middle East and North Africa	-	-	-	-	-	89	92	92	92	-	-	-	-	-	86	87	85	-	-	136	-
North America	-	-	-	-	-	100	100	100	100	-	-	-	-	-	-	-	-	-	-	77	133
South Asia	-	-	-	28	4	67	70	70	70	-	-	-	39	40	-	-	-	-	2	77	24
Sub-Saharan Africa	26	27	25	35	4	41	47	46	45	35	16	72	34	43	84	84	83	-	5	-	-
Eastern and Southern Africa	26	28	24	32	5	32	40	37	36	44	-	-	34	44	-	-	-	-	4	104	-
West and Central Africa	26	26	26	37	4	48	53	54	52	27	19	67	35	42	86	87	85	-	7	-	-
Least developed countries	22	23	21	37	6	41	46	46	45	-	-	-	41	46	83	84	83	-	5	68	30
World	**-**	**-**	**-**	**19**	**3**	**72**	**76**	**76**	**75**	**-**	**-**	**-**	**35**	**36**	**-**	**-**	**-**	**-**	**-**	**123**	**36**

For a complete list of countries and areas in the regions, subregions and country categories, see page on Regional Classifications or visit <data,unicef,org/regionalclassifications>,

It is not advisable to compare data from consecutive editions of *The State of the World's Children* report,

NOTES

- Data not available.

Italicized data are from older sources than data presented for other indicators on the same topic within this table. Such discrepancies may be due to an indicator being unavailable in the latest data source, or to the databases for each indicator having been updated as of different dates

[Y] Data differ from the standard definition or refer to only part of a country. If they fall within the noted reference period, such data are included in the calculation of regional and global averages.

[P] Based on small denominators (typically 25–49 unweighted cases). No data based on fewer than 25 unweighted cases are displayed.

[X] Data refer to years or periods other than those specified in the column heading. Such data are not included in the calculation of regional and global averages. Estimates from data years prior to 2000 are not displayed.

[V] Estimates of 100% were assumed given that civil registration systems in these countries are complete and all vital events (including births) are registered. Source: United Nations, Department of Economic and Social Affairs, Statistics Division, last update January 2021.

[H] A more detailed explanation of the methodology and the changes in calculating these estimates can be found in the section titled, General note on the data.

[R] Data refer to the most recent year available during the period specified in the column heading.

MAIN DATA SOURCES

Child labour – Demographic and Health Surveys (DHS), Multiple Indicator Cluster Surveys (MICS) and other national surveys. Last update: March 2022.

Child marriage – DHS, MICS and other national surveys. Last update: March 2022.

Birth registration – DHS, MICS, other national surveys, censuses and vital registration systems. Last update: March 2022.

Female genital mutilation – DHS, MICS and other national surveys. Last update: March 2022.

Justification of wife-beating among adolescents – DHS, MICS and other national surveys. Last update: March 2022.

Violent discipline – DHS, MICS and other national surveys. Last update: March 2022.

Sexual violence in childhood – DHS, MICS and other national surveys. Last update: March 2022.

Children in residential care – Administrative records. Last update: June 2022.

Children in detention – Administrative records. Last update: June 2022.

DEFINITIONS OF THE INDICATORS

Child labour – Percentage of children 5–17 years old involved in child labour at the moment of the survey. A child is considered to be involved in child labour under the following conditions: (a) children 5–11 years old who, during the reference week, did at least one hour of economic activity and/ or more than 21 hours of unpaid household services, (b) children 12–14 years old who, during the reference week, did at least 14 hours of economic activity and/or more than 21 hours of unpaid household services, (c) children 15–17 years old who, during the reference week, did at least 43 hours of economic activity.

Child marriage – Percentage of women 20–24 years old who were first married or in union before they were 18 years old; percentage of men 20–24 years old who were first married or in union before they were 18 years old.

Birth registration – Percentage of children under age 5 and under age 1 who were registered at the moment of the survey. The numerator of this indicator includes children reported to have a birth certificate, regardless of whether or not it was seen by the interviewer, and those without a birth certificate whose mother or caregiver says the birth has been registered.

Female genital mutilation (FGM) – (Fa) Women: percentage of women 15–49 years old who have undergone FGM; (Fb) girls: percentage of girls 0–14 years old who have undergone FGM (as reported by their mothers); (Fc) want the practice to stop: percentage of women 15–49 years old who have heard about FGM and think the practice should stop.

Justification of wife-beating among adolescents – Percentage of girls and boys 15–19 years old who consider a husband to be justified in hitting or beating his wife for at least one of the specified reasons, i.e., if his wife burns the food, argues with him, goes out without telling him, neglects the children or refuses sexual relations.

Violent discipline – Percentage of children 1–14 years old who experience any violent discipline (psychological aggression and/or physical punishment) in the past month.

Sexual violence in childhood – Percentage of women and men 18–29 years old who experienced sexual violence by age 18.

Children in residential care – Rate of children 0–17 years old in residential care per 100,000. Residential care is defined in the Guidelines for the Alternative Care of Children (para 29 (c) iv) as: 'care provided in any non-family-based group setting, such as places of safety for emergency care, transit centres in emergency situations, and all other short- and long-term residential care facilities, including group homes'. This includes 'orphanages', and small group homes.

Children in detention – Rate of children under age 18 years in detention per 100,000. The definition of 'detention' includes children detained pre-trial, pre-sentence and post–sentencing in any type of facility (including police custody).

TABLE 13. SOCIAL PROTECTION AND EQUITY

Countries and areas	Mothers with newborns receiving cash benefit (%) 2010–2019 [R]	Proportion of children covered by social protection 2010–2019 [R]	Distribution of social protection benefits (%) 2010–2019 [R]			Share of household income (%) 2010–2019 [R]			Gini Coefficient 2010–2019 [R]	Palma Index of income inequality 2010–2019 [R]	VMIR (vast majority income ratio) 2010–2019 [R]	GDP per capita (current US$) 2010–2019 [R]
			Bottom 40%	Top 20%	Bottom 20%	Bottom 40%	Top 20%	Bottom 20%				
Afghanistan	2	0	-	-	-	-	-	-	31	-	-	507
Albania	-	-	46	14	28	20	41	8	33	1.3	0.8	5,353
Algeria	11	-	-	-	-	23	37	9	28	1.0	0.8	3,974
Andorra	-	-	-	-	-	-	-	-	28	1.0	-	40,886
Angola	-	-	-	-	-	12	56	4	51	3.5	0.6	2,791
Anguilla	73	2	-	-	-	-	-	-	-	-	-	-
Antigua and Barbuda	37	-	-	-	-	-	-	-	-	-	-	17,113
Argentina	32	80	75	6	49	14	48	5	42	2.1	0.7	9,912
Armenia	62	30	58	9	36	22	39	9	34	1.4	0.7	4,623
Australia	100	100	-	-	-	20	42	7	33	1.3	0.7	55,057
Austria	100	100	-	-	-	21	39	8	28	1.0	0.8	50,122
Azerbaijan	16	17	29	33	17	-	-	-	27	0.7	0.8	4,793
Bahamas	47	-	-	-	-	-	-	-	41	2.0	-	34,864
Bahrain	-	57	-	-	-	-	-	-	60	-	-	23,504
Bangladesh	21	29	44	18	24	21	41	9	48	2.9	0.7	1,856
Barbados	-	-	-	-	-	-	-	-	32	3.1	-	18,148
Belarus	100	-	50	17	27	24	35	10	25	0.9	0.8	6,698
Belgium	100	100	-	-	-	23	36	9	25	0.9	0.8	46,345
Belize	20	3	-	-	-	-	-	-	53	3.9	0.5	4,815
Benin	41	12	-	-	-	13	52	3	48	2.9	0.6	1,219
Bhutan	10	14	-	-	-	18	44	7	37	1.6	0.7	3,316
Bolivia (Plurinational State of)	59	66	43	24	25	15	47	5	43	2.2	0.6	3,552
Bosnia and Herzegovina	100	-	37	25	16	20	41	8	33	1.3	0.7	6,109
Botswana	24	4	22	36	7	11	59	4	53	3.8	0.5	7,961
Brazil	48	68	59	4	33	11	58	3	54	4.1	0.5	8,717
British Virgin Islands	-	-	-	-	-	-	-	-	-	-	-	-
Brunei Darussalam	63	-	-	-	-	-	-	-	56	5.0	-	31,087
Bulgaria	100	49	-	-	-	17	48	6	41	2.0	0.7	9,828
Burkina Faso	0	-	3	68	2	20	44	8	35	1.5	0.7	787
Burundi	-	-	-	-	-	18	46	7	39	1.7	0.7	261
Cabo Verde	19	38	-	-	-	15	49	6	46	2.1	0.6	3,604
Cambodia	2	5	-	-	-	-	-	-	31	1.2	0.7	1,643
Cameroon	1	2	1	51	0	13	52	5	47	2.7	0.6	1,507
Canada	100	40	-	-	-	20	41	7	30	1.1	0.7	46,190
Central African Republic	0	0	-	-	-	-	-	-	56	4.5	0.5	468
Chad	-	-	3	65	1	15	49	5	43	2.2	0.6	710
Chile	47	69	42	11	19	16	51	6	48	2.9	0.6	14,896
China	69	3	48	16	24	17	45	7	47	1.7	0.7	10,217
Colombia	-	36	68	3	39	12	56	4	53	3.9	0.6	6,429
Comoros	-	-	-	-	-	14	50	5	45	2.5	0.6	1,370
Congo	-	-	-	-	-	12	54	4	49	3.1	0.6	2,280
Cook Islands	-	100	-	-	-	-	-	-	-	-	-	-
Costa Rica	23	39	64	3	30	13	54	4	50	3.1	0.6	12,244
Côte d'Ivoire	-	-	4	57	1	16	48	6	61	6.4	0.7	2,276
Croatia	100	-	61	12	39	21	38	8	29	1.0	0.8	14,944
Cuba	43	0	-	-	-	-	-	-	27	0.9	-	8,822
Cyprus	100	60	-	-	-	21	41	8	31	1.2	0.7	27,858
Czechia	100	-	-	-	-	25	36	10	24	0.8	0.8	23,490
Democratic People's Republic of Korea	-	-	-	-	-	-	-	-	-	-	-	-
Democratic Republic of the Congo	-	1	8	64	3	16	48	6	42	2.1	0.6	581
Denmark	100	100	-	-	-	23	38	9	28	1.0	0.8	60,213
Djibouti	5	4	74	9	54	16	48	5	42	2.0	0.7	3,415
Dominica	39	-	-	-	-	-	-	-	44	2.5	-	8,111
Dominican Republic	17	62	45	12	21	16	49	6	43	2.2	0.6	8,282
Ecuador	7	9	60	6	32	14	51	5	46	2.5	0.6	6,184
Egypt	100	-	-	-	-	22	41	9	32	1.2	0.7	3,019
El Salvador	11	9	57	10	28	17	46	6	41	1.9	0.7	4,187
Equatorial Guinea	-	-	-	-	-	-	-	-	50	-	-	8,132
Eritrea	-	0	-	-	-	-	-	-	-	-	-	643
Estonia	100	100	-	-	-	21	38	8	31	1.1	0.7	23,718
Eswatini	14	-	47	13	23	11	60	4	55	4.1	0.5	3,895
Ethiopia	-	5	39	27	17	19	43	7	33	1.5	0.7	856
Fiji	25	3	35	24	17	19	45	8	37	1.6	0.7	6,176

TABLE 13. SOCIAL PROTECTION AND EQUITY

Countries and areas	Mothers with newborns receiving cash benefit (%) 2010–2019 [R]	Proportion of children covered by social protection 2010–2019 [R]	Distribution of social protection benefits (%) 2010–2019 [R]			Share of household income (%) 2010–2019 [R]			Gini Coefficient 2010–2019 [R]	Palma Index of income inequality 2010–2019 [R]	VMIR (vast majority income ratio) 2010–2019 [R]	GDP per capita (current US$) 2010–2019 [R]
			Bottom 40%	Top 20%	Bottom 20%	Bottom 40%	Top 20%	Bottom 20%				
Finland	100	100	-	-	-	23	37	9	26	0.9	0.8	48,771
France	100	100	-	-	-	21	41	8	29	1.1	0.7	40,496
Gabon	-	-	-	-	-	17	44	6	38	1.6	0.7	7,767
Gambia	-	-	87	8	4	19	44	7	36	1.5	0.7	778
Georgia	26	48	66	8	44	19	43	7	36	1.5	0.7	4,698
Germany	100	100	-	-	-	20	40	8	30	1.1	0.8	46,468
Ghana	42	26	82	4	58	14	49	5	44	2.3	0.6	2,202
Greece	100	-	-	-	-	20	40	7	31	1.1	0.7	19,581
Grenada	85	-	-	-	-	-	-	-	37	1.6	-	10,809
Guatemala	18	3	56	10	30	13	54	5	45	2.4	0.6	4,620
Guinea	-	-	-	-	-	20	42	8	34	1.3	0.7	963
Guinea-Bissau	-	-	-	-	-	-	-	-	51	3.3	0.5	697
Guyana	30	-	-	-	-	-	-	-	35	2.4	0.6	6,610
Haiti	-	4	-	-	-	16	47	6	61	6.5	0.4	1,272
Holy See	-	-	-	-	-	-	-	-	-	-	-	-
Honduras	-	19	55	16	28	12	52	4	49	3.1	0.6	2,575
Hungary	100	100	-	-	-	22	38	8	28	1.0	0.8	16,730
Iceland	100	-	-	-	-	24	36	10	23	0.8	0.8	67,084
India	42	24	43	17	23	20	44	8	52	3.6	0.7	2,100
Indonesia	28	26	58	6	31	18	46	7	38	1.7	0.7	4,136
Iran (Islamic Republic of)	13	16	-	-	-	16	49	6	41	1.9	0.7	5,550
Iraq	-	-	27	35	12	22	39	9	41	2.0	0.8	5,955
Ireland	100	100	-	-	-	21	40	8	28	1.0	0.7	78,779
Israel	100	-	-	-	-	16	44	5	35	1.4	0.7	43,589
Italy	100	-	-	-	-	18	42	6	33	1.3	0.7	33,226
Jamaica	7	27	52	2	32	16	48	6	37	1.7	0.6	5,582
Japan	-	85	-	-	-	21	41	8	34	1.3	0.8	40,247
Jordan	5	9	-	-	-	-	-	-	40	1.9	0.7	4,405
Kazakhstan	44	57	39	20	19	23	38	10	27	1.0	0.8	9,813
Kenya	30	4	38	24	20	17	48	6	41	1.9	0.7	1,817
Kiribati	-	1	-	-	-	-	-	-	37	1.6	0.7	1,655
Kuwait	-	-	-	-	-	-	-	-	36	2.4	-	32,000
Kyrgyzstan	24	17	62	7	35	23	40	10	28	1.0	0.8	1,310
Lao People's Democratic Republic	13	-	-	-	-	18	46	7	36	1.6	0.7	2,535
Latvia	100	100	-	-	-	19	42	7	35	1.4	0.7	17,819
Lebanon	-	-	-	-	-	21	40	8	32	1.2	0.8	7,584
Lesotho	-	10	48	10	23	14	50	5	45	2.4	0.5	1,118
Liberia	-	6	40	16	23	19	43	7	35	1.4	0.7	622
Libya	-	-	-	-	-	-	-	-	30	-	-	7,686
Liechtenstein	100	100	-	-	-	-	-	-	-	-	-	181,403
Lithuania	100	-	-	-	-	19	43	7	35	1.5	0.7	19,551
Luxembourg	100	100	-	-	-	19	42	7	32	1.2	0.7	114,685
Madagascar	-	-	-	-	-	16	49	6	43	2.1	0.6	523
Malawi	-	10	37	17	18	16	52	6	45	2.4	0.6	412
Malaysia	47	3	48	12	25	16	47	6	41	2.0	0.7	11,414
Maldives	26	8	35	23	15	21	40	8	31	1.2	0.7	10,627
Mali	-	5	-	-	-	-	-	-	33	1.3	0.7	879
Malta	100	-	-	-	-	22	38	9	28	1.0	0.8	29,737
Marshall Islands	-	-	-	-	-	-	-	-	-	-	-	3,788
Mauritania	-	-	-	-	-	20	40	8	33	1.3	0.7	1,679
Mauritius	-	-	29	27	12	19	45	7	37	1.6	0.7	11,099
Mexico	11	23	51	16	28	15	52	5	46	2.6	0.6	9,946
Micronesia (Federated States of)	-	7	-	-	-	16	46	6	40	1.8	0.7	3,568
Monaco	-	-	-	-	-	-	-	-	-	-	-	185,829
Mongolia	100	85	45	18	24	20	41	8	33	1.3	0.7	4,340
Montenegro	100	-	61	11	43	16	44	5	34	1.3	0.7	8,910
Montserrat	-	-	-	-	-	-	-	-	-	-	-	-
Morocco	-	-	-	-	-	17	47	7	40	1.8	0.7	3,204
Mozambique	0	0	-	-	-	12	60	4	47	3.8	0.5	504
Myanmar	2	2	50	13	33	22	40	9	31	1.2	0.7	1,408
Namibia	25	23	35	26	18	9	64	3	56	6.2	0.5	4,957
Nauru	-	-	-	-	-	19	43	8	-	1.9	-	9,397
Nepal	10	23	-	-	-	-	-	-	33	1.3	0.7	1,071

TABLE 13. SOCIAL PROTECTION AND EQUITY

Countries and areas	Mothers with newborns receiving cash benefit (%) 2010–2019 [R]	Proportion of children covered by social protection 2010–2019 [R]	Distribution of social protection benefits (%) 2010–2019 [R]			Share of household income (%) 2010–2019 [R]			Gini Coefficient 2010–2019 [R]	Palma Index of income inequality 2010–2019 [R]	VMIR (vast majority income ratio) 2010–2019 [R]	GDP per capita (current US$) 2010–2019 [R]
			Bottom 40%	Top 20%	Bottom 20%	Bottom 40%	Top 20%	Bottom 20%				
Netherlands (Kingdom of the)	100	100	-	-	-	23	37	9	28	1.0	0.8	52,295
New Zealand	100	67				-	-	-	34	1.4		41,558
Nicaragua	18	3	-	-	-	14	52	5	46	2.6	0.6	1,913
Niger	-	4	29	17	13	20	42	8	34	1.4	0.7	554
Nigeria	0	12	45	16	21	19	42	7	35	1.4	0.6	2,230
Niue	-	-				-	-	-	-	-	-	-
North Macedonia	100	-	-		-	19	39	6	31	1.1	0.7	6,022
Norway	100	100				23	37	9	25	0.9	0.8	75,420
Oman	-	-	-	-	-	-	-	-	40	-	-	15,343
Pakistan	-	5	60	8	33	22	41	9	33	1.4	0.7	1,285
Palau	-	60	-	-	-	-	-	-	51	3.8	-	14,902
Panama	19	22	51	12	25	12	54	4	51	3.4	0.6	15,731
Papua New Guinea	-	-	-	-	-	-	-	-	42	2.1	0.7	2,829
Paraguay	8	19	58	4	28	14	51	5	47	2.8	0.6	5,415
Peru	9	16	81	2	51	15	47	5	43	2.2	0.6	6,978
Philippines	12	31	55	13	28	16	49	6	44	2.3	0.6	3,485
Poland	100	100	62	9	38	22	39	8	29	1.0	0.8	15,695
Portugal	100	93	-	-	-	20	41	7	32	1.2	0.7	23,214
Qatar	-	-	-	-	-	-	-	-	40	-	-	62,088
Republic of Korea	-	40	-	-	-	21	39	8	35	1.4	0.8	31,846
Republic of Moldova	100	-	51	13	30	24	36	10	26	0.9	0.8	4,494
Romania	100	100	52	15	32	17	41	5	35	1.4	0.8	12,913
Russian Federation	63	100	34	22	13	18	45	7	35	1.4	0.7	11,585
Rwanda	1	5	31	34	14	16	51	6	44	2.3	0.6	820
Saint Kitts and Nevis	78	-	-	-	-	-	-	-	40	-	-	19,935
Saint Lucia	39	-	-	-	-	11	55	3	51	3.5	0.6	11,611
Saint Vincent and the Grenadines	29	-	-	-	-	-	-	-	40	-	-	7,458
Samoa	29	0	-	-	-	18	46	7	39	1.8	0.7	4,324
San Marino	100	-	-	-	-	-	-	-	28	-	-	48,995
Sao Tome and Principe	2	-	-	-	-	12	61	4	56	4.2	0.8	1,947
Saudi Arabia	-	3	-	-	-	-	-	-	42	-	-	23,140
Senegal	3	1	7	69	3	17	47	6	40	1.9	0.7	1,447
Serbia	-	-	51	18	35	17	42	5	33	1.3	0.7	7,412
Seychelles				-	-	20	39	7	47	2.6	0.6	17,448
Sierra Leone	-	1	-	-	-	20	44	8	36	1.5	0.7	528
Singapore	89	-	-	-	-	-	-	-	47	1.9	-	65,233
Slovakia	100	100	-	-	-	24	34	9	23	0.7	0.8	19,266
Slovenia	96	79	-	-	-	25	35	10	24	0.8	0.8	25,941
Solomon Islands	24	-	-	-	-	18	45	7	37	1.6	0.7	2,374
Somalia	-	-	-	-	-	-	-	-	41	1.9	-	127
South Africa	8	77	50	10	25	7	68	2	67	10.1	0.4	6,001
South Sudan	-	18	-	-	-	-	-	-	46	2.7	0.6	1,120
Spain	100	100	-	-	-	18	41	6	33	1.3	0.7	29,565
Sri Lanka	29	32	59	7	33	18	47	7	45	2.5	0.7	3,853
State of Palestine	7	12	30	29	15	19	41	7	45	2.5	0.7	3,562
Sudan	-	-	-	-	-	20	42	8	34	1.4	0.7	442
Suriname	0	58	-	-	-	-	-	-	38	5.8	0.5	6,360
Sweden	100	100	-	-	-	21	38	8	28	1.0	0.8	51,648
Switzerland	100	100	-	-	-	20	41	8	31	1.2	0.7	81,989
Syrian Arab Republic	-	-	-	-	-	-	-	-	34	1.2	0.7	1,178
Tajikistan	67	14	15	43	8	19	42	7	34	1.4	0.7	871
Thailand	40	21	52	12	26	19	43	8	36	1.5	0.7	7,807
Timor-Leste	-	38	42	25	14	23	38	9	29	1.1	0.8	1,561
Togo	-	49	-	-	-	15	49	5	43	2.2	0.6	679
Tokelau	-	-	-	-	-	-	-	-	-	-	-	-
Tonga	26	3	-	-	-	18	45	7	38	1.6	0.7	4,903
Trinidad and Tobago	40	15	-	-	-	-	-	-	40	1.9	0.7	17,398
Tunisia	25	29	-	-	-	20	41	8	33	1.3	0.7	3,317
Türkiye	-	-	64	6	38	16	48	5	42	2.0	0.6	9,127
Turkmenistan	-	-	-	-	-	-	-	-	27	2.0	0.7	6,967
Turks and Caicos Islands	58	-	-	-	-	-	-	-	-	-	-	31,353
Tuvalu	-	-	-	-	-	-	-	-	39	1.8	0.7	4,059
Uganda	5	-	10	79	3	16	50	6	43	2.1	0.6	794
Ukraine	100	100	46	16	22	24	37	10	26	0.9	0.8	3,659

TABLE 13. SOCIAL PROTECTION AND EQUITY

Countries and areas	Mothers with newborns receiving cash benefit (%) 2010–2019 R	Proportion of children covered by social protection 2010–2019 R	Distribution of social protection benefits (%) 2010–2019 R			Share of household income (%) 2010–2019 R			Gini Coefficient 2010–2019 R	Palma Index of income inequality 2010–2019 R	VMIR (vast majority income ratio) 2010–2019 R	GDP per capita (current US$) 2010–2019 R
			Bottom 40%	Top 20%	Bottom 20%	Bottom 40%	Top 20%	Bottom 20%				
United Arab Emirates	-	1	-	-	-	23	35	9	33	1.2	-	43,103
United Kingdom	100	66	-	-	-	19	42	7	35	1.3	0.7	42,329
United Republic of Tanzania	0	-	54	9	18	17	48	7	40	1.9	0.7	1,122
United States	-	-	-	-	-	16	47	5	42	2.0	0.7	65,298
Uruguay	100	-	59	13	37	16	46	6	39	1.8	0.7	16,190
Uzbekistan	16	29	49	14	30	19	44	7	40	1.5	0.7	1,725
Vanuatu	-	13	-	-	-	-	-	-	38	1.6	0.7	3,115
Venezuela (Bolivarian Republic of)	-	-	-	-	-	-	-	-	38	1.6	0.6	16,054
Viet Nam	44	1	83	3	64	19	43	7	42	1.5	0.7	2,715
Yemen	-	-	-	-	-	19	45	7	37	1.6	0.7	774
Zambia	4	21	9	59	1	9	61	3	57	5.0	0.5	1,305
Zimbabwe	-	7	61	16	49	15	51	6	44	2.3	0.6	1,464
SUMMARY												
East Asia and Pacific	57	14	51	14	27	18	45	7	43	1.7	0.7	11,386
Europe and Central Asia	85	91	47	16	25	20	42	7	32	1.3	0.7	24,694
Eastern Europe and Central Asia	66	81	45	17	24	19	43	7	34	1.4	0.7	8,437
Western Europe	100	100	-	-	-	20	40	7	30	1.1	0.8	38,421
Latin America and Caribbean	31	45	59	8	33	13	53	4	48	3.1	0.6	8,810
Middle East and North Africa	49	-	-	-	-	20	43	8	36	1.5	0.7	7,756
North America	-	-	-	-	-	16	46	5	40	1.9	0.7	63,369
South Asia	38	22	46	16	24	20	44	8	49	3.2	0.7	1,961
Sub-Saharan Africa	7	14	34	31	17	16	48	6	42	2.6	0.6	1,604
Eastern and Southern Africa	9	19	39	28	18	15	51	6	44	3.0	0.6	1,628
West and Central Africa	6	10	31	35	15	17	45	6	40	2.0	0.7	1,578
Least developed countries	9	12	33	33	16	18	46	7	40	2.2	0.7	1,078
World	**48**	**27**	**47**	**17**	**25**	**18**	**45**	**7**	**43**	**2.2**	**0.7**	**11,562**

For a complete list of countries and areas in the regions, subregions and country categories, see page on Regional Classifications or visit <data.unicef.org/regionalclassifications>.

It is not advisable to compare data from consecutive editions of *The State of the World's Children* report.

NOTES

- Data not available.

R Data refer to the most recent year available during the period specified in the column heading.

MAIN DATA SOURCES

Mothers with newborns receiving cash benefit (%) – ILO World Social Protection Report, 2017–2020. Last update: May 2021.

Proportion of children covered by social protection – ILO World Social Protection Report, 2017–2020. Last update: May 2021.

Distribution of Social Protection Benefits – The Atlas of Social Protection: Indicators of Resilience and Equity. Last update: May 2021.

Share of household income – World Development Indicators. Last update: February 2021.

Gini Coefficient – World Income Inequality Database. Last update: May 2020.

Palma Index of income inequality – World Income Inequality Database. Last update: May 2020.

GDP per capita (current US$) – World Development Indicators. Last update: February 2021.

VMIR (vast majority income ratio) - UNICEF estimates based on World Development Indicators. Last update: February 2021.

DEFINITIONS OF THE INDICATORS

Mothers with newborns receiving cash benefit (%) – Proportion of women giving birth covered by maternity benefits: ratio of women receiving cash maternity benefits to women giving birth in the same year (estimated based on age-specific fertility rates published in the UN's World Population Prospects or on the number of live births corrected for the share of twin and triplet births).

Proportion of children covered by social protection – Proportion of children covered by social protection benefits: ratio of children/households receiving child or family cash benefits to the total number of children/households with children.

Distribution of Social Protection Benefits – Percentage of benefits going to the 1st quintile, bottom 40% and 5th quintile relative to the total benefits going to the population. social protection coverage includes: providing social assistance through cash transfers to those who need them, especially children; benefits and support for people of working age in case of maternity, disability; and pension coverage for the elderly.

Share of household income – Percentage of income received by the 20 per cent of households with the highest income, by the 40 per cent of households with the lowest income and by the 20 per cent of households with the lowest income.

Gini Coefficient – Gini index measures the extent to which the distribution of income (or, in some cases, consumption expenditure) among individuals or households within an economy deviates from a perfectly equal distribution. A Lorenz curve plots the cumulative percentages of total income received against the cumulative number of recipients, starting with the poorest individual or household. The Gini index measures the area between the Lorenz curve and a hypothetical line of absolute equality, expressed as a percentage of the maximum area under the line. Thus a Gini index of 0 represents perfect equality, while an index of 100 implies perfect inequality.

Palma Index of income inequality – Palma index is defined as the ratio of the richest 10% of the population's share of gross national income divided by the poorest 40%'s share.

GDP per capita (current US$) – GDP per capita is gross domestic product divided by midyear population. GDP is the sum of gross value added by all resident producers in the economy plus any product taxes and minus any subsidies not included in the value of the products. It is calculated without making deductions for depreciation of fabricated assets or for depletion and degradation of natural resources. Data are in current US dollars.

VMIR (vast majority income ratio) - The Vast Majority Income Ratio measures the income ratio of the first 80% (vast majority) in the income ranking.

TABLE 14. WASH

Countries and areas	Households 2020									Schools 2021									Healthcare facilities 2021			
	At least basic drinking water services (%)			At least basic sanitation services (%)			Basic hygiene facilities (%)			Basic water services (%)			Basic sanitation services (%)			Basic hygiene services (%)			Basic water services (%)	Basic sanitation services (%)	Basic hygiene services (%)	Basic waste management services (%)
	Total	Urban	Rural	Total	Urban	Rural	Total	Urban	Rural	Total	Primary	Secondary	Total	Primary	Secondary	Total	Primary	Secondary				
Afghanistan	75	100	66	50	67	45	38	64	29	66	58	75	38	26	65	8	5	11	-	-	-	-
Albania	95	96	94	99	99	99	-	-	-	64	56	73	89	79	92	84	69	90	-	-	-	-
Algeria	94	96	90	86	88	79	85	88	75	90	85	92	-	-	100	-	-	-	-	-	-	-
Andorra	100	100	100	100	100	100	-	-	-	100	100	100	100	100	100	100	100	100	100	-	-	100
Angola	57	72	28	52	65	24	27	34	13	-	-	-	-	-	-	-	-	-	-	-	-	-
Anguilla	-	-	-	-	-	-	-	-	-	100	100	100	100	100	100	100	100	100	-	-	-	-
Antigua and Barbuda	-	-	-	-	-	-	-	-	-	100	99	100	100	100	100	100	99	100	-	-	-	-
Argentina	-	100	-	-	99	-	-	-	-	-	-	-	-	-	-	-	-	-	-	-	-	-
Armenia	100	100	100	94	100	83	95	97	91	98	99	97	-	-	-	98	98	97	97	41	69	97
Australia	100	100	100	100	-	-	-	-	-	100	100	100	100	100	100	100	100	100	-	-	-	-
Austria	100	100	100	100	100	100	-	-	-	-	-	-	-	-	-	-	-	-	-	-	-	-
Azerbaijan	96	100	91	-	96	-	-	-	-	100	100	100	100	100	100	100	100	100	100	48	100	-
Bahamas	-	-	-	-	-	-	-	-	-	-	-	-	-	-	-	-	-	-	-	-	-	-
Bahrain	100	-	-	100	-	-	-	-	-	100	100	100	100	100	100	100	100	100	-	-	-	88
Bangladesh	98	97	98	54	53	55	58	66	54	81	80	95	57	48	58	56	85	28	64	31	38	34
Barbados	99	-	-	98	-	-	-	-	-	100	100	100	100	100	100	100	100	100	-	-	-	-
Belarus	97	96	99	98	98	97	-	-	-	100	100	100	100	100	100	100	100	100	-	-	-	-
Belgium	100	100	100	99	99	99	-	-	-	100	100	100	-	-	-	100	100	100	-	-	-	-
Belize	98	99	98	88	94	84	90	92	89	-	-	-	-	-	-	-	-	-	-	-	-	-
Benin	65	73	58	17	27	8	12	17	8	43	43	-	-	-	73	49	51	47	-	-	-	-
Bhutan	97	98	97	77	77	76	92	89	93	72	-	-	76	-	-	-	-	-	95	16	73	36
Bolivia (Plurinational State of)	93	99	80	66	75	44	27	29	22	-	-	-	-	-	-	-	-	-	-	-	-	-
Bosnia and Herzegovina	96	95	97	-	99	-	-	-	-	-	-	-	-	-	-	-	-	-	-	-	-	-
Botswana	92	98	79	80	91	52	-	-	-	-	-	-	-	-	-	-	-	-	-	-	-	-
Brazil	99	100	96	90	94	63	-	-	-	-	-	-	-	-	-	-	-	-	-	-	45	-
British Virgin Islands	100	-	-	-	-	-	-	-	-	91	94	88	87	94	80	91	100	80	-	-	-	-
Brunei Darussalam	100	100	-	-	-	-	-	-	-	-	-	-	100	100	-	100	100	100	-	-	-	-
Bulgaria	99	100	97	86	87	84	-	-	-	-	-	-	-	-	-	-	-	-	-	-	-	-
Burkina Faso	47	80	33	22	40	13	9	17	5	61	62	46	52	58	56	32	33	16	74	-	-	21
Burundi	62	91	58	46	41	46	6	19	4	46	45	52	45	35	93	18	18	14	-	48	-	82
Cabo Verde	89	93	80	79	83	72	-	-	-	-	-	100	93	92	93	86	83	100	-	-	-	-
Cambodia	71	90	65	69	93	61	74	83	71	76	83	82	32	41	47	68	73	67	-	-	-	-
Cameroon	66	82	44	45	61	23	36	47	22	37	37	-	39	39	-	-	-	-	-	-	-	-
Canada	99	99	99	99	99	99	-	-	-	-	-	-	-	-	-	-	-	-	-	-	-	-
Central African Republic	37	50	28	14	25	6	22	34	12	16	16	-	-	-	-	-	-	-	-	-	-	-
Chad	46	74	38	12	40	4	25	35	22	37	30	-	-	-	-	20	20	-	-	-	-	75
Chile	100	100	100	100	100	100	-	-	-	-	-	-	-	-	-	-	-	-	-	-	-	-
China	94	97	90	92	95	88	-	-	-	-	-	-	-	-	-	-	-	-	91	-	36	-
Colombia	97	100	87	94	96	84	68	76	32	-	-	-	-	-	-	-	-	-	-	-	-	-
Comoros	-	-	-	-	-	-	-	-	-	-	-	-	-	-	-	-	-	-	-	-	2	-
Congo	74	87	46	20	27	6	-	-	-	54	54	-	-	-	-	-	-	-	-	-	-	-
Cook Islands	100	-	-	99	-	-	-	-	-	100	100	100	100	100	100	100	100	100	100	60	-	20
Costa Rica	100	100	100	98	98	97	86	87	83	84	86	76	81	77	94	81	79	89	100	-	-	-
Côte d'Ivoire	71	85	56	35	48	21	22	31	11	-	-	-	-	-	-	-	-	-	27	-	-	14
Croatia	-	100	-	97	98	95	-	-	-	95	-	-	95	-	-	99	-	-	-	-	-	-
Cuba	97	98	94	91	93	86	92	94	86	100	100	100	100	100	100	100	100	100	-	-	-	-
Cyprus	100	100	100	99	100	99	-	-	-	-	-	-	-	-	-	-	-	-	-	-	-	-
Czechia	100	100	100	99	99	99	-	-	-	-	-	-	-	-	-	-	-	-	100	-	100	100
Democratic People's Republic of Korea	94	97	89	85	92	73	-	-	-	-	-	-	-	-	-	-	-	-	-	-	-	-
Democratic Republic of the Congo	46	75	22	15	20	11	19	27	12	-	-	-	-	-	-	-	-	-	30	-	-	0
Denmark	100	100	100	100	100	100	-	-	-	100	100	100	100	100	100	100	100	100	-	-	-	-
Djibouti	76	84	47	67	79	22	-	-	-	-	-	-	-	-	-	94	91	-	-	-	-	-
Dominica	-	-	-	-	-	-	-	-	-	100	100	100	100	100	100	100	100	100	-	-	-	-
Dominican Republic	97	98	90	87	89	77	47	50	33	-	-	-	-	-	-	-	-	-	-	-	-	-
Ecuador	95	100	87	92	93	89	87	92	79	79	82	93	59	59	68	51	50	33	-	-	-	49
Egypt	99	100	99	97	100	96	90	93	88	-	-	-	100	100	100	100	100	100	84	68	60	-
El Salvador	98	100	93	82	87	70	-	-	-	82	80	84	88	87	92	-	-	-	-	-	-	-
Equatorial Guinea	-	-	-	-	-	-	-	-	-	-	-	-	-	-	-	-	-	-	-	-	-	-
Eritrea	-	-	-	-	-	-	-	-	-	-	-	-	33	26	46	5	3	8	-	-	-	-
Estonia	100	100	-	99	99	99	-	-	-	100	100	100	100	100	100	100	100	100	100	-	100	100
Eswatini	71	97	62	64	52	68	24	48	17	-	-	-	-	-	-	-	-	-	-	-	-	73
Ethiopia	50	84	40	9	21	5	8	20	5	15	15	22	40	39	61	20	16	29	-	-	-	64

FOR EVERY CHILD, VACCINATION 187

TABLE 14. WASH

Countries and areas	Households 2020									Schools 2021									Healthcare facilities 2021			
	At least basic drinking water services (%)			At least basic sanitation services (%)			Basic hygiene facilities (%)			Basic water services (%)			Basic sanitation services (%)			Basic hygiene services (%)			Basic water services (%)	Basic sanitation services (%)	Basic hygiene services (%)	Basic waste management services (%)
	Total	Urban	Rural	Total	Urban	Rural	Total	Urban	Rural	Total	Primary	Secondary	Total	Primary	Secondary	Total	Primary	Secondary				
Fiji	94	98	89	99	99	99	-	-	-	87	87	90	76	83	80	70	76	45	69	9	42	56
Finland	100	100	100	99	99	99	-	-	-	100	100	100	100	100	100	100	100	100	-	-	-	-
France	100	100	100	99	99	99	-	-	-	100	100	100	100	100	100	100	100	100	-	-	-	-
Gabon	85	90	45	50	51	40	-	-	-	60	59	57	-	-	-	59	57	69	-	-	-	-
Gambia	81	88	69	47	60	26	18	18	18	-	-	-	63	83	78	-	-	-	-	-	-	-
Georgia	97	99	94	86	95	72	92	95	87	-	-	-	-	-	-	-	-	-	-	-	-	-
Germany	100	100	100	99	99	99	-	-	-	100	100	100	100	100	100	100	100	100	-	-	-	-
Ghana	86	96	72	24	28	17	42	47	35	78	78	79	59	62	65	54	52	52	67	-	62	51
Greece	100	100	100	99	99	98	-	-	-	-	-	-	-	-	-	-	-	-	-	-	-	-
Grenada	-	-	-	-	-	-	-	-	-	99	100	99	-	-	-	100	100	100	-	-	-	-
Guatemala	94	98	90	68	79	56	-	-	-	-	-	-	76	76	-	-	-	-	67	-	-	-
Guinea	64	87	51	30	46	21	20	33	13	-	37	-	52	52	-	-	-	-	-	-	-	45
Guinea-Bissau	59	71	50	18	35	5	18	23	14	63	-	-	37	-	-	75	-	-	74	17	47	2
Guyana	96	100	94	86	92	84	-	-	-	-	-	-	-	-	-	-	-	-	-	-	-	-
Haiti	67	85	43	37	46	25	22	28	15	-	-	-	-	-	-	-	-	-	64	-	-	6
Holy See	-	-	-	-	-	-	-	-	-	-	-	-	-	-	-	-	-	-	-	-	-	-
Honduras	96	100	90	84	86	80	-	-	-	100	76	71	-	-	-	-	-	-	55	4	30	28
Hungary	100	100	100	98	98	99	-	-	-	100	100	100	100	100	100	100	100	100	-	-	-	-
Iceland	100	100	100	99	99	100	-	-	-	-	-	-	-	-	-	-	-	-	-	-	-	-
India	90	94	89	71	79	67	68	82	60	74	67	75	86	86	84	53	53	53	-	-	-	-
Indonesia	92	98	86	86	92	80	94	96	91	73	72	75	47	43	55	66	66	64	-	-	-	74
Iran (Islamic Republic of)	97	99	94	90	93	82	-	-	-	-	-	-	-	-	-	-	-	-	88	22	93	52
Iraq	98	100	95	100	100	100	97	98	97	60	-	-	57	-	-	66	-	-	67	-	49	21
Ireland	97	97	98	91	90	94	-	-	-	-	-	-	-	-	-	-	-	-	-	-	-	-
Israel	100	100	100	100	100	99	-	-	-	100	100	100	100	100	100	100	100	100	-	-	-	-
Italy	100	-	-	100	100	100	-	-	-	100	100	100	100	100	100	100	100	100	-	-	-	-
Jamaica	91	95	85	87	83	91	-	-	-	95	93	97	96	94	97	97	97	98	-	-	-	-
Japan	99	-	-	100	-	-	-	-	-	-	-	-	-	-	-	-	-	-	-	-	-	-
Jordan	99	99	97	97	97	95	-	-	-	100	100	100	-	-	-	-	-	-	55	41	50	-
Kazakhstan	95	98	92	98	97	99	-	-	-	-	-	-	-	-	-	-	-	-	-	-	-	-
Kenya	62	87	52	33	36	32	27	33	24	-	-	-	-	-	-	-	-	-	68	4	45	47
Kiribati	78	92	61	46	51	39	56	59	51	76	67	86	66	72	60	-	-	-	65	-	-	17
Kuwait	100	-	-	100	-	-	-	-	-	100	100	100	100	100	100	100	100	100	100	100	100	-
Kyrgyzstan	92	99	87	98	95	100	100	100	100	-	-	-	-	-	-	-	-	-	45	-	-	-
Lao People's Democratic Republic	85	97	78	79	98	69	56	73	46	56	56	-	32	32	-	35	35	-	80	4	16	19
Latvia	99	99	99	92	96	84	-	-	-	100	100	100	100	100	100	100	100	100	-	-	-	-
Lebanon	93	-	-	99	-	-	-	-	-	59	60	61	93	92	95	36	34	46	61	16	-	64
Lesotho	72	93	64	50	47	52	6	10	4	-	-	-	-	-	-	-	-	-	-	-	-	-
Liberia	75	86	64	18	29	6	-	-	-	50	44	65	27	24	35	-	-	-	-	-	-	31
Libya	100	-	-	92	-	-	-	-	-	17	-	-	61	-	-	13	-	-	-	-	-	43
Liechtenstein	100	-	-	100	-	-	-	-	-	-	-	-	-	-	-	-	-	-	-	-	-	-
Lithuania	98	100	94	94	98	86	-	-	-	-	-	-	-	-	-	-	-	-	100	-	99	93
Luxembourg	100	100	99	98	97	99	-	-	-	-	-	-	-	-	-	-	-	-	-	-	-	-
Madagascar	53	80	36	12	19	8	27	38	20	37	37	-	-	-	-	-	-	-	-	-	-	-
Malawi	70	86	67	27	34	25	8	14	7	78	87	82	66	79	53	21	28	-	76	3	27	42
Malaysia	97	99	90	-	100	-	-	-	-	97	95	99	99	99	100	98	97	99	-	-	-	-
Maldives	100	99	100	99	100	99	96	97	95	100	100	100	96	-	-	-	-	-	55	15	80	30
Mali	83	96	72	45	56	37	17	27	9	70	70	-	30	30	20	63	63	-	-	-	-	57
Malta	100	100	100	100	100	100	-	-	-	-	-	-	-	-	-	-	-	-	-	-	-	-
Marshall Islands	89	87	94	84	91	59	85	86	80	63	68	57	78	65	92	69	63	74	-	-	-	-
Mauritania	72	89	50	50	75	19	-	-	-	51	51	-	31	27	32	-	-	-	-	-	-	44
Mauritius	100	100	100	-	96	-	-	-	-	100	100	100	100	100	100	93	94	91	-	-	-	-
Mexico	100	100	98	92	94	86	-	-	-	-	-	-	74	74	80	-	-	82	-	-	-	-
Micronesia (Federated States of)	-	-	-	-	-	-	-	-	-	-	-	-	-	-	-	-	-	-	39	18	42	35
Monaco	100	100	-	100	100	-	-	-	-	100	100	100	100	100	100	100	100	100	-	-	-	-
Mongolia	85	97	61	68	76	51	86	89	81	74	73	73	63	70	63	41	44	66	-	-	-	-
Montenegro	99	99	98	98	100	94	99	99	99	-	-	-	-	-	-	-	-	-	100	85	100	100
Montserrat	98	-	-	89	-	-	-	-	-	100	100	100	100	100	100	100	100	100	-	-	-	-
Morocco	90	98	77	87	96	71	-	-	-	85	75	94	82	81	96	88	81	96	-	-	-	-
Mozambique	63	88	49	37	61	23	-	-	-	-	-	-	-	-	-	-	-	-	56	43	-	-
Myanmar	84	95	78	74	79	71	75	83	71	77	74	82	74	72	71	59	54	62	-	-	-	-
Namibia	84	96	71	35	50	20	-	-	-	-	-	-	-	-	-	-	-	-	-	-	-	-

188
THE STATE OF THE WORLD'S CHILDREN 2023

TABLE 14. WASH

Countries and areas	Households 2020									Schools 2021									Healthcare facilities 2021			
	At least basic drinking water services (%)			At least basic sanitation services (%)			Basic hygiene facilities (%)			Basic water services (%)			Basic sanitation services (%)			Basic hygiene services (%)			Basic water services (%)	Basic sanitation services (%)	Basic hygiene services (%)	Basic waste management services (%)
	Total	Urban	Rural	Total	Urban	Rural	Total	Urban	Rural	Total	Primary	Secondary	Total	Primary	Secondary	Total	Primary	Secondary				
Nauru	100	100	-	-	-	-	-	-	-	100	100	100	93	100	83	80	75	86	-	-	-	-
Nepal	90	90	90	77	76	77	62	75	59	47	39	76	-	-	-	-	-	-	-	-	-	-
Netherlands (Kingdom of the)	100	100	100	98	98	100	-	-	-	100	100	100	100	100	100	100	100	100	-	-	-	-
New Zealand	100	100	100	100	100	100	-	-	-	-	-	-	-	-	-	-	-	-	-	-	-	-
Nicaragua	82	97	59	73	81	61	-	-	-	54	-	-	12	-	-	40	-	-	58	-	-	31
Niger	47	86	39	15	52	7	23	39	20	-	-	48	25	26	-	15	15	16	25	0	4	36
Nigeria	78	92	62	43	52	33	33	41	25	35	31	49	38	35	41	19	18	20	52	14	35	35
Niue	97	-	-	96	-	-	-	-	-	100	100	100	100	100	100	100	100	100	-	-	-	-
North Macedonia	98	98	97	98	99	97	100	100	100	-	-	-	-	-	-	-	-	-	100	100	100	100
Norway	100	100	100	98	98	98	-	-	-	100	100	100	100	100	100	100	100	100	-	-	-	-
Oman	92	95	76	99	99	99	97	-	-	100	-	-	98	-	-	100	100	100	100	95	100	98
Pakistan	90	93	89	68	82	60	80	90	74	-	63	85	-	34	60	-	-	-	-	16	55	14
Palau	100	100	100	100	100	99	-	-	-	89	84	95	89	84	95	89	84	95	-	-	-	-
Panama	94	98	86	85	93	65	-	-	-	34	27	41	-	-	-	55	53	56	-	-	-	-
Papua New Guinea	45	86	39	19	49	15	30	62	25	47	46	65	46	46	69	12	11	16	-	-	-	-
Paraguay	100	100	99	93	95	88	80	85	72	72	-	-	-	-	-	-	-	-	85	26	-	6
Peru	93	97	81	79	84	60	-	-	55	77	77	75	80	80	85	-	-	-	46	7	-	28
Philippines	94	97	91	82	82	82	82	85	79	45	45	46	74	70	90	61	64	52	-	-	-	-
Poland	100	100	100	100	100	100	-	-	-	100	100	100	100	100	100	100	100	100	-	-	-	-
Portugal	100	100	100	100	100	100	-	-	-	100	100	100	100	100	100	100	100	100	-	-	-	-
Qatar	100	-	-	100	-	-	-	-	-	100	100	100	100	100	100	100	100	100	-	-	-	-
Republic of Korea	100	-	-	100	-	-	-	-	-	100	100	100	100	100	100	100	100	100	-	-	-	-
Republic of Moldova	91	97	85	79	87	73	-	-	-	92	-	-	-	-	-	100	100	100	-	-	-	-
Romania	100	100	100	87	97	76	-	-	-	72	64	85	72	64	87	72	64	87	-	-	-	-
Russian Federation	97	99	92	89	95	72	-	-	-	-	-	-	-	-	-	-	-	-	-	-	-	-
Rwanda	60	83	56	69	50	73	5	13	3	64	59	77	68	66	73	52	50	49	73	6	65	52
Saint Kitts and Nevis	-	-	-	-	-	-	-	-	-	-	-	100	-	-	-	-	-	100	-	-	-	-
Saint Lucia	97	97	97	83	79	84	-	-	-	100	100	100	100	100	100	97	100	94	-	-	-	-
Saint Vincent and the Grenadines	-	-	-	-	-	-	-	-	-	99	100	99	99	100	99	99	100	99	-	-	-	-
Samoa	92	92	92	97	95	97	79	-	-	100	100	100	100	99	100	100	100	100	-	-	-	-
San Marino	100	-	-	100	-	-	-	-	-	100	100	100	100	100	100	100	100	100	100	-	100	100
Sao Tome and Principe	78	80	74	48	51	39	55	59	44	-	-	-	76	70	-	-	-	-	-	-	-	-
Saudi Arabia	100	-	-	100	-	-	-	-	-	100	100	100	100	100	100	100	100	100	-	-	-	-
Senegal	85	95	75	57	68	46	22	35	10	-	-	-	16	9	40	22	25	9	82	-	-	25
Serbia	95	95	96	98	100	96	-	-	-	98	-	-	99	-	-	98	-	-	98	6	86	85
Seychelles	-	-	-	100	-	-	-	-	-	100	100	100	100	100	100	100	100	100	-	-	-	80
Sierra Leone	64	78	53	17	25	10	21	24	19	49	52	66	20	46	25	-	-	-	25	15	39	64
Singapore	100	100	-	100	100	-	-	-	-	100	100	100	100	100	100	100	100	100	-	-	-	-
Slovakia	100	100	100	98	99	96	-	-	-	100	100	100	100	100	100	100	100	100	-	-	-	-
Slovenia	100	-	-	98	-	-	-	-	-	100	100	100	100	100	100	100	100	100	-	-	-	-
Solomon Islands	67	91	59	35	78	21	-	-	28	36	43	59	17	10	22	12	3	3	69	5	23	19
Somalia	56	79	37	39	56	25	25	32	19	-	-	-	-	-	-	-	-	-	-	-	-	-
South Africa	94	99	83	78	77	81	44	53	27	-	-	-	-	-	-	-	-	-	-	-	-	-
South Sudan	41	70	34	16	42	9	-	-	-	51	51	-	37	37	-	18	18	-	-	-	-	-
Spain	100	100	100	100	100	100	-	-	-	100	100	100	100	100	100	100	100	100	-	-	-	-
Sri Lanka	92	100	91	94	93	94	-	-	-	85	82	87	92	91	93	-	-	-	99	-	-	27
State of Palestine	98	98	99	99	99	98	92	92	92	100	100	100	96	99	99	21	-	-	93	4	87	57
Sudan	60	74	53	37	60	24	13	-	-	43	43	-	-	-	-	8	8	-	27	7	17	3
Suriname	98	99	97	90	94	82	72	75	67	-	-	-	-	-	-	-	-	-	-	-	-	-
Sweden	100	100	100	99	99	100	-	-	-	-	-	-	-	-	-	-	-	-	-	-	-	-
Switzerland	100	100	100	100	100	100	-	-	-	100	100	100	100	100	100	100	100	100	-	-	-	-
Syrian Arab Republic	94	95	92	90	90	90	83	85	80	49	49	49	49	51	47	21	22	23	68	-	-	-
Tajikistan	82	96	77	97	94	98	73	87	68	79	-	-	47	-	-	26	-	-	-	-	-	-
Thailand	100	100	100	99	99	98	85	87	83	100	100	100	100	100	100	100	100	100	88	81	93	-
Timor-Leste	85	96	80	57	74	49	28	43	22	70	71	62	-	-	-	60	61	52	-	-	-	9
Togo	69	91	52	19	33	8	17	27	10	38	33	54	79	78	68	18	19	16	-	-	-	-
Tokelau	100	-	100	97	-	97	-	-	-	100	100	100	100	100	100	100	100	100	100	100	-	67
Tonga	99	100	98	93	95	92	70	80	66	99	98	99	98	97	99	91	86	95	92	-	-	63
Trinidad and Tobago	99	-	-	94	-	-	-	-	-	-	-	-	-	-	-	-	-	-	-	-	-	-
Tunisia	98	99	94	97	98	97	84	91	67	-	-	-	-	-	-	-	-	-	-	-	-	-
Türkiye	97	97	96	99	100	97	-	-	-	-	-	-	-	-	-	-	-	-	-	-	-	-
Turkmenistan	100	100	100	99	99	100	100	100	100	100	100	100	100	100	100	100	100	100	-	-	-	-

FOR EVERY CHILD, VACCINATION

TABLE 14. WASH

Countries and areas	Households 2020									Schools 2021									Healthcare facilities 2021			
	At least basic drinking water services (%)			At least basic sanitation services (%)			Basic hygiene facilities (%)			Basic water services (%)			Basic sanitation services (%)			Basic hygiene services (%)			Basic water services (%)	Basic sanitation services (%)	Basic hygiene services (%)	Basic waste management services (%)
	Total	Urban	Rural	Total	Urban	Rural	Total	Urban	Rural	Total	Primary	Secondary	Total	Primary	Secondary	Total	Primary	Secondary				
Turks and Caicos Islands	-	-	-	-	-	-	-	-	-	100	100	100	100	100	100	100	100	100	-	-	-	-
Tuvalu	100	100	100	-	-	-	-	-	-	76	75	76	86	80	92	100	100	100	-	-	-	-
Uganda	56	79	48	20	28	17	23	36	18	73	73	-	75	77	-	32	30	56	52	-	24	47
Ukraine	94	91	100	98	98	97	-	-	-	-	-	-	-	-	-	82	87	96	-	-	-	-
United Arab Emirates	100	-	-	99	-	-	-	-	-	100	100	100	100	100	100	100	100	100	-	-	-	-
United Kingdom	100	100	100	99	99	99	-	-	-	-	-	-	-	-	-	-	-	-	-	-	-	-
United Republic of Tanzania	61	89	45	32	47	23	48	63	40	56	50	70	44	31	66	15	15	18	55	6	42	28
United States	100	100	100	100	100	99	-	-	-	100	100	100	100	100	100	100	100	100	-	-	-	-
Uruguay	99	100	95	98	98	99	-	-	-	100	100	100	-	-	-	-	-	-	-	-	-	-
Uzbekistan	98	100	96	100	100	100	-	-	-	79	90	89	75	80	71	87	87	87	-	-	-	-
Vanuatu	91	100	88	53	65	49	-	-	-	-	-	-	-	-	-	-	-	-	72	9	27	13
Venezuela (Bolivarian Republic of)	94	-	-	96	-	-	-	-	-	-	-	-	-	-	-	-	-	-	-	-	-	-
Viet Nam	97	99	96	89	96	85	86	93	82	96	96	-	97	97	-	-	-	-	-	-	-	-
Yemen	61	77	51	54	79	39	-	-	-	-	-	-	-	-	-	-	-	-	-	-	-	13
Zambia	65	87	48	32	41	25	18	29	9	79	78	-	-	-	-	57	55	58	-	-	-	-
Zimbabwe	63	93	48	35	42	32	42	56	36	61	60	63	-	-	-	-	-	-	81	17	58	78

SUMMARY

East Asia and Pacific	94	98	89	91	95	85	-	-	-	76	74	76	69	66	73	70	70	68	90	-	38	-
Europe and Central Asia	98	99	97	97	98	93	-	-	-	95	97	98	94	96	96	94	97	98	-	-	-	-
Eastern Europe and Central Asia	96	98	94	94	97	88	-	-	-	-	-	-	-	-	-	81	-	-	-	-	-	-
Western Europe	100	100	100	99	99	99	-	-	-	100	100	100	100	100	100	100	100	100	-	-	-	-
Latin America and Caribbean	97	99	90	89	93	73	-	-	-	-	-	-	74	75	81	-	-	-	-	-	-	-
Middle East and North Africa	95	98	89	92	95	84	-	-	83	79	84	90	86	93	95	82	89	91	81	47	71	40
North America	100	100	100	100	100	99	-	-	-	100	100	100	100	100	100	100	100	100	-	-	-	-
South Asia	91	94	89	69	77	65	68	81	60	74	67	79	81	72	78	52	54	49	-	-	-	-
Sub-Saharan Africa	64	86	49	33	47	23	28	39	21	45	44	50	44	42	52	25	24	28	51	12	36	37
Eastern and Southern Africa	62	86	48	33	50	24	30	43	22	47	47	47	51	48	64	23	22	33	56	13	36	47
West and Central Africa	68	87	50	32	44	22	27	36	19	44	40	53	39	38	44	27	26	23	47	12	36	30
Least developed countries	67	85	57	37	48	31	37	47	31	56	53	67	49	45	59	32	34	31	53	21	32	34
World	**90**	**96**	**82**	**78**	**88**	**66**	**71**	**-**	**60**	**71**	**67**	**76**	**72**	**68**	**75**	**58**	**58**	**60**	**78**	**-**	**51**	**-**

For a complete list of countries and areas in the regions, subregions and country categories, see page on Regional Classifications or visit <data.unicef.org/regionalclassifications>.

It is not advisable to compare data from consecutive editions of *The State of the World's Children* report.

NOTES

- Data not available.

MAIN DATA SOURCES

Basic drinking water, sanitation and hygiene services in households – WHO/UNICEF Joint Monitoring Programme for Water Supply, Sanitation and Hygiene (JMP). Last update: July 2021.

Basic water, sanitation and hygiene services in schools – WHO/UNICEF Joint Monitoring Programme for Water Supply, Sanitation and Hygiene (JMP). Last update: June 2022.

Basic water, sanitation and hygiene services in healthcare facilities – WHO/UNICEF Joint Monitoring Programme for Water Supply, Sanitation and Hygiene (JMP). Last update: August 2022.

DEFINITIONS OF THE INDICATORS

Population using at least basic drinking water services – Percentage of the population using an improved drinking water source, where collection time is not more than 30 minutes for a round trip including queuing (improved sources include: piped water; boreholes or tubewells; protected dug wells; protected springs; rainwater; and packaged or delivered water).

Population using at least basic sanitation services – Percentage of the population using an improved sanitation facility that is not shared with other households. Improved facilities include: flush/pour flush to piped sewerage systems, septic tanks or pit latrines; ventilated improved pit latrines; composting toilets or pit latrines with slabs.

Population with basic hygiene facilities – Percentage of the population with a handwashing facility with water and soap available at home.

Proportion of schools with basic water services – Percentage of schools with drinking water from an improved source available at the school at the time of the survey.

Proportion of schools with basic sanitation services – Percentage of schools with improved sanitation facilities at the school that are single-sex and usable (available, functional and private) at the time of the survey.

Proportion of schools with basic hygiene services – Percentage of schools with handwashing facilities with water and soap available at the school at the time of the survey.

Proportion of health care facilities with basic water services – Percentage of health care facilities with water available from an improved source located on premises.

Proportion of health care facilities with basic sanitation services – Percentage of health care facilities with improved sanitation facilities that are usable with at least one toilet dedicated for staff, at least one sex-separated toilet with menstrual hygiene facilities, and at least one toilet accessible for people with limited mobility.

Proportion of health care facilities with basic hygiene services – Percentage of health care facilities with functional hand hygiene facilities (with water and soap and/or alcohol-based hand rub) available at points of care, and within five metres of toilets.

Proportion of health care facilities with basic waste management services – Percentage of health care facilities where waste is safely segregated into at least three bins, and sharps and infectious waste are treated and disposed of safely.

TABLE 15. ADOLESCENTS

Countries and areas	Adolescent population 2021		Nutrition		Protection			Education and learning				Transition to work (%) 2013–2021 [R]					
	Aged 10–19 (thousands)	Proportion of total population (%)	Thinness 2016	Overweight 2016	Intimate partner violence (%) 2013–2020 [R]	Bullying (%) 2011–2018 [R]		Proficiency in math		Proficiency in reading		Not in education, employment, or training		Unemployment		Engagement in household chores	
	Total	Total	Total	Total	Female	Male	Female	Male	Female	Male	Female	Male	Female	Male	Female	Male	Female
Afghanistan	9,809	24	17	9	29	42	45	-	-	-	-	51	82	9	9	9	22
Albania	349	12	1	24	-	17	18	56	59	38	58	21	17	34	19	1 x	3 x
Algeria	7,107	16	6	29	-	48	55	18	21	15	28	-	-	32	38	1	1
Andorra	8	11	1	34	-	-	-	-	-	-	-	-	-	-	-	-	-
Angola	7,990	23	8	11	24	-	-	-	-	-	-	18	27	17	15	15	19
Anguilla	2	12	-	-	-	22	30	-	-	-	-	-	-	-	-	-	-
Antigua and Barbuda	13	14	3	25	-	24 x	27 x	-	-	-	-	-	-	-	-	-	-
Argentina	7,043	16	1	34	-	25	24	35	27	45	51	10 y	12 y	24 y	39 y	0 x	1 x
Armenia	341	12	2	18	0 p	19	15	48	52	-	-	26	11	27	24	0	1
Australia	3,105	12	1	33	-	-	-	78	77	76	85	-	-	18	13	-	-
Austria	856	10	2	26	-	20	21	79	78	71	82	14 y	8 y	17 y	16 y	-	-
Azerbaijan	1,533	15	3	18	12 x	25	26	-	-	-	-	-	-	12 y	17 y	-	-
Bahamas	64	16	3	34	-	25	22	-	-	-	-	-	-	38 x	46 x	-	-
Bahrain	173	12	6	34	-	36	23	36	43	-	-	-	-	10 x	21 x	-	-
Bangladesh	32,305	19	18	8	28 y	27	17	-	-	-	-	10	30	12	18	0	4
Barbados	36	13	4	26	-	15	11	-	-	-	-	26	23	50	29	0 x	0 x
Belarus	1,023	11	2	22	-	-	-	71	70	72	82	6	5	32	29	0	0
Belgium	1,331	11	1	23	-	16	18	82	79	75	82	-	-	29	20	-	-
Belize	76	19	4	27	-	30	31	-	-	-	-	20	32	16	29	1	3
Benin	2,925	23	7	11	14	47	52	-	-	-	-	32	38	-	-	15	26
Bhutan	137	18	15	9	-	31	29	-	-	-	-	3	2	22	-	2 x	5 x
Bolivia (Plurinational State of)	2,404	20	1	27	-	32	28	-	-	-	-	6	10	6	6	-	-
Bosnia and Herzegovina	338	10	2	21	-	-	-	-	-	38	55	10 y	7 y	48 y	53 y	-	-
Botswana	512	20	6	16	-	53 x	52 x	-	-	-	-	28	29	45	56	-	-
Brazil	30,986	14	3	26	-	-	-	34	30	44	56	13	18	34	46	1	1
British Virgin Islands	4	13	-	-	-	18 x	17 x	-	-	-	-	-	-	-	-	-	-
Brunei Darussalam	67	15	6	25	-	25	22	50	54	42	55	17	14	22	35	-	-
Bulgaria	653	9	2	27	-	35	33	55	56	45	62	-	-	-	-	-	-
Burkina Faso	5,296	24	8	8	5 x	-	-	-	-	-	-	31	44	9	8	9 x	29 x
Burundi	3,072	24	7	10	38	-	-	-	-	-	-	13	11	2	1	21	30
Cabo Verde	107	18	7	12	-	-	-	-	-	-	-	-	-	27 y	47 y	-	-
Cambodia	3,058	18	11	10	7	23	22	11	9	6	9	12	11	3	2	2 x	6 x
Cameroon	6,272	23	6	12	20	-	-	-	-	-	-	9	18	3	5	8	22
Canada	4,128	11	1	31	-	36	40	84	84	82	90	12	10	16	15	-	-
Central African Republic	1,453	27	8	10	32 x	-	-	-	-	-	-	-	-	-	-	17	23
Chad	4,101	24	9	8	15	-	-	-	-	-	-	27	44	3	-	20	40
Chile	2,448	13	1	34	-	16	14	32	24	64	73	8	10	21	32	8 x	10 x
China	166,138	12	4	25	-	-	-	-	-	-	-	-	-	-	-	-	-
Colombia	7,870	15	2	24	-	-	-	40	30	48	52	18	26	20	34	1	2
Comoros	174	21	7	12	4 x	-	-	-	-	-	-	18	24	22	-	15 x	28 x
Congo	1,336	23	8	11	-	-	-	-	-	-	-	-	-	-	-	8	9
Cook Islands	3	15	<1	62	6 x,y	29	32	-	-	-	-	7	14	2	5	-	-
Costa Rica	741	14	2	30	-	18 x	20 x	45	35	55	61	15	16	52	69	1	0
Côte d'Ivoire	6,553	24	6	12	20 x,y	-	-	-	-	-	-	11	23	4	-	11	22
Croatia	399	10	2	26	-	23	21	70	68	72	85	-	-	36	37	-	-
Cuba	1,244	11	4	28	-	-	-	-	-	-	-	-	-	-	-	-	-
Cyprus	127	10	1	32	-	-	-	-	-	46	67	9	10	28	34	-	-
Czechia	1,072	10	2	26	-	17	19	79	80	74	85	4	4	29	21	-	-
Democratic People's Republic of Korea	3,330	13	5	22	-	-	-	-	-	-	-	-	-	-	-	-	-
Democratic Republic of the Congo	22,086	23	10	10	36	-	-	-	-	-	-	25	30	-	-	7	17
Denmark	679	12	1	24	-	12	15	85	86	79	89	-	-	14	13	-	-
Djibouti	226	20	6	16	-	44 x	36 x	-	-	-	-	17	24	88	85	-	-
Dominica	11	15	3	31	-	29 x	26 x	-	-	-	-	-	-	-	-	-	-
Dominican Republic	1,975	18	3	31	22	26	22	10	9	16	26	25	29	12	29	1	2
Ecuador	3,164	18	1	27	-	-	-	34	24	47	52	10	20	5	10	-	-
Egypt	20,530	19	3	35	17	70	70	20	23	-	-	7	22	10	32	1	5
El Salvador	1,149	18	2	29	7 y	21	24	-	-	-	-	14	27	8	15	5	13
Equatorial Guinea	331	20	8	10	56 x,p	-	-	-	-	-	-	-	-	-	-	-	-
Eritrea	909	25	8	10	-	-	-	-	-	-	-	-	-	-	-	-	-
Estonia	143	11	2	19	-	30	30	90	90	86	92	5	3	37	33	-	-

FOR EVERY CHILD, VACCINATION

191

TABLE 15. ADOLESCENTS

Countries and areas	Adolescent population 2021 Aged 10–19 (thousands) Total	Proportion of total population (%) Total	Nutrition Thinness 2016 Total	Overweight 2016 Total	Protection Intimate partner violence (%) 2013–2020 [R] Female	Bullying (%) 2011–2018 [R] Male	Bullying (%) Female	Education and learning Proficiency in math Male	Proficiency in math Female	Proficiency in reading Male	Proficiency in reading Female	Transition to work (%) 2013–2021 [R] Not in education, employment, or training Male	NEET Female	Unemployment Male	Unemployment Female	Engagement in household chores Male	Engagement in household chores Female
Eswatini	259	22	4	16	-	33	31	-	-	-	-	17	25	37	43	2 x	3 x
Ethiopia	28,114	23	10	8	24	-	-	-	-	-	-	9	18	3	6	14	21
Fiji	167	18	4	33	47 x,y	33	26	-	-	-	-	8	13	16	32	3	2
Finland	614	11	1	25	-	27	24	83	87	80	93	-	-	22	25	-	-
France	7,911	12	1	29	-	13	16	79	79	75	84	7 y	5 y	21 y	29 y	-	-
Gabon	468	20	6	15	40 x	-	-	-	-	-	-	-	-	27 x	38 x	6 x	7 x
Gambia	639	24	7	11	14	-	-	-	-	-	-	25	22	6	4	3	17
Georgia	462	12	3	19	-	17	20	38	40	28	44	17	14	31	32	0	0
Germany	7,602	9	1	25	-	21	21	79	79	76	84	-	-	8	9	-	-
Ghana	7,079	22	6	10	23 x,y	-	-	-	-	-	-	17	21	3	4	13	19
Greece	1,100	11	1	35	-	18	21	63	65	61	78	6	5	46	56	-	-
Grenada	18	15	4	25	-	29 x	26 x	-	-	-	-	-	-	-	-	-	-
Guatemala	3,787	22	1	27	9	26	20	12	10	28	33	10	40	4	4	-	-
Guinea	3,146	23	7	9	-	-	-	-	-	-	-	27	40	-	-	11	18
Guinea-Bissau	483	23	7	10	-	-	-	-	-	-	-	13	22	2	-	4	9
Guyana	148	18	6	24	-	40 x	37 x				-	40	49	30	47	2	3
Haiti	2,336	20	4	26	28	-	-				-	8 x	17 x	-	-	19 x	13 x
Holy See	-	-	-	-	-						-	-		-		-	
Honduras	2,124	21	2	26	8	13 y	12 y	19	12	28	31	13	37	12	27	4	12
Hungary	973	10	2	27	-	27	28	69	65	70	79	6	6	29	30	-	-
Iceland	47	13	1	27	-	12	11	77	82	66	81	-	-	15	12	-	-
India	253,718	18	27	6	18	-	-	-	-	-	-	13	28	26	15	-	-
Indonesia	45,844	17	10	14	-	24	19	26	30	24	36	14	15	16	15	-	-
Iran (Islamic Republic of)	12,194	14	9	25	-	-	-	-	-	-	-	12	24	17	21	-	-
Iraq	9,609	22	5	30	-	32	22	-	-	-	-	17	38	36	52	1	6
Ireland	683	14	<1	29	-	32	32	84	84	85	91	-	-	18	23	-	-
Israel	1,458	16	1	34	-	29	18	63	69	60	77	-	-	8	6	-	-
Italy	5,656	10	1	34	-	11	12	64	61	72	81	-	-	48	55	-	-
Jamaica	441	16	2	28	11 y	26	25	-	-	-	-	26	25	26	35	1	0
Japan	10,966	9	2	13	-	-	-	-	-	-	-	-	-	4	4	-	-
Jordan	2,288	21	4	30	15	47 x	37 x	40	41	46	71	22	21	54	41	0	2
Kazakhstan	3,033	16	2	19	-	15	16	51	51	29	43	-	-	3 y	3 y	-	-
Kenya	12,725	24	8	11	23	57 x	57 x	-	-	-	-	9	13	8	7	-	-
Kiribati	25	20	<1	54	67 p	42	32	-	-	-	-	43	26	29	-	17	19
Kuwait	536	13	4	43	-	36	28	20	16	-	-	-	-	-	-	-	-
Kyrgyzstan	1,185	18	3	15	3 x	-	-	-	-	-	-	8	9	10	10	5	11
Lao People's Democratic Republic	1,472	20	9	13	14 y	15	11	-	-	-	-	20	21	4	4	5	11
Latvia	190	10	2	20	-	44	49	83	83	71	84	-	-	-	-	-	-
Lebanon	1,038	19	5	31	-	24	12	36	34	28	36	15	20	28	29	-	-
Lesotho	470	21	6	15	-	-	-	-	-	-	-	22	30	10	35	11	16
Liberia	1,250	24	7	10	58	43	51	-	-	-	-	37	36	9	5	18	21
Libya	1,309	19	6	31	-	40 x	31 x	-	-	-	-	-	-	-	-	-	-
Liechtenstein	4	10	-	-	-	-	-	-	-	-	-	-	-	-	-	-	-
Lithuania	264	9	3	19	-	51	51	73	76	68	83	-	-	-	-	-	-
Luxembourg	67	11	1	25	-	21	23	74	72	66	76	-	-	37	29	-	-
Madagascar	6,583	23	7	10	19	-	-	-	-	-	-	3 x	3 x	3	2	17	26
Malawi	5,044	25	6	10	28	43 x	47 x	-	-	-	-	10	16	-	-	5	12
Malaysia	5,224	16	8	25	-	19 y	14 y	56	60	47	61	-	-	15 y	16 y	-	-
Maldives	67	13	14	16	4	30	30	-	-	-	-	30	26	29	16	-	-
Mali	5,366	24	8	10	21 y	-	-	-	-	-	-	16	36	7	11	2	8
Malta	44	8	1	35	-	29	21	61	63	55	74	17	22	22	17	-	-
Marshall Islands	8	19	<1	58	27 y	-	-	-	-	-	-	31	23	-	-	-	-
Mauritania	1,105	24	8	13	-	48 x	46 x	-	-	-	-	29	44	18	23	13	23
Mauritius	175	13	7	14	-	29	22	-	-	-	-	-	-	-	-	-	-
Mexico	21,813	17	2	34	-	-	-	47	41	52	58	9	19	7	9	2	3
Micronesia (Federated States of)	24	21	<1	50	35 y	-	-	-	-	-	-	18	23	-	29	-	-
Monaco	3	8	<1	<1	-	-	-	-	-	-	-	-	-	-	-	-	-
Mongolia	534	16	2	17	8 y	36	25	-	-	-	-	11	7	17	-	18	14
Montenegro	78	12	2	24	-	-	-	55	52	48	63	12	10	44	-	0	0
Montserrat	1	13	-	-	-	32 x	25 x	-	-	-	-	-	-	-	-	-	-

192

THE STATE OF THE WORLD'S CHILDREN 2023

TABLE 15. ADOLESCENTS

Countries and areas	Adolescent population 2021 Aged 10–19 (thousands) Total	Proportion of total population (%) Total	Nutrition Thinness 2016 Total	Nutrition Overweight 2016 Total	Protection Intimate partner violence (%) 2013–2020 [R] Female	Protection Bullying (%) 2011–2018 [R] Male	Bullying (%) Female	Education and learning Proficiency in math Male	Proficiency in math Female	Proficiency in reading Male	Proficiency in reading Female	Transition to work (%) 2013–2021 [R] Not in education, employment, or training Male	Not in education, employment, or training Female	Unemployment Male	Unemployment Female	Engagement in household chores Male	Engagement in household chores Female
Morocco	6,255	17	6	26	-	44	32	14	15	22	32	-	-	17 x	11 x	-	-
Mozambique	7,583	24	4	12	10 y	45	46	-	-	-	-	-	-	7	5	-	-
Myanmar	9,069	17	13	11	22	51	49	-	-	-	-	9	12	6	6	-	-
Namibia	509	20	8	14	52 p	48	45	-	-	-	-	17	20	37	39	-	-
Nauru	3	21	<1	64	-	40	38	-	-	-	-	22 y	39 y	33 y	61 y	-	-
Nepal	6,171	21	16	7	17	56	45	-	-	-	-	16	30	22	24	7	17
Netherlands (Kingdom of the)	1,974	11	1	24	-	12	12	84	85	71	81	-	-	12	13	-	-
New Zealand	654	13	<1	38	-	-	-	79	78	77	86	-	-	17	16	-	-
Nicaragua	1,319	19	2	28	-	-	-	-	-	-	-	7	32	6	11	-	-
Niger	6,072	24	10	8	-	-	-	-	-	-	-	57 y	72 y	19 y	17 y	18 x	25 x
Nigeria	49,904	23	10	8	13	-	-	-	-	-	-	24	34	27	40	17	19
Niue	0	16	<1	58	-	38 x	-	-	-	-	-	-	-	-	-	-	-
North Macedonia	240	11	2	25	-	18	18	37	41	34	57	9	8	40	62	1	1
Norway	645	12	1	27	-	16	14	79	83	74	88	-	-	20	19	-	-
Oman	590	13	7	30	-	45	39	20	27	-	-	-	-	50 y	40 y	-	-
Pakistan	51,846	22	19	9	17 y	45 x	35 x	-	-	-	-	14	46	10	8	-	-
Palau	2	14	<1	62	8 y	-	-	-	-	-	-	-	-	-	-	-	-
Panama	731	17	2	28	-	-	-	21	17	33	39	12	12	17	26	0	1
Papua New Guinea	2,094	21	1	31	60	-	-	-	-	-	-	26 x	30 x	3 x	2 x	-	-
Paraguay	1,214	18	2	27	-	19	15	11	6	30	34	11	23	13	27	4	9
Peru	5,918	18	1	26	18	47 x	48 x	-	-	-	-	19	23	7	9	3	5
Philippines	22,156	19	10	12	11	53	49	-	-	15	23	9	9	5	8	-	-
Poland	3,882	10	2	24	-	23	18	85	86	80	90	-	-	18	23	-	-
Portugal	1,034	10	1	30	-	17	19	77	77	76	84	-	-	32	41	-	-
Qatar	205	8	5	37	-	49	35	36	37	36	62	-	-	0 y	0 y	-	-
Republic of Korea	4,658	9	2	25	-	-	-	84	86	81	89	-	-	7	8	-	-
Republic of Moldova	354	12	3	17	15 x	43	44	49	50	49	66	5	4	-	-	-	-
Romania	2,083	11	3	23	-	31	30	54	53	52	67	-	-	43	45	-	-
Russian Federation	15,631	11	2	19	-	31	35	78	78	73	83	-	-	26	32	-	-
Rwanda	3,120	23	6	11	-	-	-	-	-	-	-	25	23	24	23	0	0
Saint Kitts and Nevis	6	14	4	27	-	25	20	-	-	-	-	-	-	-	-	-	-
Saint Lucia	25	14	4	22	-	24	29	-	-	-	-	34 y	30 y	65 y	54 y	3 x	1 x
Saint Vincent and the Grenadines	15	15	4	28	-	31 x	29 x	-	-	-	-	-	-	-	-	-	-
Samoa	46	21	<1	51	-	43	34	-	-	-	-	17	19	12	35	3	2
San Marino	3	10	<1	<1	-	-	-	-	-	-	-	-	-	-	-	-	-
Sao Tome and Principe	53	24	6	13	28 x	-	-	-	-	-	-	-	-	-	-	4	11
Saudi Arabia	5,735	16	8	35	-	-	-	12	11	34	62	-	-	27	44	-	-
Senegal	3,915	23	10	9	3	-	-	8	7	8	9	21	37	-	5	6	23
Serbia	714	10	2	26	-	17	19	60	61	55	70	11	10	28	38	1	2
Seychelles	15	14	6	21	-	45	50	-	-	-	-	31	23	31	27	-	-
Sierra Leone	1,950	23	7	10	43	60	57	-	-	-	-	24	28	-	-	12	20
Singapore	498	8	2	21	-	-	-	92	95	86	92	4	2	2	11	-	-
Slovakia	551	10	1	22	-	20	19	75	75	62	75	6 y	5 y	41 y	56 y	-	-
Slovenia	208	10	1	25	-	26	23	83	84	75	89	3	4	17	21	-	-
Solomon Islands	155	22	1	24	-	64	68	-	-	-	-	5 y	6 y	-	-	6	9
Somalia	4,051	24	7	12	-	-	-	-	-	-	-	34	40	40	37	-	-
South Africa	10,222	17	4	26	12 y	-	-	-	-	-	-	11	11	23	34	1	2
South Sudan	2,858	27	<1	<1	-	-	-	-	-	-	-	-	-	-	-	-	-
Spain	4,998	11	1	32	-	10	9	75	75	80	87	-	-	50	52	-	-
Sri Lanka	3,535	16	15	12	-	50	29	-	-	-	-	11	12	29	35	0	0
State of Palestine	1,147	22	-	-	-	-	-	-	-	-	-	21	14	42	-	1	2
Sudan	10,079	22	<1	<1	-	-	-	-	-	-	-	17 x	33 x	29 x	33 x	4	8
Suriname	109	18	4	30	-	25	25	-	-	-	-	11	11	23	62	1	2
Sweden	1,225	12	2	23	-	18	19	81	82	77	86	-	-	42	38	-	-
Switzerland	852	10	<1	21	-	14	18	84	83	72	82	11	10	9	11	-	-
Syrian Arab Republic	5,576	26	6	27	-	-	-	-	-	-	-	-	-	19 x	27 x	-	-
Tajikistan	1,945	20	4	14	6	7 x	7 x	-	-	-	-	-	-	12 y	7 y	-	-
Thailand	8,219	11	8	20	-	38	28	43	51	31	49	8	9	5	5	-	-
Timor-Leste	312	24	11	11	38	39	25	-	-	-	-	11	15	-	13	4	6
Togo	1,954	23	7	10	13	-	-	-	-	-	-	15	25	11	2	19	31
Tokelau	0	21	-	-	-	39	39	-	-	-	-	-	-	-	-	-	-

FOR EVERY CHILD, VACCINATION

193

TABLE 15. ADOLESCENTS

Countries and areas	Adolescent population 2021 Aged 10–19 (thousands) Total	Proportion of total population (%) Total	Nutrition Thinness 2016 Total	Overweight 2016 Total	Protection Intimate partner violence (%) 2013–2020 [R] Female	Bullying (%) 2011–2018 [R] Male	Bullying Female	Education and learning Proficiency in math Male	Proficiency in math Female	Proficiency in reading Male	Proficiency in reading Female	Transition to work (%) 2013–2021 [R] Not in education, employment, or training Male	NEET Female	Unemployment Male	Unemployment Female	Engagement in household chores Male	Engagement in household chores Female
Tonga	23	22	<1	57	-	46	31	-	-	-	-	20	16	1	14	3	0
Trinidad and Tobago	200	13	6	23	-	13	18	43	52	48	67	10	11	-	30	0 x	0 x
Tunisia	1,782	15	7	24	-	37 x	24 x	27	24	23	33	19	18	33	26	1 x	1 x
Türkiye	12,767	15	5	28	18 y	39	33	41	43	68	79	13	21	17	22	-	-
Turkmenistan	1,085	17	3	17	-	-	-	-	-	-	-	-	-	-	-	0	0
Turks and Caicos Islands	5	11	-	-	-	-	-	-	-	-	-	-	-	-	-	5	2
Tuvalu	2	18	<1	57	-	40	15	-	-	-	-	17 y	29 y	-	-	0	0
Uganda	11,645	25	6	10	31	50 x	41 x	49	34	50	49	14	18	5	4	7	18
Ukraine	4,485	10	2	20	2 x	40	41	-	-	68	81	-	-	29 y	27 y	2 x	2 x
United Arab Emirates	744	8	5	34	-	33	22	45	48	46	68	-	-	32	30	-	-
United Kingdom	7,876	12	1	30	-	38	37	82	80	79	86	-	-	19	13	-	-
United Republic of Tanzania	15,031	24	7	11	30	25 y	28 y	-	-	-	-	8	14	2	3	4	7
United States	43,810	13	1	41	-	26 x,y	25 x,y	74	72	77	85	-	-	-	-	-	-
Uruguay	478	14	2	32	-	18	20	51	48	53	63	9	10	39	52	1 x	2 x
Uzbekistan	5,611	16	3	16	-	-	-	-	-	-	-	-	-	22	21	-	-
Vanuatu	68	21	2	29	-	60	46	-	-	-	-	25	30	14	15	1	0
Venezuela (Bolivarian Republic of)	5,420	19	2	33	-	-	-	-	-	-	-	16	25	21 y	24 y	-	-
Viet Nam	14,107	14	14	9	16 x,y	26	26	79	83	81	91	13	13	7	6	3	4
Yemen	7,580	23	14	18	-	47	33	-	-	-	-	18	58	25	29	-	-
Zambia	4,697	24	6	12	27	63 x	67 x	2	3	4	6	19	24	6	8	8 x	9 x
Zimbabwe	3,788	24	6	14	31	-	-	-	-	-	-	16	28	7	9	4	10

SUMMARY

East Asia and Pacific	302,032	13	-	-	-	-	-	-	-	-	-	-	-	-	-	-	-
Europe and Central Asia	106,929	12	-	-	-	26	26	-	-	-	-	-	-	24	26	-	-
Eastern Europe and Central Asia	54,309	13	-	-	-	33	32	-	-	-	-	-	-	22	25	-	-
Western Europe	52,619	11	-	-	-	20	20	-	-	-	-	-	-	25	27	-	-
Latin America and Caribbean	105,350	16	-	-	-	-	-	-	-	-	-	13	21	20	28	-	-
Middle East and North Africa	85,858	18	-	-	-	51	46	-	-	-	-	13	29	23	33	-	-
North America	47,938	13	-	-	-	-	-	-	-	-	-	8	8	13	11	-	-
South Asia	357,589	19	-	-	19	-	-	-	-	-	-	14	32	22	15	-	-
Sub-Saharan Africa	273,695	23	-	-	22	-	-	-	-	-	-	19	27	13	17	9	15
Eastern and Southern Africa	139,851	23	-	-	24	-	-	-	-	-	-	12	18	9	10	8	13
West and Central Africa	133,844	23	-	-	20	-	-	-	-	-	-	24	34	19	27	9	16
Least developed countries	245,872	22	-	-	26	-	-	-	-	-	-	19	30	10	11	8	16
World	**1,283,495**	**16**	**-**	**-**	**19**	**-**	**-**	**-**	**-**	**-**	**-**	**13**	**22**	**17**	**17**	**-**	**-**

For a complete list of countries and areas in the regions, subregions and country categories, see page on Regional Classifications or visit <data.unicef.org/regionalclassifications>.

It is not advisable to compare data from consecutive editions of *The State of the World's Children* report.

NOTES

- Data not available.

y Data differ from the standard definition or refer to only part of a country. If they fall within the noted reference period, such data are included in the calculation of regional and global averages.

p Based on small denominators (typically 25–49 unweighted cases). No data based on fewer than 25 unweighted cases are displayed.

x Data refer to years or periods other than those specified in the column heading. Such data are not included in the calculation of regional and global averages. Estimates from data years prior to 2000 are not displayed.

R Data refer to the most recent year available during the period specified in the column heading.

MAIN DATA SOURCES

Adolescent population – United Nations, Department of Economic and Social Affairs, Population Division (2019). *2019 Revision of World Population Prospects.*

Thinness and overweight – NCD Risk Factor Collaboration (NCD-RisC), based on Worldwide trends in body mass index, underweight, overweight and obesity from 1975 to 2016: a pooled analysis of 2416 population-based measurement studies in 128.9 million children, adolescents, and adults. The Lancet 2017, 390 (10113): 2627–2642. Last update: August 2019.

Intimate partner violence – DHS, MICS and other national surveys. Last update: March 2022.

Bullying – Health Behaviour in School-aged Children Study (HBSC), Global School-based Student Health Surveys (GSHS) and other national surveys. Last update: March 2022.

Proficiency in math and reading – United Nations Statistics Division. Last update: April 2019.

NEET – International Labour Organization. Last update: December 2022.

Unemployment – International Labour Organization. Last update: December 2022.

Engagement in household chores – DHS, MICS and other national surveys. Last update: March 2022.

DEFINITIONS OF THE INDICATORS

Thinness – Percentage of adolescents aged 10–19 years with BMI < –2 standard deviations of the median according to the WHO growth reference for school-age children and adolescents.

Overweight – Percentage of adolescents aged 10–19 years with BMI > 1 standard deviations of the median according to the WHO growth reference for school-age children and adolescents.

Intimate partner violence – Percentage of ever-partnered girls aged 15–19 years who have experienced physical and/or sexual violence by a current or former intimate partner during the last twelve months.

Bullying – Percentage of students aged 13–15 years who reported being bullied on one or more days in the past 30 days.

Proficiency in math – Percentage of children and young people at the end of lower secondary achieving at least a minimum proficiency level in math.

Proficiency in reading – Percentage of children and young people at the end of lower secondary achieving at least a minimum proficiency level in reading.

Not in education, employment or training (NEET) – Percentage of adolescents aged 15–19 years not in education, employment or training.

Unemployment – Percentage of adolescents aged 15–19 years in the labour force who are unemployed.

Engagement in household chores – Percentage of adolescents aged 10–14 years who, during the reference week, spent at least 21 hours on unpaid household services.

TABLE 16. CHILDREN WITH DISABILITIES

Countries and areas	Children with disabilities (%) 2015–2021 [R]			Child nutrition 2015–2021 [R]				Early childhood development 2015–2021 [R]				Education				Child protection 2015–2021 [R]		WASH 2015–2021 [R]		Social protection and equity 2017–2021 [R]	
				Moderate and severe underweight (%)		Moderate and severe stunting (%)		Early stimulation and responsive care (%)		Early childhood education (%)		Never attended school (%) 2015–2021 [R]		Foundational learning skills (%) 2017–2021 [R]		Severe physical punishment (%)		Basic sanitation services on premises (%)		Social transfers (%)	
	Aged 2–17	Aged 2–4	Aged 5–17	With dis-abilities	With-out dis-abilities	With dis-abilities	With-out dis-abilities	With dis-abilities	With-out dis-abilities	With dis-abilities	With-out dis-abilities	With dis-abilities	With-out dis-abilities	With dis-abilities	With-out dis-abilities	With dis-abilities	With-out dis-abilities	With dis-abilities	With-out dis-abilities	With dis-abilities	With-out dis-abilities
Afghanistan	-	-	-	-		-		-	-			-	-		-	-		-		-	
Albania	-	-	-	-		-		-	-		-	-		-		-		-		-	-
Algeria	17	3	20	7	2	14	10	46	62	7	15	3	1	-	-	23	17	86	86	34	26
Andorra	-	-	-	-		-		-	-			-	-		-	-		-		-	
Angola	-	-	-	-		-		-	-			-	-		-	-		-		-	
Anguilla	-	-	-	-		-		-	-			-	-		-	-		-		-	
Antigua and Barbuda	-	-	-	-		-		-	-			-	-		-	-		-		-	
Argentina	11	4	14	4	3	13	10	85	85	57	65	0	0	-	-	12	6	95	96	-	-
Armenia	-	-	-	-		-		-	-			-	-		-	-		-		-	
Australia	-	-	-	-		-		-	-			-	-		-	-		-		-	
Austria	-	-	-	-		-		-	-			-	-		-	-		-		-	
Azerbaijan	-	-	-	-		-		-	-			-	-		-	-		-		-	
Bahamas	-	-	-	-		-		-	-			-	-		-	-		-		-	
Bahrain	-	-	-	-		-		-	-			-	-		-	-		-		-	
Bangladesh	7	3	8	33	25	42	30	58	63	13	19	8	2	19	25	42	30	56	63	72	70
Barbados	-	-	-	-		-		-	-			-	-		-	-		-		-	
Belarus	4	2	5	-	-	-	-	96 p	97	73	91	2	0	60	67	0	0	98	99	76	63
Belgium	-	-	-	-		-		-	-			-	-		-	-		-		-	
Belize	-	-	-	-		-		-	-			-	-		-	-		-		-	
Benin	-	-	-	-		-		-	-			-	-		-	-		-		-	
Bhutan	-	-	-	-		-		-	-			-	-		-	-		-		-	
Bolivia (Plurinational State of)	-	-	-	-		-		-	-			-	-		-	-		-		-	
Bosnia and Herzegovina	-	-	-	-		-		-	-			-	-		-	-		-		-	
Botswana	-	-	-	-		-		-	-			-	-		-	-		-		-	
Brazil	-	-	-	-		-		-	-			-	-		-	-		-		-	
British Virgin Islands	-	-	-	-		-		-	-			-	-		-	-		-		-	
Brunei Darussalam	-	-	-	-		-		-	-			-	-		-	-		-		-	
Bulgaria	-	-	-	-		-		-	-			-	-		-	-		-		-	
Burkina Faso	-	-	-	-		-		-	-			-	-		-	-		-		-	
Burundi	-	-	-	-		-		-	-			-	-		-	-		-		-	
Cabo Verde	-	-	-	-		-		-	-			-	-		-	-		-		-	
Cambodia	-	-	-	-		-		-	-			-	-		-	-		-		-	
Cameroon	-	-	-	-		-		-	-			-	-		-	-		-		-	
Canada	-	-	-	-		-		-	-			-	-		-	-		-		-	
Central African Republic	27	15	31	30	23	54	47	34 y	40 y	4	7	13	10	0	1	48	35	8	10	40	37
Chad	24	10	29	36	29	48	42	55	55	1	1	48	41	4	3	35	31	9	10	2	2
Chile	-	-	-	-		-		-	-			-	-		-	-		-		-	
China	-	-	-	-		-		-	-			-	-		-	-		-		-	
Colombia	-	-	-	-		-		-	-			-	-		-	-		-		-	
Comoros	-	-	-	-		-		-	-			-	-		-	-		-		-	
Congo	-	-	-	-		-		-	-			-	-		-	-		-		-	
Cook Islands	-	-	-	-		-		-	-			-	-		-	-		-		-	
Costa Rica	18	7	21	7	3	10	8	71	76	40	44	0	0	-	-	5	2	94	96	49	44
Côte d'Ivoire	-	-	-	-		-		-	-			-	-		-	-		-		-	
Croatia	-	-	-	-		-		-	-		-	-		-		-		-		-	-
Cuba	8	2	11	0	3	38	7	87	90	29	50	0	0	-	-	6	1	83	86	-	-
Cyprus	-	-	-	-		-		-	-			-	-		-	-		-		-	
Czechia	-	-	-	-		-		-	-			-	-		-	-		-		-	
Democratic People's Republic of Korea	1	2	1	-		-		-	-			-	-		-	-		-		-	
Democratic Republic of the Congo	16	7	20	32	25	57	47	33	45	4	5	7	5	0	1	47	42	14	13	-	-
Denmark	-	-	-	-		-		-	-			-	-		-	-		-		-	
Djibouti	-	-	-	-		-		-	-			-	-		-	-		-		-	
Dominica	-	-	-	-		-		-	-			-	-		-	-		-		-	
Dominican Republic	10	5	11	7	2	11	5	53	64	32	49	0	0	-	-	7	4	83	86	-	-
Ecuador	-	-	-	-		-		-	-			-	-		-	-		-		-	
Egypt	-	-	-	-		-		-	-			-	-		-	-		-		-	
El Salvador	-	-	-	-		-		-	-			-	-		-	-		-		-	
Equatorial Guinea	-	-	-	-		-		-	-			-	-		-	-		-		-	
Eritrea	-	-	-	-		-		-	-			-	-		-	-		-		-	
Estonia	-	-	-	-		-		-	-			-	-		-	-		-		-	
Eswatini	-	-	-	-		-		-	-			-	-		-	-		-		-	

FOR EVERY CHILD, VACCINATION

TABLE 16. CHILDREN WITH DISABILITIES

Countries and areas	Children with disabilities (%) 2015–2021 R			Child nutrition 2015–2021 R				Early childhood development 2015–2021 R				Education				Child protection 2015–2021 R		WASH 2015–2021 R		Social protection and equity 2017–2021 R	
				Moderate and severe underweight (%)		Moderate and severe stunting (%)		Early stimulation and responsive care (%)		Early childhood education (%)		Never attended school (%) 2015–2021 R		Foundational learning skills (%) 2017–2021 R		Severe physical punishment (%)		Basic sanitation services on premises (%)		Social transfers (%)	
	Aged 2–17	Aged 2–4	Aged 5–17	With disabilities	Without disabilities	With disabilities	Without disabilities	With disabilities	Without disabilities	With disabilities	Without disabilities	With disabilities	Without disabilities	With disabilities	Without disabilities	With disabilities	Without disabilities	With disabilities	Without disabilities	With disabilities	Without disabilities
Ethiopia	–	–	–	–	–	–	–	–	–	–	–	–	–	–	–	–	–	–	–	–	–
Fiji	9	6	9	6	5	10	8	98	97	15 p	22	4	0	21	43	17	13	85	86	86	89
Finland	–	–	–	–	–	–	–	–	–	–	–	–	–	–	–	–	–	–	–	–	–
France	–	–	–	–	–	–	–	–	–	–	–	–	–	–	–	–	–	–	–	–	–
Gabon	–	–	–	–	–	–	–	–	–	–	–	–	–	–	–	–	–	–	–	–	–
Gambia	9	5	10	20	14	31	20	8	17	20	25	18	15	4	5	21	16	41	45	–	–
Georgia	8	2	10	3 p	2	9 p	7	83 p	78	–	78	4	0	–	–	13	4	97	98	96	89
Germany	–	–	–	–	–	–	–	–	–	–	–	–	–	–	–	–	–	–	–	–	–
Ghana	19	11	21	8	12	19	20	27	35	72	71	4	3	5	9	24	16	16	16	–	–
Greece	–	–	–	–	–	–	–	–	–	–	–	–	–	–	–	–	–	–	–	–	–
Grenada	–	–	–	–	–	–	–	–	–	–	–	–	–	–	–	–	–	–	–	–	–
Guatemala	–	–	–	–	–	–	–	–	–	–	–	–	–	–	–	–	–	–	–	–	–
Guinea	–	–	–	–	–	–	–	–	–	–	–	–	–	–	–	–	–	–	–	–	–
Guinea-Bissau	14	5	16	16	17	37	29	47	43	12	15	17	11	1	4	20	21	12	13	–	–
Guyana	–	–	–	–	–	–	–	–	–	–	–	–	–	–	–	–	–	–	–	–	–
Haiti	–	–	–	–	–	–	–	–	–	–	–	–	–	–	–	–	–	–	–	–	–
Holy See	–	–	–	–	–	–	–	–	–	–	–	–	–	–	–	–	–	–	–	–	–
Honduras	14	6	16	16	7	31	21	34	36	9	14	0	0	–	–	8	4	80	81	–	–
Hungary	–	–	–	–	–	–	–	–	–	–	–	–	–	–	–	–	–	–	–	–	–
Iceland	–	–	–	–	–	–	–	–	–	–	–	–	–	–	–	–	–	–	–	–	–
India	–	–	–	–	–	–	–	–	–	–	–	–	–	–	–	–	–	–	–	–	–
Indonesia	–	–	–	–	–	–	–	–	–	–	–	–	–	–	–	–	–	–	–	–	–
Iran (Islamic Republic of)	–	–	–	–	–	–	–	–	–	–	–	–	–	–	–	–	–	–	–	–	–
Iraq	18	3	22	11	3	18	10	35	45	3	2	7	3	–	–	40	30	90	91	36	29
Ireland	–	–	–	–	–	–	–	–	–	–	–	–	–	–	–	–	–	–	–	–	–
Israel	–	–	–	–	–	–	–	–	–	–	–	–	–	–	–	–	–	–	–	–	–
Italy	–	–	–	–	–	–	–	–	–	–	–	–	–	–	–	–	–	–	–	–	–
Jamaica	–	–	–	–	–	–	–	–	–	–	–	–	–	–	–	–	–	–	–	–	–
Japan	–	–	–	–	–	–	–	–	–	–	–	–	–	–	–	–	–	–	–	–	–
Jordan	–	–	–	–	–	–	–	–	–	–	–	–	–	–	–	–	–	–	–	–	–
Kazakhstan	–	–	–	–	–	–	–	–	–	–	–	–	–	–	–	–	–	–	–	–	–
Kenya	–	–	–	–	–	–	–	–	–	–	–	–	–	–	–	–	–	–	–	–	–
Kiribati	21	13	22	12	5	27	18	77	77	62	73	2	0	15	14	31	24	38	41	84	81
Kuwait	–	–	–	–	–	–	–	–	–	–	–	–	–	–	–	–	–	–	–	–	–
Kyrgyzstan	7	1	9	6 p	1	16 p	12	81 p	87	–	39	3	0	8	17	12	5	96	98	60	49
Lao People's Democratic Republic	2 y	2	–	37	24	58	37	24 y	45 y	11	33	–	–	–	–	6	5	50	65	6	9
Latvia	–	–	–	–	–	–	–	–	–	–	–	–	–	–	–	–	–	–	–	–	–
Lebanon	–	–	–	–	–	–	–	–	–	–	–	–	–	–	–	–	–	–	–	–	–
Lesotho	8	8	8	9	10	40	34	28	28	52	45	2	0	6	9	12	7	50	49	–	–
Liberia	–	–	–	–	–	–	–	–	–	–	–	–	–	–	–	–	–	–	–	–	–
Libya	–	–	–	–	–	–	–	–	–	–	–	–	–	–	–	–	–	–	–	–	–
Liechtenstein	–	–	–	–	–	–	–	–	–	–	–	–	–	–	–	–	–	–	–	–	–
Lithuania	–	–	–	–	–	–	–	–	–	–	–	–	–	–	–	–	–	–	–	–	–
Luxembourg	–	–	–	–	–	–	–	–	–	–	–	–	–	–	–	–	–	–	–	–	–
Madagascar	13	10	14	32	29	49	46	27	25	13	15	13	11	3	6	16	9	4	4	28	30
Malawi	12	5	14	19	13	43	38	37	35	27	34	2	1	5	7	20	17	42	45	49	50
Malaysia	–	–	–	–	–	–	–	–	–	–	–	–	–	–	–	–	–	–	–	–	–
Maldives	–	–	–	–	–	–	–	–	–	–	–	–	–	–	–	–	–	–	–	–	–
Mali	–	–	–	–	–	–	–	–	–	–	–	–	–	–	–	–	–	–	–	–	–
Malta	–	–	–	–	–	–	–	–	–	–	–	–	–	–	–	–	–	–	–	–	–
Marshall Islands	–	–	–	–	–	–	–	–	–	–	–	–	–	–	–	–	–	–	–	–	–
Mauritania	–	–	–	–	–	–	–	–	–	–	–	–	–	–	–	–	–	–	–	–	–
Mauritius	–	–	–	–	–	–	–	–	–	–	–	–	–	–	–	–	–	–	–	–	–
Mexico	8	2	11	11	3	13	12	52 y	76 y	53	61	2	1	–	–	8	5	0	0	–	–
Micronesia (Federated States of)	–	–	–	–	–	–	–	–	–	–	–	–	–	–	–	–	–	–	–	–	–
Monaco	–	–	–	–	–	–	–	–	–	–	–	–	–	–	–	–	–	–	–	–	–
Mongolia	5	2	6	4	2	13	11	40	58	55 p	74	6	0	34	36	9	5	59	65	–	–
Montenegro	6	1	7	–	0	–	8	–	91	–	53	7	0	–	–	5	5	96	94	–	–
Montserrat	–	–	–	–	–	–	–	–	–	–	–	–	–	–	–	–	–	–	–	–	–
Morocco	–	–	–	–	–	–	–	–	–	–	–	–	–	–	–	–	–	–	–	–	–
Mozambique	–	–	–	–	–	–	–	–	–	–	–	–	–	–	–	–	–	–	–	–	–

TABLE 16. CHILDREN WITH DISABILITIES

Countries and areas	Children with disabilities (%) 2015–2021 [R]			Child nutrition 2015–2021 [R]				Early childhood development 2015–2021 [R]				Education				Child protection 2015–2021 [R]		WASH 2015–2021 [R]		Social protection and equity 2017–2021 [R]	
				Moderate and severe underweight (%)		Moderate and severe stunting (%)		Early stimulation and responsive care (%)		Early childhood education (%)		Never attended school (%) 2015–2021 [R]		Foundational learning skills (%) 2017–2021 [R]		Severe physical punishment (%)		Basic sanitation services on premises (%)		Social transfers (%)	
	Aged 2–17	Aged 2–4	Aged 5–17	With disabilities	Without disabilities	With disabilities	Without disabilities	With disabilities	Without disabilities	With disabilities	Without disabilities	With disabilities	Without disabilities	With disabilities	Without disabilities	With disabilities	Without disabilities	With disabilities	Without disabilities	With disabilities	Without disabilities
Myanmar	-	-	-	-	-	-	-	-	-	-	-	-	-	-	-	-	-	-	-	-	-
Namibia	-	-	-	-	-	-	-	-	-	-	-	-	-	-	-	-	-	-	-	-	-
Nauru	-	-	-	-	-	-	-	-	-	-	-	-	-	-	-	-	-	-	-	-	-
Nepal	11	2	13	56	26	51	35	53	74	34 p	62	5	2	23	29	23	21	72	74	43	37
Netherlands (Kingdom of the)	-	-	-	-	-	-	-	-	-	-	-	-	-	-	-	-	-	-	-	-	-
New Zealand	-	-	-	-	-	-	-	-	-	-	-	-	-	-	-	-	-	-	-	-	-
Nicaragua	-	-	-	-	-	-	-	-	-	-	-	-	-	-	-	-	-	-	-	-	-
Niger	-	-	-	-	-	-	-	-	-	-	-	-	-	-	-	-	-	-	-	-	-
Nigeria	-	-	-	-	-	-	-	-	-	-	-	-	-	-	-	-	-	-	-	-	-
Niue	-	-	-	-	-	-	-	-	-	-	-	-	-	-	-	-	-	-	-	-	-
North Macedonia	9	2	11	-	1	-	4	-	88	-	37	1	0	22	35	13	7	88	95	61	53
Norway	-	-	-	-	-	-	-	-	-	-	-	-	-	-	-	-	-	-	-	-	-
Oman	-	-	-	-	-	-	-	-	-	-	-	-	-	-	-	-	-	-	-	-	-
Pakistan	-	-	-	-	-	-	-	-	-	-	-	-	-	-	-	-	-	-	-	-	-
Palau	-	-	-	-	-	-	-	-	-	-	-	-	-	-	-	-	-	-	-	-	-
Panama	-	-	-	-	-	-	-	-	-	-	-	-	-	-	-	-	-	-	-	-	-
Papua New Guinea	-	-	-	-	-	-	-	-	-	-	-	-	-	-	-	-	-	-	-	-	-
Paraguay	-	-	-	-	-	-	-	-	-	-	-	-	-	-	-	-	-	-	-	-	-
Peru	-	-	-	-	-	-	-	-	-	-	-	-	-	-	-	-	-	-	-	-	-
Philippines	-	-	-	-	-	-	-	-	-	-	-	-	-	-	-	-	-	-	-	-	-
Poland	-	-	-	-	-	-	-	-	-	-	-	-	-	-	-	-	-	-	-	-	-
Portugal	-	-	-	-	-	-	-	-	-	-	-	-	-	-	-	-	-	-	-	-	-
Qatar	-	-	-	-	-	-	-	-	-	-	-	-	-	-	-	-	-	-	-	-	-
Republic of Korea	-	-	-	-	-	-	-	-	-	-	-	-	-	-	-	-	-	-	-	-	-
Republic of Moldova	-	-	-	-	-	-	-	-	-	-	-	-	-	-	-	-	-	-	-	-	-
Romania	-	-	-	-	-	-	-	-	-	-	-	-	-	-	-	-	-	-	-	-	-
Russian Federation	-	-	-	-	-	-	-	-	-	-	-	-	-	-	-	-	-	-	-	-	-
Rwanda	-	-	-	-	-	-	-	-	-	-	-	-	-	-	-	-	-	-	-	-	-
Saint Kitts and Nevis	-	-	-	-	-	-	-	-	-	-	-	-	-	-	-	-	-	-	-	-	-
Saint Lucia	-	-	-	-	-	-	-	-	-	-	-	-	-	-	-	-	-	-	-	-	-
Saint Vincent and the Grenadines	-	-	-	-	-	-	-	-	-	-	-	-	-	-	-	-	-	-	-	-	-
Samoa	19	7	23	3	3	13	7	74	88	11	27	0	0	18	22	28	19	96	96	61	62
San Marino	-	-	-	-	-	-	-	-	-	-	-	-	-	-	-	-	-	-	-	-	-
Sao Tome and Principe	17	5	20	5	5	11	12	34	43	24	35	2	0	16	27	17	14	36	44	9	8
Saudi Arabia	-	-	-	-	-	-	-	-	-	-	-	-	-	-	-	-	-	-	-	-	-
Senegal	-	-	-	-	-	-	-	-	-	-	-	-	-	-	-	-	-	-	-	-	-
Serbia	4	2	5	-	1	-	5	85 p	96	-	61	-	0	-	-	0	1	99	98	67	54
Seychelles	-	-	-	-	-	-	-	-	-	-	-	-	-	-	-	-	-	-	-	-	-
Sierra Leone	20	7	23	13	11	38	30	27 y	28 y	11	12	13	12	-	-	30	26	16	15	35	27
Singapore	-	-	-	-	-	-	-	-	-	-	-	-	-	-	-	-	-	-	-	-	-
Slovakia	-	-	-	-	-	-	-	-	-	-	-	-	-	-	-	-	-	-	-	-	-
Slovenia	-	-	-	-	-	-	-	-	-	-	-	-	-	-	-	-	-	-	-	-	-
Solomon Islands	-	-	-	-	-	-	-	-	-	-	-	-	-	-	-	-	-	-	-	-	-
Somalia	-	-	-	-	-	-	-	-	-	-	-	-	-	-	-	-	-	-	-	-	-
South Africa	-	-	-	-	-	-	-	-	-	-	-	-	-	-	-	-	-	-	-	-	-
South Sudan	-	-	-	-	-	-	-	-	-	-	-	-	-	-	-	-	-	-	-	-	-
Spain	-	-	-	-	-	-	-	-	-	-	-	-	-	-	-	-	-	-	-	-	-
Sri Lanka	-	-	-	-	-	-	-	-	-	-	-	-	-	-	-	-	-	-	-	-	-
State of Palestine	12	2	15	5	2	9	8	57	76	22	35	1	0	26	37	24	21	96	97	37	34
Sudan	-	-	-	-	-	-	-	-	-	-	-	-	-	-	-	-	-	-	-	-	-
Suriname	11	5	14	1	7	18	9	53	67	31 p	46	2	1	11	18	13	8	77	84	41	35
Sweden	-	-	-	-	-	-	-	-	-	-	-	-	-	-	-	-	-	-	-	-	-
Switzerland	-	-	-	-	-	-	-	-	-	-	-	-	-	-	-	-	-	-	-	-	-
Syrian Arab Republic	-	-	-	-	-	-	-	-	-	-	-	-	-	-	-	-	-	-	-	-	-
Tajikistan	-	-	-	-	-	-	-	-	-	-	-	-	-	-	-	-	-	-	-	-	-
Thailand	-	-	-	-	-	-	-	-	-	-	-	-	-	-	-	-	-	-	-	-	-
Timor-Leste	-	-	-	-	-	-	-	-	-	-	-	-	-	-	-	-	-	-	-	-	-
Togo	19	8	21	19	15	28	27	24 y	28 y	14	21	3	3	3	6	30	21	18	16	-	-
Tokelau	-	-	-	-	-	-	-	-	-	-	-	-	-	-	-	-	-	-	-	-	-
Tonga	9	7	10	1	1	2	2	86	88	14 p	37	1	0	-	-	30	23	86	89	49	36
Trinidad and Tobago	-	-	-	-	-	-	-	-	-	-	-	-	-	-	-	-	-	-	-	-	-

FOR EVERY CHILD, VACCINATION

197

TABLE 16. CHILDREN WITH DISABILITIES

Countries and areas	Children with disabilities (%) 2015–2021 [R]			Child nutrition 2015–2021 [R]				Early childhood development 2015–2021 [R]				Education				Child protection 2015–2021 [R]		WASH 2015–2021 [R]		Social protection and equity 2017–2021 [R]	
				Moderate and severe underweight (%)		Moderate and severe stunting (%)		Early stimulation and responsive care (%)		Early childhood education (%)		Never attended school (%) 2015–2021 [R]		Foundational learning skills (%) 2017–2021 [R]		Severe physical punishment (%)		Basic sanitation services on premises (%)		Social transfers (%)	
	Aged 2–17	Aged 2–4	Aged 5–17	With disabilities	Without disabilities	With disabilities	Without disabilities	With disabilities	Without disabilities	With disabilities	Without disabilities	With disabilities	Without disabilities	With disabilities	Without disabilities	With disabilities	Without disabilities	With disabilities	Without disabilities	With disabilities	Without disabilities
Tunisia	20	3	24	1	1	13	8	52	74	31 p	51	2	0	19	26	36	21	95	96	15	10
Türkiye	-	-	-	-	-	-	-	-	-	-	-	-	-	-	-	-	-	-	-	-	-
Turkmenistan	2	1	3	0 p	2	-	5	74 p	90	-	41	7 p	0	58 p	66	1	1	98	98	69	62
Turks and Caicos Islands	6	2	7	-	1	-	0	-	87	-	93	0	0	-	57	24 p	5	95 p	95	8 p	8
Tuvalu	12	9	13	-	4	-	6	-	88	-	73	0	0	18 p	32	14	5	82	82	47	37
Uganda	-	-	-	-	-	-	-	-	-	-	-	-	-	-	-	-	-	-	-	-	-
Ukraine	-	-	-	-	-	-	-	-	-	-	-	-	-	-	-	-	-	-	-	-	-
United Arab Emirates	-	-	-	-	-	-	-	-	-	-	-	-	-	-	-	-	-	-	-	-	-
United Kingdom	-	-	-	-	-	-	-	-	-	-	-	-	-	-	-	-	-	-	-	-	-
United Republic of Tanzania	-	-	-	-	-	-	-	-	-	-	-	-	-	-	-	-	-	-	-	-	-
United States	-	-	-	-	-	-	-	-	-	-	-	-	-	-	-	-	-	-	-	-	-
Uruguay	-	-	-	-	-	-	-	-	-	-	-	-	-	-	-	-	-	-	-	-	-
Uzbekistan	-	-	-	-	-	-	-	-	-	-	-	-	-	-	-	-	-	-	-	-	-
Vanuatu	-	-	-	-	-	-	-	-	-	-	-	-	-	-	-	-	-	-	-	-	-
Venezuela (Bolivarian Republic of)	-	-	-	-	-	-	-	-	-	-	-	-	-	-	-	-	-	-	-	-	-
Viet Nam	2	1	2	-	-	-	-	45 p	65	-	81	8	0	61	68	5	2	72	86	41	32
Yemen	-	-	-	-	-	-	-	-	-	-	-	-	-	-	-	-	-	-	-	-	-
Zambia	-	-	-	-	-	-	-	-	-	-	-	-	-	-	-	-	-	-	-	-	-
Zimbabwe	9	4	10	13	9	30	25	31	38	19	29	1	0	4	3	12	6	33	35	49	44
SUMMARY																					
East Asia and Pacific	-	-	-	-	-	-	-	-	-	-	-	-	-	-	-	-	-	-	-	-	-
Europe and Central Asia	-	-	-	-	-	-	-	-	-	-	-	-	-	-	-	-	-	-	-	-	-
Eastern Europe and Central Asia	-	-	-	-	-	-	-	-	-	-	-	-	-	-	-	-	-	-	-	-	-
Western Europe	-	-	-	-	-	-	-	-	-	-	-	-	-	-	-	-	-	-	-	-	-
Latin America and Caribbean	-	-	-	-	-	-	-	-	-	-	-	-	-	-	-	-	-	-	-	-	-
Middle East and North Africa	-	-	-	-	-	-	-	-	-	-	-	-	-	-	-	-	-	-	-	-	-
North America	-	-	-	-	-	-	-	-	-	-	-	-	-	-	-	-	-	-	-	-	-
South Asia	-	-	-	-	-	-	-	-	-	-	-	-	-	-	-	-	-	-	-	-	-
Sub-Saharan Africa	-	-	-	-	-	-	-	-	-	-	-	-	-	-	-	-	-	-	-	-	-
Eastern and Southern Africa	-	-	-	-	-	-	-	-	-	-	-	-	-	-	-	-	-	-	-	-	-
West and Central Africa	-	-	-	-	-	-	-	-	-	-	-	-	-	-	-	-	-	-	-	-	-
Least developed countries	-	-	-	-	-	-	-	-	-	-	-	-	-	-	-	-	-	-	-	-	-
World	-	-	-	-	-	-	-	-	-	-	-	-	-	-	-	-	-	-	-	-	-

For a complete list of countries and areas in the regions, subregions and country categories, see page on Regional Classifications or visit <data.unicef.org/regionalclassifications>.

It is not advisable to compare data from consecutive editions of *The State of the World's Children* report.

NOTES

- Data not available.

y Data differ from the standard definition or refer to only part of a country. If they fall within the noted reference period, such data are included in the calculation of regional and global averages.

p Based on small denominators (typically 25–49 unweighted cases). No data based on fewer than 25 unweighted cases are displayed.

R Data refer to the most recent year available during the period specified in the column heading.

MAIN DATA SOURCES

For all indicators in the table – Multiple Indicator Cluster Surveys (MICS). Last update: September 2022.

DEFINITIONS OF THE INDICATORS

Children with disabilities – Children aged 2–17 years who have one or more difficulties in at least one functional domain.

Moderate and severe underweight – Percentage of children aged 24–59 months who are below minus two standard deviations of the median weight-for-age of the WHO Child Growth Standards.

Moderate and severe stunting – Percentage of children aged 24–59 months who are below minus two standard deviations of the median height-for-age of the WHO Child Growth Standards.

Early stimulation and responsive care – Percentage of children aged 24–59 months with whom an adult has engaged in four or more of the following activities to provide early stimulation and responsive care in the past three days: a) reading books to the child, b) telling stories to the child, c) singing songs to the child, d) taking the child outside the home, e) playing with the child, and f) spending time with the child naming, counting or drawing things.

Early childhood education – Percentage of children aged 36–59 months who are attending an early childhood education programme.

Never attended school – Percentage of children aged 10–17 years who have never attended school.

Foundational learning skills – Percentage of children aged 7–14 years who demonstrate foundational numeracy skills and foundational reading skills.

Severe physical punishment – Percentage of children aged 2–14 years who experienced severe physical punishment by caregivers in the past month.

Basic sanitation services on premises – Percentage of children aged 2–17 years living in a household with improved sanitation facilities not shared with other households and located in their own dwelling or in their own yard/plot.

Social transfers – Percentage of children aged 2–17 years living in a household that received any type of social transfers and benefits in the last three months.

TABLE 17. WOMEN'S ECONOMIC EMPOWERMENT

Countries and areas	Social Institutions and Gender Index (SIGI) 2019	Legal frameworks on gender equality in employment 2018–2020 R	Maternity leave benefits 2022	Paternity leave benefits 2022	Educational attainment (%) 2008–2021 R Upper secondary Male	Female	Labour force participation rate (%) 2010–2020 R Male Rural	Male Urban	Male Total	Female Rural	Female Urban	Female Total	Unemployment rate (%) 2010–2020 R Male Rural	Male Urban	Male Total	Female Rural	Female Urban	Female Total	Mobile phone ownership (%) 2014–2020 R Male	Female	Financial inclusion (%) 2014–2020 R Male	Female	Time use (%) 2013–2020 R Male	Female
Afghanistan	Very high	-	No	Yes	12	5	75	72	75	24	17	22	10	12	10	8	35	14	-	-	23	7	-	-
Albania	Low	-	Yes	Yes	46	44	64	70	68	50	54	53	10	13	12	9	12	11	-	-	-	-	-	-
Algeria	-	-	Yes	Yes	28	23	74	65	68	13	19	17	8	11	10	19	21	20	93	83	56	29	-	-
Andorra	-	-	-	-	48	47	-	-	-	-	-	-	-	-	-	-	-	-	-	-	-	-	-	-
Angola	-	-	No	Yes	20	12	87	73	79	90	66	76	2	11	7	1	14	7	78	80	36	22	-	-
Anguilla	-	-	-	-	-	-	-	-	-	-	-	-	-	-	-	-	-	-	-	-	-	-	-	-
Antigua and Barbuda	-	-	No	No	-	-	-	-	-	-	-	-	-	-	-	-	-	-	-	-	-	-	-	-
Argentina	-	-	No	Yes	32 x	36 x	69	75	73	49	53	51	7	10	9	9	12	11	-	-	-	-	-	-
Armenia	Low	80	Yes	No	90	90	68	63	65	49	39	43	11	23	18	11	27	20	76	77	56	41	-	-
Australia	Very low	-	Yes	Yes	81	79	68	73	71	58	62	61	4	6	5	4	6	5	-	-	-	-	-	-
Austria	Very low	-	Yes	Yes	86	75	67	67	67	56	55	55	2	6	5	2	6	4	-	-	-	-	-	-
Azerbaijan	Low	-	Yes	No	92	85	66	72	70	60	65	63	3	5	4	4	7	6	88	80	29	28	-	-
Bahamas	-	-	No	No	81	82	79	83	82	68	71	70	10	10	10	10	10	10	-	-	-	-	-	-
Bahrain	-	-	No	Yes	69	67	84	89	87	44	46	45	0	1	1	4	5	5	100	100	86	75	-	-
Bangladesh	Very high	-	Yes	No	42	32	81	82	82	39	31	36	3	4	3	6	9	7	-	-	-	-	-	-
Barbados	-	-	No	No	23 x	25 x	67	70	69	60	63	62	10	10	10	10	10	10	-	-	-	-	-	-
Belarus	Low	50	Yes	No	96	94	68	74	72	55	60	58	4	7	6	2	4	4	95	97	81	81	-	-
Belgium	Very low	-	Yes	Yes	72	71	60	59	59	52	49	49	4	6	6	4	5	5	-	-	-	-	-	-
Belize	-	-	Yes	No	41	46	83	79	81	43	58	50	3	6	4	9	10	10	-	-	-	-	-	-
Benin	Medium	-	Yes	Yes	2 x	0 x	76	69	73	72	65	69	1	4	2	1	4	3	-	-	-	-	-	-
Bhutan	-	-	No	Yes	20	14	73	76	74	64	49	60	1	3	2	2	6	3	-	-	-	-	-	-
Bolivia (Plurinational State of)	Low	-	No	Yes	81	79	93	75	81	78	58	64	1	5	3	1	5	4	-	-	-	-	-	-
Bosnia and Herzegovina	Low	-	Yes	Yes	80	59	58	58	58	34	42	37	12	16	14	19	18	19	-	-	-	-	-	-
Botswana	-	-	No	No	2 x	1 x	78	75	76	63	67	65	13	15	14	20	21	21	-	-	-	-	-	-
Brazil	Low	80	Yes	Yes	45	50	68	76	74	38	58	55	8	11	10	13	14	14	88	90	73	68	5	12
British Virgin Islands	-	-	-	-	19 x	21 x	-	-	-	-	-	-	-	-	-	-	-	-	76	77	-	-	-	-
Brunei Darussalam	-	-	No	No	64	62	68	74	73	53	57	56	11	5	6	13	7	8	91	99	-	-	-	-
Bulgaria	Low	-	Yes	Yes	79	77	56	67	64	40	55	50	8	3	5	8	3	4	-	-	-	-	-	-
Burkina Faso	Medium	-	Yes	Yes	9	4	77	70	75	60	56	59	4	7	5	3	10	5	-	-	-	-	-	-
Burundi	-	-	No	Yes	8	4	79	70	78	84	58	81	1	8	2	0	8	1	25	12	7	7	-	-
Cabo Verde	-	70	No	Yes	20	20	61	71	67	40	60	53	9	14	13	8	13	12	73	71	-	-	-	-
Cambodia	Low	-	No	No	15	5	89	84	85	80	69	77	0	0	0	0	0	0	62	62	22	22	-	-
Cameroon	Very high	50	Yes	Yes	25	11	84	78	81	78	63	71	1	5	3	1	8	4	-	-	39	30	5	16
Canada	Very low	-	Yes	Yes	84	85	68	71	70	59	62	61	6	6	6	5	5	5	-	-	-	-	-	-
Central African Republic	High	-	Yes	Yes	3 x	0 x	85	68	80	69	55	65	2	8	4	3	9	4	-	-	-	-	-	-
Chad	High	-	Yes	Yes	9	2	82	66	77	68	55	64	1	4	2	1	4	2	-	-	-	-	-	-
Chile	Medium	80	Yes	Yes	60	58	75	73	73	43	53	52	5	7	7	7	8	8	87	97	78	71	-	-
China	-	-	Yes	Pas	25	19	85	70	76	68	56	61	4	6	5	3	5	4	-	-	-	-	-	-
Colombia	Very low	90	Yes	Yes	52	54	85	79	80	43	59	56	4	9	8	10	13	13	72	74	49	42	3	5
Comoros	-	-	Yes	No	-	-	57	57	57	35	34	34	5	8	6	9	12	10	-	-	-	-	-	-
Congo	-	-	Yes	No	14 x	4 x	78	67	71	77	61	68	3	14	9	3	17	10	-	-	-	-	-	-
Cook Islands	-	-	-	-	-	-	-	-	-	-	-	-	-	-	-	-	-	-	-	-	-	-	-	-
Costa Rica	Low	60	Yes	No	39	42	79	77	77	43	55	52	8	10	9	16	15	15	86	86	75	61	8	22
Côte d'Ivoire	High	80	Yes	Yes	16	12	68	59	63	45	44	45	1	5	3	1	6	4	71	64	47	36	-	-
Croatia	Very low	-	Yes	Yes	79	63	58	58	58	41	48	45	6	6	6	8	7	7	-	-	-	-	-	-
Cuba	-	-	-	-	58	57	63	68	66	39	42	41	1	2	2	1	2	2	-	-	-	-	12	21
Cyprus	Low	90	Yes	Yes	76	73	63	71	70	51	60	58	6	6	6	9	8	8	99	98	87	90	-	-
Czechia	Very low	90	Yes	Yes	94	87	68	69	69	51	54	53	2	2	2	2	2	2	97	97	84	79	-	-
Democratic People's Republic of Korea	-	-	-	-	-	-	94	75	88	78	63	74	1	7	3	1	5	2	-	-	-	-	-	-
Democratic Republic of the Congo	Medium	-	-	-	39	17	72	59	66	73	46	61	2	10	5	1	8	3	-	-	-	-	-	-
Denmark	Very low	90	Yes	Yes	78	80	64	68	67	55	60	58	4	5	5	4	6	5	82	83	100	100	-	-
Djibouti	-	-	Yes	Yes	-	-	72	65	69	53	48	51	9	13	11	9	14	11	61	52	-	-	-	-
Dominica	-	-	No	No	11 x	10 x	-	-	-	-	-	-	-	-	-	-	-	-	-	-	-	-	-	-
Dominican Republic	Very low	90	Yes	Yes	46	51	82	79	80	46	56	54	3	5	4	10	10	10	71	70	58	54	4	17
Ecuador	Low	80	No	Yes	43	44	87	78	81	64	52	55	1	4	3	2	6	5	65	61	60	43	-	-
Egypt	-	-	No	No	67	67	73	69	71	18	20	19	6	8	7	18	26	21	99	100	39	27	-	-
El Salvador	Low	90	Yes	Yes	37	31	79	74	76	35	51	45	3	5	4	4	4	4	81	78	38	24	7	20
Equatorial Guinea	-	-	No	Yes	-	-	64	69	67	52	56	55	6	9	8	6	9	8	-	-	-	-	-	-
Eritrea	-	-	No	No	-	-	92	74	86	76	62	72	4	13	6	4	13	7	-	-	-	-	-	-
Estonia	Very low	-	Yes	Yes	85	86	65	74	71	52	60	58	5	4	4	5	5	5	-	-	-	-	-	-
Eswatini	-	-	No	No	7 x	13 x	52	71	57	43	64	49	23	15	21	25	22	24	-	-	-	-	-	-

FOR EVERY CHILD, VACCINATION

TABLE 17. WOMEN'S ECONOMIC EMPOWERMENT

Countries and areas	Social Institutions and Gender Index (SIGI) 2019	Legal frameworks on gender equality in employment 2018–2020 [R]	Maternity leave benefits 2022	Paternity leave benefits 2022	Educational attainment (%) 2008–2021 [R] Upper secondary Male	Female	Labour force participation rate (%) 2010–2020 [R] Male Rural	Urban	Total	Female Rural	Urban	Total	Unemployment rate (%) 2010–2020 [R] Male Rural	Urban	Total	Female Rural	Urban	Total	Mobile phone ownership (%) 2014–2020 [R] Male	Female	Financial inclusion (%) 2014–2020 [R] Male	Female	Time use (%) 2013–2020 [R] Male	Female
Ethiopia	Low	30	Yes	Yes	13	6	89	73	85	77	63	73	1	4	2	2	6	3	-	-	41	29	-	-
Fiji	-	-	Yes	Yes	42	47	81	72	77	37	39	38	2	5	4	4	6	5	-	-	-	-	-	-
Finland	Very low	100	Yes	Yes	76	78	59	65	63	52	57	56	6	8	7	5	7	6	99	98	100	100	-	-
France	Very low	90	Yes	Yes	75	70	59	60	60	51	51	51	6	10	9	7	9	8	80	78	97	91	-	-
Gabon	High	-	Yes	Yes	-	-	59	64	62	41	45	43	12	15	14	27	28	28	-	-	-	-	-	-
Gambia	-	-	Yes	Yes	2 x	1 x	66	69	68	53	50	51	4	9	7	10	14	12	-	-	-	-	-	-
Georgia	Low	-	Yes	No	93	92	80	67	73	66	48	55	6	19	13	5	16	10	93	90	58	64	-	-
Germany	Very low	-	Yes	Yes	87	80	68	67	67	57	55	56	2	4	4	2	3	3	-	-	-	-	-	-
Ghana	Medium	-	No	No	27	15	72	71	72	65	63	64	2	6	4	3	6	4	-	-	-	-	-	-
Greece	Low	-	Yes	Yes	68	62	58	61	60	41	46	45	12	15	14	19	22	22	-	-	-	-	-	-
Grenada	-	-	No	No	-	-	-	-	-	-	-	-	-	-	-	-	-	-	90	95	-	-	-	-
Guatemala	Low	60	No	No	26	22	90	83	86	32	48	41	1	3	2	3	4	3	64	57	46	42	3	19
Guinea	Very high	50	Yes	No	12	3	64	51	60	67	54	63	3	11	5	2	7	3	86	69	27	20	-	-
Guinea-Bissau	-	-	No	No	-	-	84	67	79	70	57	66	2	6	3	2	6	3	-	-	-	-	-	-
Guyana	-	-	No	No	-	-	69	62	67	40	50	43	12	12	12	17	16	17	-	-	-	-	-	-
Haiti	Medium	-	No	No	1 x	0 x	78	67	73	70	58	64	6	17	11	10	23	16	-	-	35	30	-	-
Holy See	-	-	-	-	-	-	-	-	-	-	-	-	-	-	-	-	-	-	-	-	-	-	-	-
Honduras	Low	-	No	No	32	28	92	81	86	43	58	52	2	8	5	5	8	7	-	-	-	-	-	-
Hungary	Low	-	Yes	Yes	84	76	67	66	66	48	49	48	5	3	3	4	3	4	-	-	-	-	-	-
Iceland	-	-	Yes	Yes	74	74	79	79	79	68	71	70	4	4	4	3	3	3	-	-	-	-	-	-
India	Medium	-	Yes	No	34	19	77	75	76	22	19	21	5	6	5	3	10	5	-	-	-	-	-	-
Indonesia	High	-	No	Yes	42	35	85	80	82	56	52	54	3	5	4	3	4	3	68	58	46	51	-	-
Iran (Islamic Republic of)	Very high	-	Yes	Yes	48	49	77	71	72	19	17	18	6	11	10	14	20	18	84	59	96	92	-	-
Iraq	Very high	70	Yes	No	34	24	76	74	74	7	13	12	10	10	10	13	34	31	63	43	26	20	-	-
Ireland	Very low	90	Yes	No	68	73	67	70	69	54	58	56	5	6	5	5	5	5	87	88	95	95	-	-
Israel	-	70	Yes	No	82	81	70	68	68	64	59	60	3	4	4	3	4	4	95	94	92	94	-	-
Italy	Very low	-	Yes	Yes	53	52	58	59	59	39	42	41	9	9	9	11	11	11	93	90	96	92	8	20
Jamaica	Low	50	No	No	-	-	76	71	73	59	61	60	5	7	6	8	11	10	96	97	79	78	-	-
Japan	Low	70	Yes	Yes	82	79	69	73	72	52	54	54	2	3	3	2	3	2	94	92	98	98	3	15
Jordan	Very high	-	No	Yes	51	50	67	61	64	15	14	15	13	18	15	21	27	24	-	-	-	-	-	-
Kazakhstan	Low	70	Yes	No	98	97	72	78	76	59	65	63	3	5	4	4	6	5	91	90	57	60	6	19
Kenya	Medium	90	No	Yes	26	18	75	79	77	74	68	72	1	4	2	1	6	3	48	47	86	78	-	-
Kiribati	-	-	No	No	-	-	-	-	-	-	-	-	-	-	-	-	-	-	-	-	-	-	-	-
Kuwait	-	-	No	No	27	39	85	89	88	48	50	50	1	1	1	5	7	6	99	100	83	73	-	-
Kyrgyzstan	Low	-	Yes	No	90	87	75	74	75	49	41	44	4	6	6	7	10	9	-	-	-	-	-	-
Lao People's Democratic Republic	Low	-	Yes	-	-	-	83	75	80	80	70	77	0	1	1	0	1	1	-	-	-	-	-	-
Latvia	Very low	-	Yes	Yes	89	93	65	70	68	52	58	56	9	6	7	7	5	5	-	-	-	-	-	-
Lebanon	Very high	-	No	No	33 x	33 x	68	75	72	22	24	23	3	6	5	7	11	10	-	-	-	-	-	-
Lesotho	Medium	-	No	No	13	14	79	72	76	63	58	60	18	23	20	26	30	28	80	83	45	46	-	-
Liberia	High	-	Yes	No	8 x	3 x	89	73	80	83	63	72	1	6	4	1	4	2	-	-	-	-	-	-
Libya	-	-	Yes	No	13 x	10 x	62	67	65	32	35	34	13	16	15	23	25	24	-	-	-	-	-	-
Liechtenstein	-	-	-	-	81 x	63 x	-	-	-	-	-	-	-	-	-	-	-	-	-	-	-	-	-	-
Lithuania	Very low	100	Yes	Yes	91	89	63	71	68	53	60	57	10	5	7	7	5	6	96	96	85	81	-	-
Luxembourg	-	-	Yes	Yes	70	68	63	67	65	52	57	55	4	7	6	4	6	6	-	-	-	-	-	-
Madagascar	High	-	Yes	No	11	9	91	80	89	87	73	83	1	5	2	1	6	2	-	-	-	-	-	-
Malawi	High	-	No	No	8 x	2 x	81	76	80	74	62	73	4	7	5	5	14	7	-	-	-	-	-	-
Malaysia	-	30	No	No	62	63	77	80	77	53	45	51	2	5	3	3	6	4	98	95	88	82	-	-
Maldives	-	-	No	Yes	6 x	4 x	83	86	85	41	42	42	5	8	6	4	7	5	-	-	-	-	-	-
Mali	High	-	Yes	No	8	3	83	76	81	62	48	58	7	6	7	7	13	8	-	-	-	-	-	-
Malta	Low	-	Yes	Yes	49	47	73	67	67	52	48	48	2	3	3	3	4	4	-	-	-	-	-	-
Marshall Islands	-	-	No	No	72	68	-	-	-	-	-	-	-	-	-	-	-	-	-	-	-	-	-	-
Mauritania	-	-	Yes	Yes	13	7	63	63	63	26	30	28	6	12	10	8	15	12	-	-	-	-	-	-
Mauritius	-	90	Yes	Yes	48	40	67	73	71	43	46	45	3	5	4	7	11	9	81	78	93	87	-	-
Mexico	Low	80	No	Yes	39	38	82	77	79	34	49	46	2	4	4	3	4	4	73	70	41	33	11	28
Micronesia (Federated States of)	-	-	No	No	-	-	-	-	-	-	-	-	-	-	-	-	-	-	-	-	-	-	-	-
Monaco	-	-	-	-	-	-	-	-	-	-	-	-	-	-	-	-	-	-	-	-	-	-	-	-
Mongolia	Low	-	Yes	No	39	50	80	66	71	69	49	55	3	8	6	3	6	5	94	95	91	95	8	19
Montenegro	-	-	Yes	No	80	65	60	66	64	45	49	48	13	16	15	14	17	16	-	-	-	-	-	-
Montserrat	-	-	-	-	-	-	-	-	-	-	-	-	-	-	-	-	-	-	-	-	-	-	-	-
Morocco	Very high	70	Yes	Yes	-	-	83	62	70	26	19	22	6	10	9	8	13	11	96	95	41	17	-	-
Mozambique	Low	70	No	Yes	12	6	83	72	79	86	63	77	1	7	3	1	11	4	37	26	51	33	-	-

TABLE 17. WOMEN'S ECONOMIC EMPOWERMENT

Countries and areas	Social Institutions and Gender Index (SIGI) 2019	Legal frameworks on gender equality in employment 2018–2020 R	Maternity leave benefits 2022	Paternity leave benefits 2022	Educational attainment (%) 2008–2021 R Upper secondary Male	Female	Labour force participation rate (%) 2010–2020 R Male Rural	Urban	Total	Female Rural	Urban	Total	Unemployment rate (%) 2010–2020 R Male Rural	Urban	Total	Female Rural	Urban	Total	Mobile phone ownership (%) 2014–2020 R Male	Female	Financial inclusion (%) 2014–2020 R Male	Female	Time use (%) 2013–2020 R Male	Female
Myanmar	High	-	Yes	Yes	24	22	78	72	76	47	45	46	0	1	0	0	1	1	68	57	26	26	-	-
Namibia	Low	-	No	No	19 x	16 x	54	71	63	49	61	56	16	24	21	13	22	19	-	-	-	-	-	-
Nauru	-	-	-	-	-	-	-	-	-	-	-	-	-	-	-	-	-	-	-	-	-	-	-	-
Nepal	Medium	-	Yes	Yes	24	10	86	75	84	86	64	82	2	7	3	1	10	3	-	-	-	-	-	-
Netherlands (Kingdom of the)	Very low	100	Yes	Yes	76	70	69	70	70	59	59	59	2	4	3	3	3	3	86	82	99	100	-	-
New Zealand	Very low	-	Yes	No	76	75	79	74	75	68	64	65	3	4	4	4	5	4	-	-	-	-	-	-
Nicaragua	Very low	-	No	Yes	-	-	91	80	85	37	58	50	2	8	5	5	5	5	-	-	-	-	-	-
Niger	-	-	Yes	Yes	5	2	88	71	84	66	40	61	0	2	1	0	2	0	77	55	20	11	-	-
Nigeria	High	30	No	No	51 x	39 x	64	63	63	47	50	49	6	14	9	5	11	8	49	32	51	27	-	-
Niue	-	-	-	-	-	-	-	-	-	-	-	-	-	-	-	-	-	-	-	-	-	-	-	-
North Macedonia	-	-	Yes	Yes	75	62	70	65	66	46	45	45	14	18	17	18	18	18	-	-	-	-	-	-
Norway	Very low	100	Yes	Yes	79	79	67	68	68	58	62	61	4	4	4	3	4	3	-	-	99	100	-	-
Oman	-	-	No	No	57	72	78	85	84	25	40	36	0	1	1	6	8	7	98	96	-	-	-	-
Pakistan	Very high	20	Yes	No	13	10	84	79	82	28	12	22	4	5	4	3	10	4	65	26	35	7	-	-
Palau	-	-	No	No	88	88	-	-	-	-	-	-	-	-	-	-	-	-	-	-	-	-	-	-
Panama	-	-	Yes	Yes	52	57	86	78	80	52	56	55	2	5	4	3	7	6	-	-	-	-	-	-
Papua New Guinea	-	-	No	No	-	-	46	54	48	46	50	46	3	6	3	1	3	1	-	-	-	-	-	-
Paraguay	Medium	-	Yes	Yes	43	42	87	84	85	55	62	60	4	6	5	8	9	8	-	-	-	-	-	-
Peru	Low	100	Yes	Yes	63	53	95	83	85	88	66	71	0	4	3	0	4	3	85	79	51	34	-	-
Philippines	Very high	100	Yes	Yes	28	33	74	72	73	45	49	47	2	3	2	2	3	3	-	-	30	39	-	-
Poland	Very low	-	Yes	Yes	90	86	66	66	66	47	50	49	3	3	3	4	3	4	-	-	-	-	-	-
Portugal	Very low	-	Yes	Yes	42	44	63	65	65	49	56	55	5	6	6	7	7	7	-	-	-	-	-	-
Qatar	-	-	No	No	37	60	92	96	95	53	58	57	0	0	0	0	1	0	100	100	-	-	2	8
Republic of Korea	Low	70	Yes	Yes	83	70	76	72	73	56	53	54	3	4	4	3	4	4	97	95	95	95	4	14
Republic of Moldova	Low	90	Yes	Yes	76	74	40	54	45	34	44	38	6	5	6	4	5	4	-	-	43	45	-	-
Romania	Very low	100	-	-	74	65	66	65	65	42	48	46	5	4	4	4	3	3	97	96	62	54	-	-
Russian Federation	Low	-	Yes	No	86	84	65	72	70	48	57	55	7	4	5	7	4	4	97	97	75	76	8	18
Rwanda	Low	-	No	Yes	12	8	85	78	83	87	71	84	0	4	1	0	5	1	-	-	-	-	-	-
Saint Kitts and Nevis	-	-	No	No	-	-	-	-	-	-	-	-	-	-	-	-	-	-	-	-	-	-	-	-
Saint Lucia	-	-	No	No	39	44	72	79	76	65	71	69	12	15	14	15	18	17	-	-	-	-	-	-
Saint Vincent and the Grenadines	-	-	No	No	-	-	73	80	77	54	59	57	19	21	20	15	18	17	-	-	-	-	-	-
Samoa	-	-	No	Yes	70	75	54	61	56	29	41	31	7	10	7	10	10	10	-	-	-	-	-	-
San Marino	-	-	Yes	No	52	56	-	-	-	-	-	-	-	-	-	-	-	-	-	-	-	-	-	-
Sao Tome and Principe	-	-	Yes	No	46	32	78	71	74	43	40	42	7	11	9	18	23	21	-	-	-	-	-	-
Saudi Arabia	-	-	No	Yes	64	59	76	79	78	22	22	22	2	3	3	24	23	23	99	97	81	58	-	-
Senegal	Medium	-	Yes	Yes	17	5	61	54	57	34	36	35	3	9	6	3	10	7	-	-	-	-	-	-
Serbia	Very low	100	Yes	Yes	79	69	67	61	63	48	48	48	8	11	10	10	12	11	97	92	73	70	9	19
Seychelles	-	-	Yes	Yes	48 x	44 x	-	-	-	-	-	-	-	-	-	-	-	-	-	-	-	-	-	-
Sierra Leone	High	-	No	No	18 x	7 x	51	63	58	48	63	58	11	3	5	6	3	4	-	-	-	-	-	-
Singapore	Low	-	Yes	Yes	77	72	76	79	78	60	63	62	2	3	3	2	4	3	89	88	100	96	-	-
Slovakia	Very low	100	Yes	No	91	84	68	68	68	51	53	52	7	5	6	7	5	6	78	74	85	83	-	-
Slovenia	Very low	90	Yes	Yes	87	79	63	62	63	53	53	53	4	4	4	5	5	5	98	97	98	97	-	-
Solomon Islands	-	-	No	No	-	-	90	81	86	86	78	82	0	1	1	0	1	1	-	-	-	-	-	-
Somalia	-	-	Yes	No	-	-	79	63	74	24	19	22	9	23	13	9	24	13	-	-	-	-	-	-
South Africa	Low	-	Yes	Yes	77	54	49	69	63	37	56	50	31	26	27	33	30	31	77	80	68	70	-	-
South Sudan	-	-	No	Yes	16	11	79	63	74	75	61	71	8	20	11	9	24	13	-	-	-	-	-	-
Spain	Very low	100	Yes	Yes	53	53	59	64	64	46	53	52	12	13	13	17	16	16	97	97	96	92	-	-
Sri Lanka	High	-	No	No	61	63	74	73	74	34	30	34	3	3	3	7	6	7	-	-	-	-	-	-
State of Palestine	-	40	-	-	45	47	76	69	70	19	18	18	12	23	21	29	44	41	79	70	34	16	3	20
Sudan	-	-	No	No	5 x	1 x	71	65	68	31	27	29	11	13	11	23	39	29	70	54	20	10	-	-
Suriname	-	-	Yes	Yes	23	26	61	66	64	37	41	39	3	5	4	9	13	11	-	-	-	-	-	-
Sweden	Very low	-	Yes	Yes	77	77	66	69	68	59	62	61	6	7	7	6	7	7	-	-	-	-	-	-
Switzerland	Very low	-	Yes	No	90	84	75	73	73	65	62	63	3	4	4	4	5	5	-	-	-	-	-	-
Syrian Arab Republic	-	-	Yes	No	25	19	78	71	74	15	14	15	4	8	6	17	24	20	-	-	-	-	-	-
Tajikistan	Medium	-	Yes	No	85	76	46	52	50	27	30	29	5	9	8	3	6	5	-	-	-	-	-	-
Thailand	Medium	60	No	No	35	35	76	75	75	58	60	59	1	1	1	1	1	1	83	84	84	80	-	-
Timor-Leste	-	-	-	-	-	-	75	66	73	65	51	62	2	8	3	3	17	6	-	-	-	-	-	-
Togo	High	-	Yes	Yes	17	3	62	61	61	58	54	56	3	7	5	1	5	3	49	39	53	38	-	-
Tokelau	-	-	-	-	-	-	-	-	-	-	-	-	-	-	-	-	-	-	-	-	-	-	-	-
Tonga	-	-	No	No	53	55	58	52	56	39	36	38	3	3	3	4	4	4	-	-	-	-	-	-
Trinidad and Tobago	Low	-	Yes	No	67	68	68	72	71	48	51	50	3	4	4	3	4	4	-	-	-	-	-	-

FOR EVERY CHILD, VACCINATION

TABLE 17. WOMEN'S ECONOMIC EMPOWERMENT

Countries and areas	Social Institutions and Gender Index (SIGI) 2019	Legal frameworks on gender equality in employment 2018–2020 R	Maternity leave benefits 2022	Paternity leave benefits 2022	Educational attainment (%) 2008–2021 R Upper secondary		Labour force participation rate (%) 2010–2020 R Male			Female			Unemployment rate (%) 2010–2020 R Male			Female			Mobile phone ownership (%) 2014–2020 R		Financial inclusion (%) 2014–2020 R		Time use (%) 2013–2020 R	
					Male	Female	Rural	Urban	Total	Rural	Urban	Total	Rural	Urban	Total	Rural	Urban	Total	Male	Female	Male	Female	Male	Female
Tunisia	High	-	No	Yes	4 x	1 x	70	69	69	17	29	25	11	13	12	22	22	22	83	77	46	28	-	-
Türkiye	Low	-	Yes	Yes	49	36	68	75	72	33	35	34	10	14	12	14	18	16	-	-	-	-	-	-
Turkmenistan	-	-	-	-	81 x	73 x	68	74	72	42	46	44	3	6	5	1	3	2	-	-	-	-	-	-
Turks and Caicos Islands	-	-	-	-	-	-	-	-	-	-	-	-	-	-	-	-	-	-	-	-	-	-	-	-
Tuvalu	-	-	-	-	-	-	-	-	-	-	-	-	-	-	-	-	-	-	-	-	-	-	-	-
Uganda	High	-	No	Yes	14	6	73	74	73	68	65	67	1	2	1	1	6	2	-	-	-	-	-	-
Ukraine	Low	50	Yes	No	78 x	71 x	61	64	63	45	48	47	10	8	9	8	8	8	89	90	65	61	-	-
United Arab Emirates	-	60	No	Yes	72	71	90	95	93	51	53	52	1	2	1	5	7	6	100	100	93	76	-	-
United Kingdom	Very Low	-	Yes	Yes	80	80	65	69	68	55	59	58	3	4	4	2	4	4	-	-	-	-	-	-
United Republic of Tanzania	High	-	No	Yes	5	2	90	83	87	85	72	80	1	3	2	1	6	3	-	-	-	-	-	-
United States	Very low	-	No	Yes	91	91	63	70	69	53	58	57	4	4	4	4	4	4	-	-	-	-	-	-
Uruguay	Low	90	Yes	Yes	27	35	77	73	73	50	56	56	2	8	8	7	12	11	82	84	68	61	8	20
Uzbekistan	-	-	Yes	No	98	96	74	76	75	48	50	49	4	7	6	4	7	6	78	66	38	36	-	-
Vanuatu	-	-	No	No	9 x	5 x	83	71	79	64	54	61	1	4	2	1	3	1	-	-	-	-	-	-
Venezuela (Bolivarian Republic of)	-	-	Yes	Yes	59	65	75	75	75	42	42	42	4	7	7	6	8	8	-	-	-	-	-	-
Viet Nam	Low	80	Yes	Yes	34	30	86	75	82	78	64	73	2	3	2	2	3	2	78	77	31	30	-	-
Yemen	Very high	-	No	No	-	-	70	72	71	5	8	6	12	10	12	24	28	25	-	-	-	-	-	-
Zambia	Medium	-	Yes	No	23 x	9 x	82	75	79	74	67	70	12	10	11	12	14	13	44	45	52	40	-	-
Zimbabwe	Medium	70	Yes	No	16	9	92	83	89	87	64	78	1	11	5	1	16	6	46	48	59	52	-	-

SUMMARY

Countries and areas					Male	Female	Rural	Urban	Total	Rural	Urban	Total	Rural	Urban	Total	Rural	Urban	Total	Male	Female	Male	Female	Male	Female
East Asia and Pacific	-	-	-	-	34	29	83	72	76	64	55	59	3	5	4	3	4	3	80	75	59	61	-	-
Europe and Central Asia	-	-	-	-	76	72	65	67	67	47	52	50	6	7	7	7	7	7	91	90	80	77	-	-
Eastern Europe and Central Asia	-	-	-	-	78	73	66	71	69	45	50	48	7	8	7	7	8	8	93	92	66	66	-	-
Western Europe	-	-	-	-	75	71	64	65	65	50	53	52	5	7	6	7	7	7	89	88	96	92	-	-
Latin America and Caribbean	-	-	-	-	45	46	80	76	77	45	54	53	4	8	7	7	10	9	81	81	59	52	-	-
Middle East and North Africa	-	-	-	-	49	47	75	72	73	17	21	19	7	9	8	17	22	20	91	81	62	47	-	-
North America	-	-	-	-	90	91	64	70	69	53	58	57	4	4	4	4	4	4	-	-	-	-	-	-
South Asia	-	-	-	-	32	20	78	76	77	25	20	24	5	6	5	4	10	5	-	-	-	-	-	-
Sub-Saharan Africa	-	-	-	-	27	17	76	68	73	66	55	61	4	11	6	4	13	7	58	49	49	36	-	-
Eastern and Southern Africa	-	-	-	-	22	14	81	73	78	71	59	67	4	12	7	6	17	9	61	58	51	43	-	-
West and Central Africa	-	-	-	-	32	21	71	64	68	58	51	55	4	10	6	3	9	5	55	39	47	27	-	-
Least developed countries	-	-	-	-	21	13	81	72	78	61	48	57	3	7	4	4	11	6	63	54	32	23	-	-
World	**-**	**-**	**-**	**-**	**43**	**38**	**78**	**72**	**74**	**47**	**48**	**47**	**4**	**7**	**5**	**4**	**8**	**6**	**80**	**73**	**60**	**54**	**-**	**-**

For a complete list of countries and areas in the regions, subregions and country categories, see page on Regional Classifications or visit <data.unicef.org/regionalclassifications>.

It is not advisable to compare data from consecutive editions of *The State of the World's Children* report.

NOTES

- Data not available.

R Data refer to the most recent year available during the period specified in the column heading.

x Data refer to years or periods other than those specified in the column heading. Such data are not included in the calculation of regional and global averages. Estimates from data years prior to 2000 are not displayed.

MAIN DATA SOURCES

Social Institutions and Gender Equality Index (SIGI) – Organisation for Economic Co-operation and Development (OECD). Last update: March 2019.

Legal frameworks that promote, enforce and monitor gender equality in employment and economic benefits – UN Women, World Bank Group, OECD Development Centre. Last update: May 2021

Maternity leave benefits – World Bank Women Business and the Law. Last update: February 2022.

Paternity leave benefits – World Bank Women Business and the Law. Last update: February 2022.

Educational attainment – UNESCO Institute for Statistics (UIS). Last update: September 2021.

Labour force participation rate – International Labour Organization (ILO). Last update: June 2021.

Unemployment rate – International Labour Organization (ILO). Last update: June 2021.

Mobile phone ownership – Global SDG Indicators Database, 2022. Last update: December 2022.

Financial inclusion – Global SDG Indicators Database, 2022. Last update: December 2022.

Time use – Global SDG Indicators Database, 2022. Last update: December 2022.

DEFINITIONS OF THE INDICATORS

Social Institutions and Gender Index (SIGI) – Level of gender discrimination in social institutions defined as discrimination in the family, restricted physical integrity, restricted access to reproductive and financial resources, and restricted liberties.

Legal frameworks that promote, enforce and monitor gender equality in employment and economic benefits – Measures as a percentage of achivement from 0 to 100 with 100 being best practice, government efforts to put in place legal frameworks that promote, enforce and monitor gender equality in the area of employment and economic benefits.

Maternity leave benfits – Whether the law provides for 14 weeks or more of paid maternity leave in accordance with the International Labour Organization standards.

Paternity leave benefits – Whether the law provides for paid paternity leave (of any length).

Educational attainment – Percentage of the population aged 25 years and older that completed at least upper secondary education (ISCED 3).

Labour force participation rate – The proportion of a country's working-age population that engages actively in the labour market, either by working or looking for work.

Unemployment rate – The percentage of persons in the labour force who are unemployed.

Mobile phone ownership – Proportion of individuals who own a mobile telephone.

Financial inclusion – The percentage of adults (ages 15+) who report having an account (by themselves or together with someone else) at a bank or another type of financial institution or personally using a mobile money service in the past 12 months.

Time use - Proportion of time spent on unpaid domestic and care work among individuals aged 15 years and older.

TABLE 18. MIGRATION

Countries and areas	International migrant stock 2020 Total (thousands)	Under 18 (thousands)	Total as share of national population (%)	Refugees by asylum country 2021 Total	Under 18	Per 1,000 population	Per 1 US$ GNI per capita	Refugees by origin country 2021 Total	Under 18	Internally displaced persons (IDPs) 2021 Total T	Under 18 Ru	Share due to conflict and violence (%) Sd	Share due to disaster (%) Sd	New internal displacements 2021 Total T	Under 18 Ru	Share due to conflict and violence (%) Sd	Share due to disaster (%) Sd
Afghanistan	144	54	<1	66,949	37,672	2	134	2,712,858	1,240,137	5,703,808	2,800,000	76	24	748,128	360,000	97	3
Albania	49	24	2	109	44	0	0	19,847	-	0	0	0	100	251	52	0	100
Algeria	250	34	<1	97,890	-	2	27	6,003	-	3,454	1,200	0	100	6,645	2,300	0	100
Andorra	46	3	59	-	-	-	-	0	-	-	-	-	-	-	-	-	-
Angola	656	128	2	26,045	14,206	1	15	11,403	-	7,464	3,900	0	100	21,727	11,000	0	100
Anguilla	6	1	38	25	-	2	-	0	-	0	0	-	-	500	0	0	100
Antigua and Barbuda	29	2	30	0	-	0	0	105	-	0	0	-	-	1,423	380	0	100
Argentina	2,282	346	5	168,672	-	4	0	124	-	0	0	0	100	709	200	0	100
Armenia	190	13	6	34,728	1,908	12	8	12,255	-	837	200	100	0	37	9	100	0
Australia	7,686	633	30	55,606	-	2	1	16	-	224	51	0	100	48,939	11,000	0	100
Austria	1,738	139	19	152,514	-	17	3	23	-	0	0	-	-	56	10	0	100
Azerbaijan	252	28	2	1,676	534	0	0	39,478	-	654,839	180,000	100	0	0	0	100	0
Bahamas	64	7	16	10	-	0	0	736	-	250	66	0	100	0	0	0	100
Bahrain	936	59	55	256	65	0	0	416	-	-	-	-	-	-	-	-	-
Bangladesh	2,115	589	1	918,907	481,775	5	351	22,672	-	468,864	150,000	91	9	98,921	31,000	0	100
Barbados	35	3	12	0	-	0	0	265	-	376	76	0	100	376	76	0	100
Belarus	1,067	46	11	2,729	882	0	0	4,632	-	-	-	-	-	-	-	-	-
Belgium	2,005	197	17	74,063	-	6	1	29	-	1,900	390	0	100	16,077	3,300	0	100
Belize	62	5	16	86	-	0	0	81	-	0	0	-	-	6,273	2,200	0	100
Benin	394	88	3	1,736	536	0	1	730	-	2,701	1,300	100	0	10,000	4,800	0	100
Bhutan	54	4	7	-	-	-	-	6,702	1,828	0	0	-	-	120	36	0	100
Bolivia (Plurinational State of)	164	62	1	12,921	-	1	0	549	-	313	110	0	100	906	320	0	100
Bosnia and Herzegovina	36	5	1	240	46	0	0	18,190	-	91,734	16,000	100	0	314	54	0	100
Botswana	110	16	5	688	305	0	0	122	-	780	300	0	100	780	300	0	100
Brazil	1,080	244	<1	237,948	-	1	8	1,954	-	46,707	12,000	44	56	470,368	120,000	5	95
British Virgin Islands	22	3	73	-	-	-	-	-	-	0	0	-	-	6,000	0	0	100
Brunei Darussalam	112	8	26	0	-	0	0	0	-	0	0	-	-	94	26	0	100
Bulgaria	184	66	3	22,830	-	3	2	455	-	0	0	-	-	25	4	0	100
Burkina Faso	724	139	3	25,010	14,023	1	29	20,209	9,913	1,579,976	810,000	100	0	682,245	350,000	100	0
Burundi	345	102	3	81,491	43,405	6	340	323,635	166,224	113,408	58,000	17	83	86,979	45,000	0	100
Cabo Verde	16	1	3	0	-	0	0	10	-	0	0	-	-	750	250	0	100
Cambodia	79	7	<1	24	-	0	0	12,072	-	5,769	2,100	0	100	14,639	5,300	0	100
Cameroon	579	207	2	457,269	253,483	17	288	125,475	57,644	936,767	460,000	97	3	133,216	64,000	99	1
Canada	8,049	633	21	130,125	26,417	3	3	60	-	1,940	370	0	100	59,673	11,000	0	100
Central African Republic	89	21	2	9,305	4,984	2	18	737,658	408,040	728,023	370,000	95	5	519,189	260,000	95	5
Chad	547	144	3	555,782	297,287	32	855	11,771	5,485	415,943	220,000	94	6	66,499	35,000	64	36
Chile	1,645	201	9	502,336	-	26	0	987	-	1,389	320	0	100	2,486	570	0	100
China	1,040	210	<1	303,436	-	0	26	170,200	-	942,638	200,000	0	100	6,037,150	1,300,000	0	100
Colombia	1,905	692	4	1,843,894	512,638	36	0	115,793	34,097	5,236,494	1,400,000	100	0	165,555	44,000	81	19
Comoros	12	2	1	27	8	0	0	1,670	-	19,000	8,600	0	100	19,372	8,800	0	100
Congo	388	88	7	40,765	17,567	7	25	14,253	-	57,173	27,000	100	0	6,653	3,200	0	100
Cook Islands	5	1	26	-	-	-	-	-	-	0	0	-	-	12	0	0	100
Costa Rica	521	78	10	31,990	-	6	1	235	-	0	0	0	100	290	71	0	100
Côte d'Ivoire	2,565	276	10	4,349	2,083	0	2	39,940	13,242	301,705	150,000	100	0	0	0	89	11
Croatia	528	7	13	1,020	351	0	0	18,085	-	3,000	520	0	100	0	0	0	100
Cuba	3	<1	<1	199	24	0	0	11,534	-	0	0	0	100	193,742	37,000	0	100
Cyprus	190	19	16	16,277	-	13	1	5	-	242,540	49,000	100	0	59	12	0	100
Czechia	541	29	5	1,910	-	0	0	758	-	460	86	0	100	2,780	520	0	100
Democratic People's Republic of Korea	50	5	<1	-	-	-	-	528	-	0	0	0	100	5,000	1,200	0	100
Democratic Republic of the Congo	953	166	1	524,148	323,851	5	904	908,401	469,755	5,540,000	2,900,000	96	4	3,599,919	1,900,000	75	25
Denmark	718	69	12	36,023	-	6	1	8	-	-	-	-	-	-	-	-	-
Djibouti	120	22	12	23,232	8,849	21	7	2,607	-	11	4	0	100	11	4	0	100
Dominica	8	2	12	0	-	0	0	54	-	0	0	-	-	350	0	0	100
Dominican Republic	604	77	6	116,162	-	10	0	635	-	0	0	0	100	10,388	3,400	0	100
Ecuador	785	305	4	560,485	167,563	31	10	1,825	-	719	230	0	100	5,651	1,800	0	100
Egypt	544	91	<1	280,686	100,931	3	80	27,498	-	1,100	430	0	100	1,100	430	0	100
El Salvador	43	6	<1	98	32	0	0	52,041	-	0	0	0	100	175,804	55,000	100	0
Equatorial Guinea	231	4	16	-	-	-	-	168	-	-	-	-	-	-	-	-	-
Eritrea	14	3	<1	121	73	0	0	511,911	161,090	10,000	4,800	100	0	0	0	0	100
Estonia	199	8	15	321	-	0	0	271	-	-	-	-	-	-	-	-	-
Eswatini	33	7	3	895	325	1	0	165	-	0	0	-	-	105	46	0	100

FOR EVERY CHILD, VACCINATION

203

TABLE 18. MIGRATION

Countries and areas	International migrant stock 2020			Refugees by asylum country 2021				Refugees by origin country 2021		Internally displaced persons (IDPs) 2021				New internal displacements 2021			
	Total (thousands)	Under 18 (thousands)	Total as share of national population (%)	Total	Under 18	Per 1,000 population	Per 1 US$ GNI per capita	Total	Under 18	Total [T]	Under 18 [Ru]	Share due to conflict and violence (%) [Sd]	Share due to disaster (%) [Sd]	Total [T]	Under 18 [Ru]	Share due to conflict and violence (%) [Sd]	Share due to disaster (%) [Sd]
Ethiopia	1,086	465	<1	821,283	491,771	7	856	149,125	46,504	4,168,513	1,900,000	86	14	5,382,365	2,500,000	96	4
Fiji	14	3	2	18	8	0	0	414	-	0	0	0	100	14,341	4,900	0	100
Finland	386	45	7	24,078	-	4	0	5	-	0	0	-	-	51	10	0	100
France	8,525	695	13	499,914	126,862	8	11	38	-	0	0	0	100	9,075	1,900	0	100
Gabon	417	103	19	272	63	0	0	620	-	2	1	0	100	2	1	0	100
Gambia	216	47	9	4,418	1,805	2	6	11,042	-	0	0	0	100	3,116	1,600	22	78
Georgia	79	15	2	1,818	478	0	0	9,754	-	333,145	78,000	92	8	85	20	0	100
Germany	15,762	1,151	19	1,255,694	407,771	15	25	59	-	740	130	0	100	17,340	2,900	0	100
Ghana	476	95	2	11,894	3,816	0	5	14,251	5,848	3,744	1,600	0	100	12,015	5,200	0	100
Greece	1,340	98	13	119,650	-	11	6	87	-	1,552	250	0	100	66,518	11,000	0	100
Grenada	7	<1	6	234	-	2	0	52	-	0	0	-	-	26	7	0	100
Guatemala	84	13	<1	1,948	-	0	0	26,927	-	264,846	110,000	92	8	15,711	6,100	1	99
Guinea	121	31	<1	5,741	2,081	0	6	34,403	-	2,562	1,300	0	100	2,562	1,300	0	100
Guinea-Bissau	18	6	<1	1,846	845	1	2	2,039	-	414	200	0	100	414	200	0	100
Guyana	31	4	4	25,840	-	32	0	285	-	0	0	-	-	216	71	0	100
Haiti	19	5	<1	0	-	0	0	29,454	-	236,343	90,000	7	93	240,714	91,000	8	92
Holy See	<1	<1	100	-	-	-	-	0	-	-	-	-	-	-	-	-	-
Honduras	39	13	<1	144	-	0	0	51,687	17,036	247,120	91,000	100	0	811	290	68	32
Hungary	585	74	6	5,676	-	1	0	4,653	-	0	0	-	-	14	2	0	100
Iceland	65	8	19	1,830	-	5	0	5	-	0	0	-	-	219	50	0	100
India	4,879	307	<1	212,413	-	0	98	14,230	-	527,873	170,000	96	4	4,916,252	1,500,000	0	100
Indonesia	356	48	<1	9,982	2,501	0	2	13,962	-	228,143	70,000	32	68	775,998	240,000	3	97
Iran (Islamic Republic of)	2,797	1,171	3	798,343	306,591	9	237	142,989	-	13,443	3,900	0	100	40,586	12,000	0	100
Iraq	366	104	<1	280,072	121,476	6	56	343,898	105,193	1,206,530	530,000	98	2	66,325	29,000	86	14
Ireland	871	153	18	9,571	2,211	2	0	5	7	0	0	-	-	25	6	0	100
Israel	1,954	83	23	1,191	-	0	0	453	-	0	0	0	100	7,045	2,300	45	55
Italy	6,387	415	11	144,862	-	2	4	61	-	7	1	0	100	2,558	400	0	100
Jamaica	24	7	<1	98	-	0	0	2,419	-	0	0	-	-	16	4	0	100
Japan	2,771	271	2	1,132	-	0	0	39	-	38,882	5,800	0	100	13,593	2,000	0	100
Jordan	3,458	1,580	34	712,823	343,027	64	159	2,981	-	0	0	-	-	138	53	0	100
Kazakhstan	3,732	361	20	352	108	0	0	3,198	-	72	24	0	100	141	47	0	100
Kenya	1,050	297	2	481,048	263,794	9	239	7,529	-	244,320	110,000	78	22	41,076	18,000	11	89
Kiribati	3	<1	3	-	-	-	-	0	-	0	0	-	-	2,520	1,000	0	100
Kuwait	3,110	591	73	720	212	0	0	1,702	-	-	-	-	-	-	-	-	-
Kyrgyzstan	199	11	3	317	109	0	0	3,035	-	0	0	100	0	46,384	17,000	100	0
Lao People's Democratic Republic	49	6	<1	-	-	-	-	6,778	-	3,605	1,300	0	100	5	2	0	100
Latvia	239	10	13	705	-	0	0	122	-	0	0	-	-	24	5	0	100
Lebanon	1,713	515	25	845,865	459,167	151	245	6,061	-	50	15	100	0	906	260	7	93
Lesotho	12	2	<1	296	71	0	0	6	-	0	0	-	-	729	280	0	100
Liberia	88	14	2	8,169	3,637	2	13	5,384	1,213	1,208	570	0	100	3,708	1,700	0	100
Libya	827	161	12	3,141	1,139	0	0	19,090	6,561	160,456	53,000	100	0	1,234	400	0	100
Liechtenstein	26	4	68	133	-	3	0	5	-	-	-	-	-	-	-	-	-
Lithuania	145	17	5	1,880	-	1	0	54	-	0	0	-	-	0	0	-	-
Luxembourg	298	27	48	6,011	-	9	0	0	-	0	0	-	-	560	110	0	100
Madagascar	36	6	<1	165	57	0	0	425	-	2,807	1,300	100	0	6,130	2,800	21	79
Malawi	191	42	1	21,529	11,084	1	34	513	-	0	0	0	100	602	300	0	100
Malaysia	3,477	426	11	132,086	37,583	4	12	1,182	-	6,983	1,900	0	100	128,536	36,000	0	100
Maldives	70	4	13	-	-	-	-	80	-	0	0	-	-	296	67	0	100
Mali	486	87	2	49,975	29,027	2	57	183,392	100,608	350,110	190,000	93	7	255,168	140,000	98	2
Malta	115	8	26	9,335	-	18	0	7	-	-	-	-	-	-	-	-	-
Marshall Islands	3	<1	6	-	-	-	-	7	-	0	0	-	-	200	0	0	100
Mauritania	182	73	4	101,942	47,884	22	59	39,279	18,085	1,560	710	0	100	1,560	710	0	100
Mauritius	29	2	2	10	-	0	0	198	-	0	0	0	100	113	24	0	100
Mexico	1,198	684	<1	136,627	30,750	1	8	16,403	-	379,269	120,000	100	0	47,555	14,000	61	39
Micronesia (Federated States of)	3	<1	2	-	-	-	-	-	-	0	0	-	-	6,760	2,700	0	100
Monaco	27	2	68	17	-	0	-	0	-	-	-	-	-	-	-	-	-
Mongolia	21	4	<1	0	-	0	0	2,508	-	6,331	2,300	0	100	6,331	2,300	0	100
Montenegro	71	4	11	175	60	0	0	623	-	0	0	-	-	6	1	0	100
Montserrat	1	<1	28	-	-	-	-	-	-	-	-	-	-	-	-	-	-
Morocco	102	20	<1	7,272	2,612	0	2	5,385	-	10	3	0	100	10	3	0	100
Mozambique	339	81	1	4,797	1,914	0	10	90	-	873,358	450,000	84	16	230,569	120,000	81	19

204   THE STATE OF THE WORLD'S CHILDREN 2023

TABLE 18. MIGRATION

Countries and areas	International migrant stock 2020			Refugees by asylum country 2021				Refugees by origin country 2021		Internally displaced persons (IDPs) 2021				New internal displacements 2021			
	Total (thousands)	Under 18 (thousands)	Total as share of national population (%)	Total	Under 18	Per 1,000 population	Per 1 US$ GNI per capita	Total	Under 18	Total [T]	Under 18 [Ru]	Share due to conflict and violence (%) [Sd]	Share due to disaster (%) [Sd]	Total [T]	Under 18 [Ru]	Share due to conflict and violence (%) [Sd]	Share due to disaster (%) [Sd]
Myanmar	76	13	<1	0	-	0	0	1,177,029	569,486	650,450	200,000	100	0	606,037	180,000	74	26
Namibia	109	12	4	3,733	1,786	1	1	441	-	0	0	-	-	255	110	0	100
Nauru	2	<1	20	953	240	76	0	5	-	-	-	-	-	-	-	-	-
Nepal	488	34	2	19,574	-	1	16	7,029	-	8,353	2,800	0	100	32,492	11,000	0	100
Netherlands (Kingdom of the)	2,358	190	14	99,586	-	6	2	58	-	0	0	-	-	51,343	9,700	0	100
New Zealand	1,382	157	29	1,794	-	0	0	33	-	50	12	0	100	4,363	1,000	0	100
Nicaragua	42	9	<1	313	-	0	0	11,041	-	9,106	3,200	0	100	231,894	81,000	0	100
Niger	348	102	1	249,945	147,577	10	424	21,901	14,031	264,257	150,000	85	15	227,950	130,000	48	52
Nigeria	1,309	363	<1	77,132	38,711	0	37	383,660	212,544	3,335,438	1,700,000	97	3	399,918	200,000	94	6
Niue	<1	<1	36	-	-	-	-	11	-	-	-	-	-	-	-	-	-
North Macedonia	131	19	6	293	102	0	0	1,842	-	108	21	100	0	80	16	0	100
Norway	852	97	16	46,042	-	9	1	5	-	4	1	0	100	783	160	0	100
Oman	2,373	279	46	295	74	0	0	53	-	0	0	-	-	5,210	1,400	0	100
Pakistan	3,277	192	1	1,491,070	801,814	6	994	132,817	56,362	173,323	71,000	60	40	69,721	28,000	0	100
Palau	5	<1	28	-	-	-	-	0	-	0	0	-	-	2,457	0	0	100
Panama	313	75	7	130,542	-	30	0	118	-	0	0	0	100	2,222	690	0	100
Papua New Guinea	31	10	<1	11,839	-	1	4	507	-	40,364	17,000	59	41	16,969	6,900	56	44
Paraguay	170	27	2	6,394	1,222	1	1	125	-	5	2	0	100	5	2	0	100
Peru	1,225	405	4	797,232	161,450	24	1	3,520	-	59,846	17,000	100	0	10,705	3,100	0	100
Philippines	226	61	<1	801	164	0	0	521	-	808,502	280,000	13	87	5,821,136	2,000,000	2	98
Poland	817	177	2	4,875	-	0	0	887	-	121	22	0	100	121	22	0	100
Portugal	1,002	63	10	2,651	-	0	0	26	-	0	0	-	-	20	3	0	100
Qatar	2,226	324	77	197	53	0	0	47	-	-	-	-	-	-	-	-	-
Republic of Korea	1,728	216	3	3,559	-	0	0	117	-	333	50	0	100	2,919	430	0	100
Republic of Moldova	104	14	3	349	47	0	0	2,190	-	0	0	-	-	0	0	0	100
Romania	705	302	4	4,200	1,188	0	0	1,417	-	0	0	-	-	412	77	0	100
Russian Federation	11,637	620	8	10,901	-	0	1	68,547	-	606	130	78	22	5,622	1,200	0	100
Rwanda	514	161	4	121,896	58,043	9	143	248,219	152,900	699	320	0	100	14,960	6,800	0	100
Saint Kitts and Nevis	8	2	15	60	-	1	0	47	-	0	0	-	-	33	0	0	100
Saint Lucia	8	2	5	0	-	0	0	457	-	8	2	0	100	25	6	0	100
Saint Vincent and the Grenadines	5	1	4	5	-	0	0	467	-	1,767	460	0	100	23,032	6,000	0	100
Samoa	4	2	2	0	-	0	0	5	-	0	0	-	-	55	24	0	100
San Marino	6	<1	16	-	-	-	-	0	-	-	-	-	-	-	-	-	-
Sao Tome and Principe	2	<1	<1	-	-	-	-	6	-	0	0	-	-	500	240	0	100
Saudi Arabia	13,455	2,329	39	333	108	0	0	2,167	-	0	0	-	-	606	170	0	100
Senegal	275	76	2	14,479	6,620	1	9	15,129	-	8,406	4,100	100	0	1,322	640	0	100
Serbia	823	19	9	25,650	-	4	3	31,737	-	0	0	100	0	34	6	0	100
Seychelles	13	1	13	-	-	-	-	14	-	0	0	-	-	20	6	0	100
Sierra Leone	54	10	<1	345	90	0	1	6,615	-	5,500	2,600	100	0	0	0	32	68
Singapore	2,524	186	43	0	-	0	0	34	-	-	-	-	-	-	-	-	-
Slovakia	197	31	4	1,046	-	0	0	1,426	-	0	0	-	-	60	11	0	100
Slovenia	278	18	13	839	-	0	0	17	-	0	0	-	-	336	59	0	100
Solomon Islands	3	<1	<1	0	-	0	0	38	-	1,000	460	100	0	1,005	460	100	0
Somalia	59	20	<1	13,804	5,898	1	31	776,678	370,545	2,967,500	1,600,000	100	0	820,189	430,000	67	33
South Africa	2,860	275	5	75,512	11,663	1	12	643	-	7,840	2,600	0	100	10,815	3,600	5	95
South Sudan	882	272	8	333,673	201,037	31	306	2,362,759	1,377,398	1,895,610	910,000	72	28	934,976	440,000	46	54
Spain	6,842	547	15	122,539	-	3	4	55	-	7,000	1,200	0	100	13,672	2,300	0	100
Sri Lanka	40	13	<1	907	297	0	0	151,107	-	12,375	3,500	100	0	121,119	34,000	0	100
State of Palestine	273	31	5	-	-	-	-	103,581	-	11,711	5,200	100	0	118,241	52,000	100	0
Sudan	1,379	600	3	1,103,918	524,161	24	1,648	825,290	445,056	3,260,522	1,500,000	97	3	541,083	250,000	82	18
Suriname	48	12	8	29	-	0	0	22	-	0	0	-	-	6,500	2,000	0	100
Sweden	2,004	234	20	240,853	-	23	4	9	-	0	0	-	-	47	10	0	100
Switzerland	2,491	171	29	118,829	36,166	14	1	0	-	13	2	0	100	144	26	0	100
Syrian Arab Republic	869	151	5	14,308	5,608	1	15	6,848,845	3,058,305	6,661,640	2,400,000	100	0	534,230	190,000	85	15
Tajikistan	276	17	3	10,724	-	1	9	2,412	-	778	330	0	100	16,167	6,900	93	7
Thailand	3,632	500	5	100,510	36,787	1	14	181	-	44,114	8,900	93	7	9,925	2,000	5	95
Timor-Leste	8	2	<1	0	-	0	0	11	-	107	46	0	100	15,876	6,900	0	100
Togo	280	100	3	10,683	5,113	1	11	7,985	-	2,000	950	100	0	2,000	950	100	0
Tokelau	1	<1	92	-	-	-	-	-	-	0	0	-	-	0	0	-	-
Tonga	4	1	4	0	-	0	0	28	-	93	38	0	100	2,678	1,100	0	100
Trinidad and Tobago	79	19	6	11,974	-	8	0	285	-	6	1	0	100	33	8	0	100

FOR EVERY CHILD, VACCINATION

205

TABLE 18. MIGRATION

Countries and areas	International migrant stock 2020			Refugees by asylum country 2021				Refugees by origin country 2021		Internally displaced persons (IDPs) 2021				New internal displacements 2021			
	Total (thousands)	Under 18 (thousands)	Total as share of national population (%)	Total	Under 18	Per 1,000 population	Per 1 US$ GNI per capita	Total	Under 18	Total ^{T}	Under 18 ^{Ru}	Share due to conflict and violence (%) ^{Sd}	Share due to disaster (%) ^{Sd}	Total ^{T}	Under 18 ^{Ru}	Share due to conflict and violence (%) ^{Sd}	Share due to disaster (%) ^{Sd}
Tunisia	60	11	<1	3,186	1,169	0	1	2,201	-	148	42	0	100	3,204	900	0	100
Türkiye	6,053	1,258	7	3,759,817	1,703,330	44	382	105,021	28,462	1,110,834	320,000	99	1	84,131	24,000	0	100
Turkmenistan	195	14	3	16	-	0	0	563	-	4,000	1,400	100	0	0	0	-	-
Turks and Caicos Islands	26	2	67	7	-	0	0	14	-	0	0	-	-	60	0	0	100
Tuvalu	<1	<1	2	-	-	-	-	0	-	0	0	-	-	400	0	0	100
Uganda	1,720	928	4	1,529,903	888,416	33	1,821	7,886	-	26,003	14,000	7	93	47,968	25,000	3	97
Ukraine	4,997	280	11	2,382	-	0	1	27,562	-	854,012	160,000	100	0	2,037	380	2	98
United Arab Emirates	8,716	1,351	88	1,355	441	0	0	160	-	0	0	0	100	40	7	0	100
United Kingdom	9,360	920	14	137,078	-	2	3	101	-	0	0	0	100	513	110	0	100
United Republic of Tanzania	426	91	<1	207,101	113,263	3	182	752	-	938	470	0	100	46,707	23,000	0	100
United States	50,633	3,325	15	339,179	-	1	5	426	-	55,568	12,000	0	100	573,078	130,000	0	100
Uruguay	108	29	3	15,872	5,594	5	0	45	-	0	0	-	-	156	38	0	100
Uzbekistan	1,162	92	3	13,032	-	0	7	3,014	-	0	0	100	0	70,000	23,000	0	100
Vanuatu	3	<1	1	0	-	0	0	0	-	63,965	28,000	0	100	80,191	36,000	0	100
Venezuela (Bolivarian Republic of)	1,324	160	5	39,328	23,306	1	3	4,605,611	1,213,905	32,392	10,000	0	100	32,592	10,000	0	100
Viet Nam	77	11	<1	0	-	0	0	317,737	-	1,816	490	0	100	779,699	210,000	0	100
Yemen	387	117	1	89,467	21,212	3	134	37,611	10,548	4,299,575	2,000,000	100	0	461,071	210,000	82	18
Zambia	188	34	1	75,154	35,326	4	72	255	-	222	110	0	100	1,325	670	0	100
Zimbabwe	416	53	3	9,483	4,634	1	7	8,115	-	42,878	21,000	0	100	2,354	1,100	0	100

SUMMARY

East Asia and Pacific	28,972	2,984	1	622,011	146,348	0	49	1,716,652	654,259	2,779,478	790,000	32	68	14,321,523	4,000,000	4	96
Europe and Central Asia	99,035	8,847	11	7,028,160	2,649,114	8	267	382,636	85,013	3,319,985	810,000	98	2	337,653	82,000	18	82
Eastern Europe and Central Asia	32,472	3,214	8	3,893,358	1,731,344	9	448	373,857	84,278	3,065,648	760,000	99	1	155,790	50,000	39	61
Western Europe	66,563	5,633	13	3,134,802	917,770	6	76	8,779	735	254,337	51,000	95	5	181,863	32,000	0	100
Latin America and Caribbean	14,795	3,603	2	4,675,622	1,236,788	7	33	4,935,937	1,304,311	6,507,581	1,900,000	95	5	1,406,546	390,000	27	73
Middle East and North Africa	44,421	9,004	9	3,137,400	1,382,145	7	440	7,668,182	3,267,776	12,358,117	5,000,000	100	0	1,245,847	500,000	81	19
North America	58,709	3,961	16	469,304	98,358	1	7	486	286	57,508	13,000	0	100	632,751	140,000	0	100
South Asia	11,066	1,197	<1	2,709,820	1,379,845	1	1,292	3,047,495	1,341,978	6,894,596	3,200,000	78	22	5,986,633	2,000,000	12	88
Sub-Saharan Africa	23,601	5,919	2	7,091,009	3,881,175	6	4,510	7,824,772	4,073,902	27,159,395	14,000,000	93	7	14,111,808	6,900,000	82	18
Eastern and Southern Africa	12,843	3,676	2	4,935,804	2,680,091	8	3,049	5,240,451	2,732,532	13,627,090	6,600,000	89	11	8,191,536	3,900,000	83	17
West and Central Africa	10,757	2,242	2	2,155,205	1,201,084	4	1,415	2,584,321	1,341,370	13,532,305	7,000,000	97	3	5,920,272	3,100,000	81	19
Least developed countries	16,185	4,899	2	7,022,880	3,827,500	6	6,065	11,241,422	5,610,728	33,592,396	16,000,000	90	10	15,723,667	7,500,000	80	20
World	**280,598**	**35,515**	**4**	**25,733,326**	**10,773,773**	**3**	**1,778**	**25,733,326**	**10,773,773**	**59,076,660**	**25,000,000**	**90**	**10**	**38,042,761**	**14,000,000**	**38**	**62**

For a complete list of countries and areas in the regions, subregions and country categories, see page on Regional Classifications or visit <data.unicef.org/regionalclassifications>.

It is not advisable to compare data from consecutive editions of *The State of the World's Children* report.

NOTES

- Data not available.

Regional and global values are based on more countries and areas than listed here. Therefore, country values do not add up to the corresponding regional and global values.

Refugees with origin listed as 'other', 'unknown', 'various' or 'stateless' are not included in the aggregates, making the global totals smaller than the comparable total of refugees by host country.

^{Sd} Share refers to total displacements.

^{T} Totals are the sum of unrounded numbers related to conflict & violence, and disasters, respectively, as published by the Internal Displacement Monitoring Centre.

^{Ru} Under 18 estimates rounded to second signficant figure (e.g., '1 234' is rounded to '1 200').

MAIN DATA SOURCES

International migrant stock: United Nations Department of Economic and Social Affairs, Population Division (2020). International Migrant Stock 2020.

Refugees: United Nations High Commissioner for Refugees, Refugee Population Statistics Database, 2022.

Internal displacement: Internal Displacement Monitoring Centre, Global Internal Displacement Database (GIDD), IDMC, 2022.

DEFINITIONS OF THE INDICATORS

International migrant stock – The number of people born in a country other than that in which they live, including refugees.

Refugees – Persons who are forced to flee their home country to escape persecution or a serious threat to their life, physical integrity or freedom. Numbers in this table refer to refugees under UNHCR

mandate only. Additional Palestine refugees registered with UNRWA are present in State of Palestine, Lebanon, the Syrian Arab Republic, and Jordan but are not listed here.

Internally displaced persons (IDPs) – Persons who have been forced or obliged to flee or to leave their homes or places of habitual residence and who have not crossed an internationally recognized state border at a given point in time.

New internal displacements – Number of movements of persons who have been forced or obliged to flee or to leave their homes or places of habitual residence and who have not crossed an internationally recognized state border in a given period.